IMMUNOTOXICITY OF METALS
AND
IMMUNOTOXICOLOGY

International Programme on Chemical Safety (UNEP-ILO-WHO) • Commission of the European
Communities • International Commission on Occupational Health • Federal Ministry for Environment,
Nature Conservation and Nuclear Safety; Federal Health Office, Federal Republic of Germany

IMMUNOTOXICITY OF METALS AND IMMUNOTOXICOLOGY

Edited by

A. D. Dayan

St. Bartholemew's Hospital Medical College
London, United Kingdom

R. F. Hertel

Fraunhofer Institute of Toxicology and Aerosol Research
Hanover, Federal Republic of Germany

E. Heseltine

Scientific Communication
Montignac, France

G. Kazantzis

London School of Hygiene and Tropical Medicine
London, United Kingdom

E. M. Smith

International Programme on Chemical Safety
World Health Organization
Geneva, Switzerland

and

M. T. Van der Venne

Health and Safety Directorate
Commission of the European Communities
Luxembourg

PLENUM PRESS • NEW YORK AND LONDON

Library of Congress Cataloging-in-Publication Data

Immunotoxicity of metals and immunotoxicology / edited by A.D. Dayan
... [et al.].
     p.   cm.
   "Proceedings of an international workshop organized with the
assistance of the Federal Health Office of the Federal Republic of
Germany and the Fraunhofer Institute for Inhalation Toxicology and
Aerosol Research held November 6-10, 1989, at the Fraunhofer
Institute and the Medical High School, Hanover, Federal Republic of
Germany"--T.p. verso.
   Includes bibliographical references and index.
   ISBN 978-1-4684-8445-8   ISBN 978-1-4684-8443-4 (eBook)
   DOI 10.1007/978-1-4684-8443-4
   1. Immunotoxicology--Congresses. 2. Immune system--Effect of
metals on--Congresses.   I. Dayan, Anthony D. II. Germany (West).
Bundesgesundheitsamt. III. Fraunhofer-Institut für Toxikologie und
Aerosolforschung (Hannover, Germany)
RC582.17.I45 1990
616.97'071--dc20   90-14178
                                                             CIP

Proceedings of an international workshop organized with the assistance of the Fraunhofer Institute for Inhalation Toxicology and Aerosol Research and the Hanover Medical High School, held November 6–10, 1989, in Hanover, Federal Republic of Germany

Publication No. EUR 12764 (EN) of the Commission of the European Communities, Scientific and Technical Communication Unit, Directorate-General Telecommunications, Information Industries and Innovation, Luxembourg

International Programme on Chemical Safety, IPCS Joint Symposia, No. 15

The authors alone are responsible for the views expressed in the signed articles in this publication. None of the organizers of the workshop nor any person acting on their behalf is responsible for the use which might be made of the following information.

PREFACE

Considerable scientific and political interest has been expressed, parallelling public concern about the effects of chemicals on the immune system and the implications of those effects for health. Coupled with speculation about the magnitude and extent of the problem is discussion of needs for predictive testing and regulatory control measures.

The first international seminar on the immunological system as a target for toxic damage was held in Luxembourg in 1984. It was organized by the International Programme on Chemical Safety (United Nations Environment Programme-International Labour Office-World Health Organization) and the Commission of the European Communities with the support of the US Environmental Protection Agency and the National Institute of Environmental Health Sciences (USA) and the participation of the International Society of Immunopharmacology. In view of the perceived importance of immunotoxicity, it was considered necessary to organize a follow-up meeting.

Thus, an international workshop on the immunotoxicity of metals and immuno-toxicology was held in Hanover, Federal Republic of Germany, on 6-10 November 1989. It was organized jointly by:
- the International Programme on Chemical Safety - a cooperative programme of the United Nations Environment Programme, the International Labour Office and the World Health Organization
- the Commission of the European Communities' Health and Safety Directorate
- the International Commission on Occupational Health, through its Scientific Committee on the Toxicology of Metals
- the Federal Ministry for Environment, Nature Conservation and Nuclear Safety, Bonn
- the Federal Health Office of the Federal Republic of Germany, Berlin (West) and
- the Fraunhofer Institute for Inhalation Toxicology and Aerosol Research, Hanover.

The workshop took place at the Fraunhofer Institute and the Medical High School in Hanover. There were 100 participants drawn from 18 countries, with a range of scientific backgrounds, who were able to share experience and opinions.

In risk assessment of chemicals, the focus was initially on acute clinical toxicity, but the effects that may occur at lower doses, such as some of the immune-mediated effects, have more recently been of increasing concern. This workshop represented the first systematic coverage of immune-related effects of metals and their compounds. The objectives of the workshop of which this volume is the proceedings were to:

    (i) review and evaluate data on metal-induced effects on the immune system in humans and animals, including autoimmune phenomena and immuno-logically induced hypersensitivity,

    (ii) compare data on the effects of the same chemical in humans and experimental animals,

    (iii) review the results of monitoring for effects on the immune system of metals in human populations,

(iv) review the current status of predictive test methods for effects on the immune system, and

(v) review histopathological changes in the immune system in experimental animals following exposure to chemical immunotoxicants and their relevance for predicting risk in human populations.

At the workshop, 29 formal presentations stimulated detailed discussions in plenary sessions and led to the formation of ad-hoc working groups. Some of these examined and discussed histopathological material and slides and new techniques that have been developed for evaluating the histopathology of the immune system. Reflecting the priorities identified, the working groups reviewed the immunotoxicology of metals, including hypersensitivity, autoimmunity, human studies and monitoring, and predictive testing. The members of the workshop concentrated on the need for defining dose-effect, dose-response relationships for metals and metallic compounds that induce immunologically mediated effects, and discussed the value of screening/predictive tests in rodents as well as the requirements for conducting appropriate epidemiological studies.

The conclusions and recommendations of their discussions are contained in the report of the workshop.

Many people assisted in the work associated with the organization and running of the workshop, in addition to those who contributed papers, and we are grateful to all of them for a most successful cooperation which brought together an impressive interdisciplinary spectrum of knowledge. Finally, the local organization at the Fraunhofer Institute and Medical High School provided a firm basis for successful international cooperation in a field of science of growing importance.

Dr M. Mercier
Manager, International
Programme on
Chemical Safety

Dr W. Hunter
Director, Health
& Safety Directorate,
Commission of the
European Communities

Dr G. Nordberg
Chairman, Scientific
Committee on the
Toxicology of Metals,
International
Commission on
Occupational Health

Dr U. Schlottman
Head, Chemical Safety,
Federal Ministry for
Environment, Nature
Conservation & Nuclear
Safety, Federal Republic
of Germany

CONTENTS

IMMUNOTOXICITY OF METALS

LIST OF ABBREVIATIONS AND ACRONYMS USED

AHTR, autoimmune hypersensitivity-type response
AIDS, acquired immunodeficiency syndrome
ALN, auricular lymph node
ALNA, auricular lymph node assay
ANA, antinucleolar antibody
BAL, bronchoalveolar lavage
BN, Brown-Norway
BSA, bovine serum albumin
CBD, chronic beryllium disease
CBETC, bis(ß-carbobutoxyethyltin) dichloride
ConA, concanavalin A
CY, cyclophosphamide
DBTC, di-n-butyltin dichloride
DETC, di-n-ethyltin dichloride
DHR, delayed hypersensitivity reaction
DHTR, direct hypersensitivity-type response
DMTC, di-n-methyltin dichloride
DNCB, dinitrochlorobenzene
DOTC, di-n-octyltin dichloride
DTH, delayed-type hypersensitivity
EDTA, ethylenediaminetetraacetic acid
ELISA, enzyme-linked immunosorbent assay
GBM, glomerular basement membrane
GN, glomerulonephritis
GPMT, guinea-pig maximization test
GVH, graft-*versus*-host
ICGN, immune complex glomerulonephropathy
IDDM, insulin-dependent diabetes mellitus
IFN, interferon
Ig, immunoglobulin
IL, interleukin
KLH, keyhole limpet haemocyanin
LPS, lipopolysaccharide
LTT, lymphocyte transformation test
MEST, mouse ear swelling test
MGC, minimal glomerular changes
MGP, membranous glomerulopathy
MHC, major histocompatibility complex
MIF, migration inhibition factor
MLR, mixed lymphocyte reaction
NK, natural killer
NOD, non-obese diabetic
OS, obese strain
PALS, periarteriolar lymphocyte sheath
PCA, passive cutaneous anaphylaxis
PCA, plaque-forming cell assay

PFC, plaque-forming cells
PHA, phytohaemagglutinin
PLN, popliteal lymph node
PLNA, popliteal lymph node assay
PPD, purified protein derivative
PUFA, polyunsaturated fat
PWM, pokeweed mitogen
RAST, radioallergosorbent test
SAFA, saturated fat
SAT, sodium aurothiomalate
SLE, systemic lupus erythematosus
SRBC, sheep red blood cells
STZ, streptozotocin
TBM, tubular basement membrane
TBTC, tri-*n*-butyltin chloride
TBTF, tri-*n*-butyltin fluoride
TBTO, bis(tri-*n*-butyltin) oxide
TCDD, 2,3,7,8-tetrachlorodibenzo-*para*-dioxin
TCR, T cell receptor
Th, T helper
TMA, trimellitic anhydride
TNF, tumour necrosis factor
TPhTA, triphenyltin acetate
TPhTC, triphenyltin chloride
TPhTH, triphenyltin hydroxide
TPTC, tripropyltin chloride
Ts, T suppressor
Ts-Ab, antibody suppressing T cells
VAA, vitamin A acetate

INTRODUCTION

IMMUNOTOXICITY OF METALS AND IMMUNOTOXICOLOGY

*Report of an International Workshop held
in Hanover, Federal Republic of Germany
on 6-10 November 1989*

INTRODUCTION

Immune response has been recognized, but not understood, for centuries. The role and function of the immune system in response to infection was perceived approximately a century ago. The hypersensitivity reaction was understood at the beginning of this century, but the recognition of autoimmune disease is comparatively recent, dating from the mid-1950s. The explosion of knowledge of the structure and function of the immune system owes most to the introduction of organ transplantation, which started, on a practical basis, at much the same time. It was found that the immune system could be modulated as a whole or in parts by chemicals used therapeutically. Observations that some non-therapeutic xenobiotic chemicals also had immunomodulatory properties raised interest in the potential risk that many biologically active chemicals might have direct primary or secondary effects on the immune system or that the system itself might mediate toxicity in other systems and organs.

The effects of chemicals, including drugs, on the human immune system are of interest to international organizations, governmental authorities, clinicians, occupational health professionals, pathologists, immunologists, toxicologists, industries, workers, consumers and other interest groups. In risk assessment of chemicals, the focus was initially on acute clinical toxicity, but effects that may occur at relatively low doses, including several of those mediated by the immune system, have become of increasing concern. Although many chemicals have been shown experimentally to cause disturbances in components of the immune system, the mechanisms and their clinical significance are not well understood. The current status of predictive testing in animals and humans for immunotoxic effects *in vitro* and *in vivo* indicates that further methods and techniques for evaluation of test results must be developed. The use of immunological assays in the monitoring of the health status of populations should be pursued and developed.

The Workshop participants discussed the following topics:

  (i) the immune system and immunotoxicology,

  (ii) immunotoxicity of metals,

  (iii) hypersensitivity induced by metals,

  (iv) autoimmunity,

  (v) studies of effects on the human immune system of occupational and environmental exposures to chemicals, and

  (vi) laboratory investigations of immunotoxicity.

THE IMMUNE SYSTEM

The primary function of the immune system is to protect the organism against infection. The development of immunology followed the observation that certain infections and molecules, perceived as foreign, confer a highly specific immunity to reinfection, an observation utilized by Jenner some 200 years ago to introduce vaccination against smallpox. The normal immune response is characterized by its memory, by which a subsequent challenge with a specific stimulus provokes a more vigorous but well regulated response. The cellular and molecular basis for these characteristics has unfolded progressively over the past thirty years.

The immune system is a dynamic and complex organ system which can be the target of chemically induced toxicity. The discipline of immunotoxicology deals with toxic manifestations resulting from chemical interaction with the immune system. Since the discipline is in its infancy, its terminology is still evolving. Clear definitions and standardization of terms (e.g., hypersensitivity, immunotoxicant, immunoenhancement) are essential to facilitate interaction and to avoid confusion among the diverse groups of scientists working within the discipline.

In addition to the inherent interactions between components of the immune system, there is also interplay between these components and those of other organ systems. Neuroendocrine interactions with the immune system are increasingly recognized as important in delineating primary and secondary immunotoxic effects of chemicals.

Immunotoxic effects of chemicals may also depend upon the immunogenetic make-up of the host; this is well established in studies in laboratory animals. Variation in susceptibility to chemical immunotoxicity observed in outbred animals and humans may thus, in part, be due to genetically based differences. Certain species and strains of laboratory animals, for example, are predisposed to developing autoimmune responses following exposure to specific chemicals. In humans in whom environmental agents induce autoimmune responses, an association with a specific major histocompatibility complex (MHC) haplotype has been described in some cases.

The uniqueness of the immune system relative to other organ systems as a target for chemical toxicity starts with the antigen component, which is required to elicit an immune response. This requirement imparts an additional level of complexity in designing immunotoxicity studies. Assessment of chemically mediated immunotoxicity cannot be based upon any single morphological or functional parameter; however, since it is not practical to evaluate all immunologically relevant parameters in a single toxicity or immunotoxicity study, the challenge facing immunotoxicology is to identify the most important predictive parameters and to suggest a practical approach to assessing immunotoxicity. The problem is further complicated by the immunological redundancy and/ or reserve which may be characteristic of the immune system and which may be an important determinant of response following exposure to immunotoxic chemicals. Further understanding of the concepts of redundancy and reserve is required, particularly in relation to the extrapolation of experimental data on immunotoxicity to humans. Molecular methods, including the use of gene probes (e.g., for measuring lymphokine/cytokine mRNA) may also provide a means for the early identification of suspected immunotoxic effects of chemicals.

IMMUNOSUPPRESSION

Disordered function of the immune system can give rise to increased susceptibility to infection, to neoplasia, to a variety of hypersensitivity states and to autoimmune disease. Increased susceptibility to infection and certain forms of neoplasia are a consequence of immune system suppression, while hypersensitivity reactions result from excessive stimulation; autoimmune disease may involve elements of both stimulation and suppression of the immune system. The realization that the immune system can be both stimulated and suppressed by chemicals, drugs and environmental chemicals led in the last decade to the rapid development of immunotoxicology. Potentially immunosuppressive chemicals may be encountered in the general environment in the form of pollution, as food contaminants and as a result of occupational exposure. In humans, a congenital deficiency of B lymphocytes, and hence of plasma cells, gives rise to agammaglobulinaemia and failure to produce antibodies against common bacterial infections. A deficiency of immunocompetent T lymphocytes, as in thymic aplasia, increases susceptibility to infection with microorganisms to which normal individuals are resistant and to a rapidly fatal outcome following infection with common viruses such as measles and chicken pox. The highly complex immune system may be impaired by a variety of extraneous factors, including certain viral infections and chemical agents. The retrovirus, human immunodeficiency virus, by its effect on CD4+ T lymphocytes gives rise to deficient cellular immunity manifested by a variety of opportunistic infections seen in acquired immune deficiency syndrome (AIDS). Studies of this virus have provided fresh insights into the functioning of the immune system. Although infectious agents are often implicated in the etiology and pathogenesis of autoimmune disease, available circumstantial data point to the likelihood that environmental chemicals may well be another set of important etiological factors in these complex disorders.

Immunosuppression has been induced with a variety of chemotherapeutic agents to enable the grafting of tissues and organs into genetically dissimilar hosts; however, such drugs suppress not only the immune response to the graft but also other immune responses. Cytotoxic drugs used in the treatment of cancer and ionizing radiation also give rise to immunosuppression. Transplant recipients who have been immunosuppressed have an increased incidence of certain cancers, in particular of lymphomas; and secondary cancers are also more common in patients treated with cytotoxic drugs.

HYPERSENSITIVITY

Immune responses, while designed to protect the individual against infection, are not always beneficial. An immune response may be inappropriate and excessive, giving rise to tissue damage. This may manifest as a type-I immediate hypersensitivity reaction, presenting commonly with urticaria, conjunctivitis, rhinorrhoea or bronchial asthma or rarely with anaphylactic shock, following exposure, for example, to insect bites, pollens, animal danders or house dust. Atopic subjects, prone to develop type-I hypersensitivity reactions, often have a family history of such disorders, although genetic factors can come into play only following the exposure to the environmental or occupational stimulus. Another common presentation is cell-mediated or delayed, type-IV hypersensitivity, manifesting with skin reactions following a variety of infections or skin contact with a wide variety of chemical agents encountered in plants, hair dyes, some drugs and in the working environment. Less common are hypersensitivity reactions characterized by cytotoxicity (type II), for example, when haemolytic anaemia, agranulocytosis or thrombocytopenia follows the administration of certain drugs. Also less common are immune complex-mediated reactions (type III) seen, for example, in allergic alveolitis, serum sickness and in some forms of glomerulonephritis.

The classification of hypersensitivity reactions as types I-IV, with reference to clinical criteria or experimental animal models, is still useful. More than one type of reaction could be manifested concomitantly, consistent with different, co-existing immune changes, all being part of a complex interaction of factors.

A number of laboratory methods are used to identify low-molecular-weight chemicals with potential to induce contact hypersensitivity reactions. Progress is being made in developing models to predict which chemicals are likely to induce anaphylactic responses after inhalation.

The guinea-pig is commonly used as an experimental animal for eliciting potential delayed-type hypersensitivity reactions, but testing is also carried out in mice. The latter include ear swelling tests and induction of lymphocyte proliferation. The advantage of the murine local lymph node assay for detecting contact allergens is its endpoint: this avoids the irrelevance of irritation or colour of the test compound. The popliteal lymph node assay (PLNA) in rodents is a possible screening test for identifying sensitizing chemicals. Recent screening of a wide variety of drugs and chemicals in the PLNA has revealed a good correlation with their potential to cause systemic autoimmune disease and contact dermatitis in humans. Predictive tests for the sensitizing chemicals as inhaled or ingested allergens are being developed. Fundamental studies of suppressor cells and tolerance induction and of modification of metals by antigen-presenting cells are under way.

Procedures for studying hypersensitivity in humans are of two kinds - those which involve the individual directly, i.e., in-vivo testing, and procedures performed *in vitro* on donated blood samples. It is not possible at present to predict susceptibility to a primary immune response. Positive results indicate that sensitization has taken place, so that provocation testing is *a posteriori* in nature. Provocation tests include skin prick and scratch tests to evaluate type-I immediate hypersensitivity reactions, and patch tests in the evaluation of type-IV delayed hypersensitivity reactions. In addition, nasal challenge and bronchial inhalation tests are used in provocation testing for type-I hypersensitivity reactions. However, such testing procedures may enhance existing sensitization or even initiate sensitization. Patch testing with beryllium sulfate provides a good example of enhancement. In-vitro testing procedures include assay of histamine release from basophils and estimation of specific immunoglobulins, in particular specific IgE. Macrophage migration inhibition and lymphocyte transformation tests, however, can give both false-negative and false-positive results.

AUTOIMMUNITY

Immune responses can give rise to serious adverse health effects as a result of an autoimmune reaction. Here, the immune response is directed against one or more of the body's own constituents, with the formation of autoantibodies and unsuppressed autoreactive T cells. A wide spectrum of disease states may result, ranging from organ-specific diseases such as primary thyroiditis with myxoedema and type-I diabetes to non-organ-specific disorders, for example, systemic lupus erythematosus with widespread lesions and complex autoantibody formation. There appears to be an inherent predisposition for the development of autoimmunity; genes both linked and unlinked to the MHC are important.

The microsomal cytochrome P450 mono-oxygenase enzyme system, its possible involvement in the induction of autoimmune reactions and its possible role in the prediction of adverse immune reactions are also important.

Experimental data indicate that cytokines play critical roles in the pathogenesis of autoimmune diseases, but it is not clear what constitutes the initiating event for the induction of autoimmune disease. In experimental animal models, there is evidence that the T-cell cytokine interleukin 4 (IL-4) plays a rôle in the activation of autoreactive B cells through the induction of increased expression of class-II MHC antigens and consequent B-cell hyperactivity with increased production of IgE. Delineation of the role that interferon gamma (IFNγ) may play in the activation of autoreactive helper T cells, through the induction of aberrant expression of class-II MHC antigens on a target organ, was proposed for two examples of organ-specific autoimmunity (i.e., autoimmune thyroiditis and insulin-dependent diabetes mellitus). Comparisons between the experimental autoimmune models and human autoimmune diseases show a good correlation in the role that cytokines play in the progression of these diseases. There are possible exploratory and therapeutic applications (e.g., the use of anti-cytokine antibody) derived from an understanding of the role that cytokines play in autoimmune diseases.

Thus, experimental allogeneic diseases represent interesting tools for investigating the rôle of T cell-derived or macrophage-derived cytokines in the triggering of autoreactive B cells and for studying the effects of cytokine synergism or antagonism. These models may be particularly relevant for understanding autoimmune phenomena in humans.

IMMUNOTOXICITY OF METALS

When a metal ion enters a biological system, it does not travel as free metal, but combines with small or large molecules, such as proteins. The strength of the binding and the structure or fold of the protein then determine the shape (stereochemistry) of the combination and the ability of the immune system to recognize the metal-altered compound as well as the nature of the response.

6

Metals may affect the immune system in several ways; several metals can induce immunosuppression in experimental situations, although the mechanisms involved have not yet been elucidated. They may bind to autologous (self) proteins (constituents) and render them immunogenic; this is probably the case in metal-induced contact dermatitis. Metals may also induce true autoimmune manifestations, such as gold-induced autoimmune nephritis. There is some evidence from experimental models that heavy metals initiate a polyclonal activation of B cells requiring the activation of CD4+ T cells. Additional mechanisms, such as inhibition of suppression, must be considered.

Some of these immunologically-related effects are observed only in susceptible individuals. Susceptibility is, both in humans and animals, under the control of genes linked to the MHC (class-II genes) and of genes located outside this complex (sulfoxydator status). Strain differences in susceptibility to metal-induced immunotoxicity have been observed in rodents. Few data are available on immunosuppressive effects of metals in humans, and limited studies on lead-exposed workers and children have provided contradictory results.

Immunosuppression

A number of immunosuppressive effects of various organotin compounds have been demonstrated in animals. Of special interest are the selective thymic effects. A rapid metabolism of trisubstituted organotin compounds to disubstituted compounds can be assumed on the basis of similarities of the observed effects on the thymus. Both dialkyl- and trialkyltin compounds exert cytotoxic and cytostatic effects on several cell types, including thymocytes. A series of tri-alkyl-substituted compounds of tin exhibited a progression in effects on the thymus gland, with maximal activity for the propyl and butyl analogues and minimal activity for shorter and longer chain derivatives. It is likely that this cytotoxicity is of importance as an early event in the development of the thymotoxic effects of organotin compounds. Effects on cytokines have also been observed and may be of importance in explaining the systemic immunotoxicity of organotin. Other studies in animals show immunosuppressive effects of lead, mercury, cadmium, cobalt and organotins (see Table 1).

Table 1. Examples of metals which in specific chemical forms give rise to immunotoxic effects

A. Effects on specific immunity

    1. Hypersensitivity reactions (humans and animals)

        Type 1   Chromium, cobalt, nickel, platinum

        Type II   Gold

        Type III   Gold, mercury

        Type IV   Beryllium, chromium, cobalt, gold, mercury, nickel, zirconium

    2. Autoimmune reactions (humans and/or animals)
        Gold, mercury

    3. Enhancement (humans and/or animals)
        Selenium, zinc

    4. Suppression (animals)
        Cadmium, cobalt, lead, mercury, tin (organotin)

B. Effects on nonspecific immunity (animals)

    1. Enhancement
        Manganese

    2. Suppression
        Cadmium, lead, mercury

Selenium is a constituent of the enzyme glutathione peroxidase. Selenium and zinc deficiency have been shown to impair both humoral and cellular immunity.

Hypersensitivity and autoimmunity

A metal must be complexed with a macromolecule in order to become an antigen and capable of inducing a hypersensitivity response. This involves the formation of covalent bonds to form a hapten-carrier conjugate. The charged halide complex salts of platinum are among the most potent sensitizers known. Metallic nickel is a potent skin sensitizer. Organogold compounds, in particular gold thiomalate, give rise to hypersensitivity reactions, and in this case there is limited evidence that metallic gold can also give rise to a delayed hypersensitivity reaction. Hexavalent chromium ions can penetrate skin and induce hypersensitivity as trivalent chromium; trivalent compounds, with their limited ability for skin penetration, are much less potent sensitizing agents.

There are extensive clinical observations of metal hypersensitivity reactions (Table 1). For example, in a general population sample in Finland, 9% of females were found to have nickel allergy with eczema of the hands. In Europe as a whole, it is estimated that about 12% of females have nickel allergy, of whom about 10% also have hand eczema. The incidence of hypersensitivity reactions in groups occupationally exposed to particular metals and their compounds is much greater than in the general population.

Anaphylactic (type I) sensitivity can be induced by platinum and delayed hypersensitivity (type IV) by nickel, chromium, cobalt and mercury. Beryllium affords a particular example of a delayed hypersensitivity response with histological changes resembling sarcoidosis.

Exposure of the public to platinum is increasing, for example, due to increasing use of platinum in catalytic converters in motor vehicles. Type-I hypersensitivity due to platinum salts is difficult to detect by laboratory methods, especially as only a few halogenated complexes have allergenic properties and the pure metal is inert. In platinum refineries possible predisposing causes of sensitization include atopy, other inhalant allergens, certain skin disorders and tobacco smoking.

The role of the oxidation state of platinum with regard to sensitization is not clear, but a parallel can be drawn between the bio-oxidation of gold and subsequent sensitization and the possible oxidation of platinum, inside and outside the body, giving rise to subsequent sensitization.

In humans, gold salts used in the treatment of rheumatoid arthritis can give rise to a number of immune-mediated side-effects such as skin reactions, thrombocytopenia and glomerulonephritis. While either toxic or immunologically mediated mechanisms might give rise to the thrombocytopenia, the glomerulonephritis is related to the development of autoimmunity, particularly in subjects who are HLA-DR3 positive. Experiments with Brown-Norway rats have demonstrated that gold salts may produce nephritis in these animals by an autoimmune mechanism. Experimental work in the mouse, which demonstrates striking differences in the T-cell sensitizing potential of trivalent and monovalent gold compounds using the PLNA, shows the role of oxidation state in T-cell immunogenicity.

Concern has been expressed concerning low-level occupational exposure to mercury, but the general population is also exposed from dental amalgam, although the concentrations are even lower. It has been demonstrated that certain strains of rats and mice develop autoimmune effects, including glomerulonephritis, after uptake of mercury at 15 µg/kg body weight (absorbed dose per day). Information is incomplete on humans concerning a possible immunological etiology of glomerulonephritis related to low-level exposure to mercury. It is possible that a small proportion of the human population may have increased sensitivity in the same way as that observed in animals.

Exposure to cobalt dichloride may cause skin sensitization in workers. An increased level of IgA has been observed in humans exposed to cobalt. Skin sensitization has also been observed in animals.

Chronic beryllium disease is an occupational disorder with an immunological pathogenesis, as shown by use of the lymphocyte blast transformation test, which can be performed on both peripheral blood and on bronchial lavage fluid. The latter is more specific, because chronic beryllium disease involves compartmentalized immune response involving primarily the lungs.

Metals can induce respiratory tract hypersensitivity. Platinum, chromium and, possibly, nickel, are responsible for IgE-mediated asthma, while other metal-induced asthmas do not seem to be IgE-mediated. Possible mechanisms of metal-induced asthma are (i) the atopic status of an individual as a predisposing factor, (ii) induction or modification of atopic status and (iii) modification of the clinical expression of atopic status, e.g., by increasing bronchial reactivity.

Evidence of immune complex formation is seen after long exposure to gold or mercury with deposits of immunoglobulin and complement in membranous glomerulonephritis, but metals are not found in the deposits. These are considered to be examples of autoimmune phenomena.

A variety of mercury compounds, including methylmercury, have been tested and comparable results always obtained in the production of autoimmunity in susceptible strains, irrespective of the route of administration. Studies in the DZB rat suggest that anti-laminin antibodies are involved in the appearance not only of linear IgG deposits but also of granular deposits. It is possible that the initial deposition of anti-laminin antibodies stimulates the production of laminin by glomerular epithelial cells.

Metal-induced autoimmunity (e.g., mercury- and gold-induced autoimmunity in rats and mice) appears to result from the development of autoreactive T cells. In the mercuric chloride-induced nephritis system, T cells have the capacity to recognize self class-II MHC antigens. Overproduction of IL-4 is then thought to result, with the eventual induction of the production of large quantities of IgE. In these models, a genetic predisposition exists which determines the development of metal-induced autoimmunities, which have multiple manifestations (e.g., anti-nuclear antibodies, anti-glomerular basement membrane antibodies). Several mechanisms may be responsible for metal-induced autoimmunity.

DOSE-RESPONSE AND RISK ASSESSMENT

Dose-effect and dose-response relationships are fundamental principles in toxicology. In the latter relationship, the proportion of a population, human or animal, exhibiting a specified toxic effect increases with the degree of exposure to the metal or other toxicant. The dose-response curve is usually a continuous function of dose, involving a "threshold" below which there is no dose-related response. Whatever the relationship may be, the slope of the curve describing the increase in response with increasing dose may be steep or shallow reflecting individual differences among responders and nonresponders. Both genetic and environmental factors determine the extent of the individual differences.

Dose-response relationships for immune effects are different from dose-response relationships observed in non-immune-mediated toxicity. Confounding factors include the preference of the mucosal immune systems to induce tolerance (i.e., non-responsiveness), dysregulation of helper:suppressor cell ratios due to previous insults, and genetic susceptibility.

A number of immune-mediated effects, such as hypersensitivity and autoimmune responses, appear to exhibit much wider individual variation to a given dose of a chemical. There must be prior or continuing exposure. Because of the wide variation, extrapolation to lower doses in large populations poses a particular problem, as illustrated by risk assessment for people with mercury amalgam tooth fillings. It is not possible without knowledge about this interindividual variability to identify a level of mercury, e.g., in blood or urine, in an individual below which a mercury-related effect will not occur. The dose-response relationship in an already "sensitized" population is quantitatively different, in the sense that immune responses are elicited at much lower doses - for example, in contact allergy to chromium and nickel.

Autoimmune phenomena induced by certain metals may exhibit 'down' regulation: continued exposure may ultimately result in disappearance of the immune effect. Repeated exposure of susceptible strains of rats or mice to mercuric chloride produces circulating immune complexes and/or autoantibodies, but with continued exposure to mercury these eventually disappear.

In general, damage to a target organ is related to the concentration of the metal in that organ. Certain immune-mediated effects may not conform to these concepts. For example, compounds of both inorganic mercury and gold damage the kidneys as a secondary consequence of their action on immunocompetent cells. Thus, despite the fact that the observed toxic response is on the kidneys, the effect is due, presumably, to interaction of the metal with immunocompetent cells.

The genetic constitution of the individual may be an important factor in determining susceptibility to the effects of metals. Individual susceptibility may be associated with genetic characteristics, such as haplotypes in the MHC. An example is the presence of the DR3 antigen in individuals who have shown an autoimmune response to gold compounds. The genotype may be involved in immune reactions in at least two ways: (i) controlling immunological reactivity *per se*, and (ii) controlling metabolism to active or inactive compounds.

Dose-response relationships for sensitization by metals may take unusual forms. In the case of nickel, low concentrations can produce sensitization but exposure to higher levels, such as in dental devices or in certain occupations, does not produce sensitization. The relationship may be paradoxical, with low-dose effects enhancing the immune system whereas higher doses cause suppression due to a toxic action on immunocompetent cells: lead is an example of the latter case. Furthermore, the route of exposure may determine whether sensitization or tolerance ocxcurs. For example, dental devices in children do not induce sensitization.

For some metallic compounds, such as nickel and chromium, which cause immunologically mediated hypersensitivity, there is sufficient information available on dose-response relationships to define those conditions of dermal exposure of the general population below which dermatitis will not occur. Reduction of percutaneous nickel exposure below 5 µg/cm² per week virtually eliminates new cases of allergy. The role of orally ingested nickel in this context is under discussion.

The chemical and physical species of a metal may be critical to determining its immunogenic potential. Platinum compounds that elicit sensitivity are confined to compounds that contain reactive halogen ligands, and only certain crystalline structures of beryllium oxide are capable of producing immune-related effects.

Metabolism of a non-reactive metal species to a reactive one can be important for immune-mediated effects. Monovalent gold has to be oxidized to the trivalent species as a necessary step before T cells can be sensitized.

In studies of immunologically mediated effects, it might be useful to characterize genetic factors in responders and nonresponders, particularly for disorders of suspected immunological etiology occurring in population groups exposed to metals and other chemical compounds. In the further exploration of immunologically mediated lung disease caused by metallic compounds, consideration should be given to the possibility of using some of the diagnostic tests successfully applied to the early diagnosis of granulomatous beryllium disease.

While important immune-mediated effects of metals have been identified by studies in humans and animals, the possible immunotoxic properties of many metals and metal compounds to which humans are exposed still need to be elucidated. Experience of studying the effects of chemicals on the human immune system is still limited. Human studies are being directed to monitoring hypersensitivity and other immune system effects (see Table 1).

PREDICTIVE TESTING AND EXTRAPOLATION FROM ANIMALS TO MAN

The induction of hypersensitivity reactions and autoimmune diseases by chemicals is an area of great concern for human health; however, there is no fully validated test to screen chemicals for their capacity to elicit adverse effects. A primary objective is to advance the development of procedures that can be employed in experimental animals to investigate the immunotoxic effects of chemicals (including drugs) on which no such data are available. Structured approaches using the rat and mouse as experimental models are being explored, with determination of the weight and histopathology of the lymphoid organs together with immunoglobulin levels as a basic approach, followed by immune function studies of nonspecific defence mechanisms and of cellular and humoral immunity. The use of in-vitro systems as complementary or alternative tests is also being developed.

Uncertainty has been expressed about the adequacy of using conventional morphological evaluation methods as a-priori indicators of immunotoxic processes. In some situations, lymphoid organ-specific effects seem not to be associated with changes in immune reactivity; conversely, some compounds affect immmune reactivity in the apparent absence of overt lymphoid organ pathology. The immune system, and the young thymus in particular, is known to be exquisitely sensitive to stress-induced hormonal/adrenal changes, and hormonal/adrenal effects must be taken into account when considering chemically induced thymic atrophy - especially in young animals.

Immunoperoxidase and monoclonal antibody techniques can be used to visualize the distribution of defined lymphocyte subsets and macrophages within frozen tissue sections. In addition to conventional histopathological approaches, video/computer-assisted morphometric and phenotypic analysis and quantification of cellular elements within tissue sections are available.

Clearly, more studies are needed that are designed to examine the normal morphology and architecture of rodent lymphoid organs. The effects of stress, diet, neuroendocrine influences and, perhaps most importantly, antigen challenge must all be accurately described and evaluated before the effect of a xenobiotic can be determined.

Current toxicity testing of chemicals includes few relevant parameters that would detect potential immunotoxicants. Inclusion of a limited number of additional parameters that could flag immunotoxicants during general assessments of toxicity, such as 28- and 90-day studies, could be done relatively economically without adding additional animals or acquiring highly specialized methodology. Strategies can be formulated for testing procedures to ensure detection of potentially immunotoxic chemicals.

Methods are available that allow assessment of immunotoxicity of chemicals in rodents. Immune system parameters (haematology, blood chemistry, organ weights and histopathology) that are or could be evaluated in 28- or 90-day repeat-dose studies in rats are listed in Table 2, with an indication of parameters already included in some guidelines and that could be included without difficulty. As experience with this group of test parameters increases, information will be accrued that will show whether it is necessary to include one or more functional assays from Table 3 to increase the predictive value of the screening procedure. This group of assays was discussed as a minimum for detecting potential immunotoxic chemicals and drugs for which no prior indication of immune-related effects is available. Some of the measurements will require standardization and validation in order to be used in routine testing programmes. Most of the observations listed in Table 2 relate to gross and microscopic morphology, and only a limited number of haematological and chemical parameters of general interest are listed in some toxicity test guidelines. In Table 3, methods for testing immune function are listed with an indication of their development to a state suitable for consideration for inclusion in routine testing. Selected assays from Table 3 are suggested for testing chemicals and drugs for which prior information indicates potential immunotoxic properties. It is believed that systematic recording of the parameters listed in Table 2, in certain instances complemented by selected tests listed in Table 3, may provide a useful basis for evaluating the potential immunotoxicity of a chemical (or drug) for humans. In studies performed to assess the toxicity of chemicals, consideration should be given to including the tests listed in Table 2.

Table 2. Immune system-related parameters that can be evaluated in repeat-dose toxicity studies in rats for chemicals and drugs for which no a-priori immunotoxic potential has been identified

Haematology	- Relative and absolute differential white blood cell counts (lymphocytes, monocytes, granulocytes, abnormal cells)[3]
	- Bone-marrow cellularity (nucleated count and smear)[1]
Blood chemistry	- Albumin/globulin ratio[3]
	- Serum immunoglobulin classes[1]
Organ weights	- Thymus[2]
	- Spleen[2]
	- Lymph nodes (local and distant to application site, e.g., for oral route, mesenteric and popliteal lymph nodes)[1]
Histopathology	- Thymus[3]
	- Spleen[3]
	- Lymph nodes (local and distant to application site)[3]
	- Bone marrow[3]
	- Peyer's patches[2] (oral) or bronchus-associated lymphoid tissue (inhalation)[2]

[1]Relevant parameters but method not yet standardized and validated.
[2]Relevant parameter not yet included in some toxicity test guidelines.
[3]Relevant parameter already included in most toxicity test guidelines.

Although not all the tests that are mentioned there are validated at present, the tests in Table 2 that are marked with superscript 2 (besides those marked with superscript 3) could be considered for inclusion in toxicity testing. Chemicals suspected of having effects on immune function on the basis of prior studies, structure-activity relationships and other appropriate information could be evaluated further by selected functional assays listed in Table 3, even if negative results are obtained in assays in Table 2. It must be realized that the predictive value of the results so obtained is not clear, and interpretation must be cautious.

Table 3. Functional methods available or requiring development for use with Table 2 in rodents to assess immunotoxicity (Selected assays would be strongly recommended for compounds for which some immunotoxic properties were implied.)

Category	Parameter assessed	Mouse	Rat
Cell-mediated immunity	Mixed leukocyte response	3,4	1
	Mitogen proliferation	3	2
	Delayed hypersensitivity response	3	2,4
	Cytotoxicity T-lymphocyte	2	1
Antibody-mediated immunity[5]	Antibody plaque-forming cell response	3,4	1
	Serum antibody titre to specific antigen (ELISA)	2	2,4
Natural resistance[6]	Natural killer cell cytotoxicity	3	2
	Macrophage: phagocytosis and intracellular killing	3	2
	Polymorphonuclear leukocyte function	1	1
Host resistance assessment models	Influenza virus	3,4	1
	Listeria monocytogenes	3,4	2,4
	Tumours	3,4	2
	Plasmodium	2	1
	Trichinella	2	2,4

[1]Further development required.
[2]Method(s) currently available, but not standardized or validated.
[3]Method standardized and validated in interlaboratory comparison (three laboratories, five compounds).
[4]Preferred method(s).
[5]These are antigen-driven responses. Antigens commonly used include sheep erythrocytes, tetanus toxoid and ovalbumin.
[6]Should consider mediator-driven responses using either interleukin-2 or interferon for in-vitro activation of natural killer cells and macrophages.

For the assessment of potential hypersensitivity, a different approach must be considered, since high, multiple dosing which promotes systemic distribution of the chemical is not appropriate for inducing or eliciting hypersensitivity reactions. More than 25 methods have been used to induce contact sensitivity in experimental animals. The guinea-pig maximization test is a widely used method, but others have also given high sensitization rates for metallic compounds with sensitizing properties in humans. There is no single method that is of proven value for predicting the sensitization of humans to chemicals, although some tests may serve a useful function in this regard.

Animal models are needed which provide information on both immunological events and functional changes in hypersensitivity reactions following exposure to chemicals *via* the respiratory tract and the gastrointestinal tract.

Concerning autoimmunity, methods exist for the detection of autoantibodies and immune complexes in man. Similar methods can be used in animal models. A link between autoimmune disease and exposure to some metals (e.g., mercury) has been established in animals genetically predisposed to develop such disease. Further studies are required in order to examine the feasibility of using animal models for predictive testing of such risks of development of similar disease in humans. New approaches like the PLNA seem promising indicators of a chemical's potential to induce immune dysregulation, but they must be validated.

The direct PLNA indicates primary and secondary T-cell responses to immunogenic compounds. The adaptive transfer of PLN T cells lends itself to detection of sensitizing metabolites during toxicity testing. The PLNA could be considered a first step in the evaluation of the immunogenicity of a substance. When the result is positive, more detailed and sophisticated methods may be applied in order to evaluate possible adverse immune reactions of the substance under test (Table 4).

The various categories of immunotoxicity (immunosuppression, immunoenhancement, hypersensitivity, autoimmunity) display different characteristics with regard to dependence on genetic variation in susceptibility, route of administration of chemical substance and biochemical mechanisms of damage. Further understanding is required before these and other factors that influence dose-response relationships can be taken into account and used in risk assessment for human populations. In order to examine the feasibility and utility of the conventional dose-effect and dose-response relationships in setting, for example, environmental safety levels, it is necessary to build up an adequate data base specifically relating the full immunomodulatory properties of a particular chemical with its conventional toxicity profile.

Table 4. A proposed tier testing system for potential autoimmunity

Phase 1: Popliteal lymph node (PLN) assay

    1. PLN weight index
    2. Number of cells in PLN
    3. ^{3}H-Thymidine incorporation
    4. Characterization of cells in PLN

Phase 2

    1. The auricular lymph node assay and topical sensitization in mice
    2. Studies involving other parenteral routes of administration of the chemical, such as inhalation, to screen for immediate-type hypersensitivity reactions
    3. Tests to detect autoantibodies
    4. Determination of serum immunoglobulin levels
    5. Quantitative and qualitative analysis of leukocytes
    6. Tests for expression of immunoregulatory cytokines in the PLN and other relevant tissues
    7. Tests for deposition of immune reactants

CONCLUSIONS AND RECOMMENDATIONS

1. For certain metallic compounds (e.g., Ni, Cr) that give rise to immunologically mediated hypersensitivity, sufficient information is available on dose-response relationships that conditions for dermal exposure can be defined such as to prevent the development of dermatitis in most cases. This information should be used widely for prevention of these dermatological disorders.

2. Dose-effect and dose-response relationships should be defined for most metals and metallic compounds that have been shown to induce effects mediated by the immune system.

3. For immunological effects other than dermal hypersensitivity, assessment of risk is difficult at present. The inclusion of immunological effects in the framework of risk assessment requires further consideration, e.g., the applicability of concepts like critical organ and critical concentration should be examined.

4. Monitoring for human immunotoxicological effects is a complex and difficult task, which deserves further study. Some important immune-mediated effects of metals have been identified in studies of humans and animals; however, for many other chemicals, metals and metal compounds, to which humans are exposed, studies to elucidate immune modulating properties need to be performed.

   Investigations in human populations should include:

   (i)   immunological studies of cases of chemical poisoning with matched controls;
   (ii)   case-control studies of patients with immunological disorders; and
   (iii) epidemiological studies of exposed persons, particularly in occupational groups, whose exposures to airborne immunoactive metallic compounds are well characterized physically and chemically.

5. In epidemiological studies of immunologically mediated effects, it is often of great importance to characterize genetic factors (e.g., MHC antigen types, enzyme polymorphism) in responders and non-responders to the effect in question. Such studies are recommended for disorders of suspected immunological etiology and occurrence in population groups exposed to metals and other chemical compounds.

6. In the further exploration of immunologically mediated lung disease caused by metallic compounds, consideration should be given to the possibility of using some of the diagnostic tests already successfully used, e.g., for the diagnosis of granulomatous beryllium disease.

7. The methods used in immunotoxicology should be standardized and subject to continuous quality control. The techniques should be validated for accuracy, reproducibility, sensitivity and specificity, preferably in international studies.

8. It is recommended that studies that are performed to screen for immunotoxicity of chemicals include the tests presented in Table 2. However, since not all the tests listed have been validated, it is recommended that only those marked with superscripts 2 and 3 be considered for inclusion in toxicity testing.

9. The induction of allergy and autoimmune diseases by xenobiotics is of great concern for human health. Tests for screening xenobiotics have been fully validated only in the field of contact hypersensitivity. Fully validated tests for screening xenobiotics for their capacity to elicit other allergic or autoimmune disorders are not available. The popliteal lymph node assay in rats and mice to monitor the ability of xenobiotics to induce immune activation leading to allergic/ autoimmune manifestations has been used successfully in several laboratories with consistent and reproducible results. Before the assay can gain international recognition and acceptance, however, international studies should be initiated to validate and further develop it.

10. Toxicity studies should be designed to examine the morphology of rodent lymphoid organs, and the value of morphometry and of specific morphological/histological methods (e.g., stepwise sections, immunohistochemistry) must be considered. Experimental parameters such as housing and diet that may influence the immune system must be accurately evaluated and described before any effect of a xenobiotic can be determined.

THE IMMUNE SYSTEM AND IMMUNOTOXICOLOGY

THE IMMUNE SYSTEM:
AN INTEGRATED OVERVIEW

J.P. Revillard

Laboratory of Immunology
INSERM U80 CNRS URA 1177 UCBL
Hôpital E. Herriot, 69437 Lyon Cedex 3, France

ABSTRACT

The immune system contributes to the maintenance of the physiological integrity of the individual by eliminating foreign material and infectious microorganisms to which the organism is exposed. Both nonspecific, or innate, immunity and specific acquired immunity participate in this function. Self and nonself discrimination are ensured by two families of highly polymorphic molecules - T-cell receptors and B-cell receptors or antibodies. The latter interact with native antigens in solid or fluid phase, whereas the former bind only to self major histocompatiblity complex molecules associated with antigenic peptides processed by antigen-presenting cells. The genetic mechanisms by which the diversity of antibodies and T-cell receptor molecules is generated are briefly summarized, and current concepts of B- and T-cell differentiation are presented. Both lineages undergo a central stage of development in fetal liver and bone marrow (B cells) or thymus (T cells), which is controlled by cellular interactions and interleukins produced within the microenvironment of these organs. A second stage of differentiation occurs in peripheral lymphatic tissues after antigenic or polyclonal mitogenic activation induced by environmental stimulants. The latter process allows adaptation of the immune response to the antigenic environment of the organisms by clonal selection of T and B cells, which are triggered to differentiate into regulatory, or effector, T cells and plasma cells, respectively. The effects of recent developments in basic immunology on immunotoxicology are discussed briefly.

INTRODUCTION

The immune system contributes to the maintenance of the physiological integrity of the individual by eliminating foreign material and infectious agents to which the organism is exposed. Two processes are involved in ensuring this biological function: nonspecific immunity and specific immunity. The two appeared successively in the evolution of species but remain closely interwoven in higher organisms. Each requires the recognition, at the molecular level, of the organism's own molecules, or 'self', and of foreign elements, or 'nonself'. Both specific and nonspecific immunity involve cells (cell-mediated immunity) and soluble molecules in biological fluids (humoral immunity). Nonspecific immunity is characterized by its innate character (not induced by an infectious agent) and by both a lack of memory of and adaptation to new pathogens. Specific or acquired immunity is triggered by the contact of an organism with a given antigen, and involves memory. Two families of antigen-recognizing molecules exist in the immune system: B-lymphocyte receptors, or antibodies, and T-lymphocyte receptors. Specific recognition is defined as a molecular interaction between a part of the antigen called the epitope (an epitope corresponds to an area of about six to 18 amino acids, or of five to six oses) and a restricted zone of the receptor, called the paratope. Antibodies recognize epitopes, present on the surface of native antigen in solution, which may be proteins or polysaccharides, whereas T-cell receptors bind to peptides processed by antigen-presenting cells. In these cells, the antigen

Immunotoxicity of Metals and Immunotoxicology, Edited by
A. D. Dayan *et al.,* Plenum Press, New York, 1990

undergoes conformational or structural changes, generating peptides, which are then presented in association with class I or class II proteins of the major histocompatibility complex (MHC, known as HLA in humans).

Experimental removal of lymphoepithelial organs led to the demonstration of two pathways for the differentiation of cells responsible for specific immunity. In chickens, ablation of the bursa of Fabricius (bursectomy) before the 12th day of development led to agamma-globulinaemia and the absence of plasmocytes in lymphoid organs, as well as the absence of antibody production. The cell-mediated response (delayed hypersensitivity, allograft rejection, graft *versus* host reaction) remains unaltered. Conversely, removal of the thymus (thymectomy) at birth, or absence of proper thymic development (e.g., in 'nude' mice), brings about aplasia of the thymo-dependent areas of the lymphoid organs. In this case, the cell-mediated response is absent. Antibodies specific for polysaccharide antigens are produced normally, but the response to antigenic stimulation by protein antigens is markedly depressed.

ANTIGENICITY AND SELF/NONSELF DISCRIMINATION

An antigen used to be defined operationally by its capacity to bind specific antibodies (and *vice versa*). An immunogen is any substance that can induce an immune response when appropriately introduced into an immunocompetent organism. A hapten is a small molecule that is not immunogenic unless linked to an antigenic carrier macromolecule. Some of the antibodies induced by immunization with hapten-carrier conjugates can bind to haptens that are linked to unrelated carriers; these are therefore considered to be hapten-specific, although the paratope of the antibody molecule interacts with a much broader molecular structure than that of the hapten itself. Carrier molecules may be components of the immunized organism; hence, application of a wide variety of substances to the skin may induce contact hypersensitivity, a form of T-cell-mediated immunity which can be considered a 'self + X' reaction, X being the chemical (e.g., dinitrochlorobenzene or oxazolone) and self (a) protein(s) of epidermal cells. This model is of great relevance to immunotoxicology because it was the first to associate reactivity to an environmental chemical with a self antigen, leading to the more recent concept of 'altered self'.

Comparison of gene sequences and protein sequences in different species shows that some parts of the molecule are relatively invariant whereas others are highly divergent. The first are involved in the three-dimensional structure of the molecule or in its biological activity (e.g., the active site of an enzyme). Comparison of the amino acid sequences of a given protein from different animal species helps to understand the concept of antigenicity. For instance, the monomorphic protein human albumin is not antigenic in the human species, but it induces antibodies when injected into nonhuman mammals or birds. Each species 'sees' human albumin in a different fashion, which to some extent reflects the difference in structure between the antigenic molecule and its counterpart in the immunized host. Despite obvious limitations owing to the fact that epitopes are associated with the tertiary structure of the molecule but only indirectly with its amino acid sequence, this approach, based on molecular evolution, may help in predicting the antigenicity of a given substance.

This concept can be extended to alloantigens, which are made up of polymorphic molecules the structure of which differs among individuals and groups of individuals within the same species. Examples of such antigens are allotypes of immunoglobulins and products of the MHC. The latter were defined by serological (alloantibodies) and cellular (mixed lymphocyte reaction) methods which provided a reasonable estimate of the number of allelic genes at each locus; however, nucleotide sequences of HLA genes and protein sequences (Parham *et al.*, 1988) showed that some polymorphism occurred within a single HLA type. Moreover, as shown in Figure 1, HLA-A1-negative individuals can recognize different structures of the HLA-A1 molecule, depending on their own HLA-A molecules.

The most polymorphic molecular structures are the molecules of the immune system that are involved in self/nonself recognition, i.e., antibodies and T-cell receptors. Each polypeptide chain of these molecules bears epitopes associated with the variable region

HLA molecule	140					145					150					155
A2-1	Q	T	T	K	H	K	W	E	A	A	H	V	A	E	Q	L
A2-3	Q	T	T	K	H	K	W	E	T	A	H	E	A	E	Q	W
A3-1	Q	I	T	K	R	K	W	E	A	A	H	E	A	E	Q	L
All	Q	I	T	K	R	K	W	E	A	A	H	A	A	E	Q	Q
Al	Q	I	T	K	R	K	W	E	A	V	H	A	A	E	Q	R
A32	Q	I	T	Q	R	K	W	E	A	A	R	V	A	E	Q	L
AW24	Q	I	T	K	R	K	W	E	A	A	H	V	A	E	Q	Q

Fig. 1. Primary structure of a part of the α_2 domain of the HLA-A molecule according to Parham *et al.* (1988); each amino acid is represented by its code letter. Note that differences appear between the two HLA-A2 molecules in positions 148, 151 and 155. Differences between pairs of various HLA-A molecules are located at various positions in the chain. Some parts of the sequence are conserved (e.g., 140-142, 145-147, 152-157).

which are called idiotopes (Kunkel *et al.*, 1963; Oudin & Michel, 1963). Each idiotope can interact with the paratope of anti-idiotypic antibodies (auto-antibodies) and/or T-cell receptors, within idiotypic networks (Jerne, 1974, 1984; Bona, 1987).

Microorganisms are endowed with a great ability to adapt to changes occurring in their environment. Adaptation is achieved by mutation/selection and regulation of the expression of their genomes. As a consequence of the immune response of their host, the pressure of selection promotes the emergence of molecular structures in the parasite that are as close as possible to those of the host. Molecular mimicry between pathogen and host structures accounts for the diversity of immunopathological manifestations of infectious diseases linked to the genetic polymorphism of individuals within a species. Sequence homologies between antigens of infectious agents (e.g., Epstein-Barr virus, peptides from mycobacteria) and polymorphic self molecules (e.g., HLA class II antigens) could account for altered host reactions to these antigens and possibly for the development of 'autoimmune' or chronic inflammatory diseases.

EPITOPES AND PARATOPES

The precise three-dimensional structure of the antibody combining site was determined recently by three groups of investigators, using X-ray diffraction analysis of crystals (Amit *et al.*, 1986; Colman *et al*, 1987; Sheriff *et al.*, 1987). These studies demonstrated the contribution of both heavy and light chains to the binding and the critical role of some residues. These data make it quite clear that point mutations involving one of the critical residues may result in a dramatic alteration of antibody affinity (and possibly in a change of specificity), whereas mutations at other positions may alter the idiotope without affecting the paratope of the antibody. In the two studies in which egg lysozyme was the antigen (Amit *et al.*, 1986; Sheriff *et al.*, 1987), no significant conformational change in antigen was observed between the native and the complexed form. With influenza neuraminidase (Colman *et al.*, 1987), more evidence of structural alteration after antigen-antibody binding was documented, suggesting that antibody may induce conformational changes of the antigen at distant sites from that of the epitope.

The three-dimensional structure of an HLA-A molecule was established by Bjorkman *et al.* (1987). The two external domains, $\alpha 1$ and $\alpha 2$, form a cavity with β sheets on the bottom and α helixes on the edges. Most of the polymorphic residues are located in this zone. The crystal contained a peptide lying in the cavity, and it was assumed that this represented a processed self or nonself antigen. Class-II HLA antigens have not been obtained as crystals as yet, but their overall structure closely resembles that of class-I antigens (Brown *et al.*, 1988). The T-cell receptor is a heterodimer with a structure similar to that of a Fab fragment of the antibody molecule (Claverie *et al.*, 1989). It is thus possible to establish models of the molecular interactions which involve the three molecules: T-cell receptor, processed antigen and HLA molecule. These interactions summarize the restriction elements of immune recognition by T cells. The T-cell receptor must interact with self HLA histotopes. This capacity is acquired by selection during intrathymic T-cell differentiation. T-Cell receptors must also interact with the antigenic peptide, a property which depends on the molecular structure of the paratope of the receptor and on the expansion or deletion of the T-cell clones which carry the appropriate receptor. Another set of restriction elements is provided by the processing of antigen and its molecular association, usually as a peptide, with self HLA class-I or class-II molecules. Because of the polymorphism of MHC molecules, different peptides from the same protein will be presented to the T-cell receptor, depending on the MHC haplotypes of the individual. By using synthetic antigens of restricted heterogeneity or natural proteins at critically low doses as immunogens, it is possible to classify animals as responders or non-responders. This property, which is the functional assay for studying immune response genes, depends on the molecular structure of the MHC l-A and l-E antigens which can or cannot bind to the appropriate peptide.

These structural data provide the background for hypotheses about the interference of environmental toxic substances with these molecular interactions. The elegant studies of Druet and coworkers on the model of mercuric chloride in the rat clearly established the genetic restriction of the immunotoxic effects of this metal and provided strong indirect evidence for an alteration of self MHC class-II antigen-T-cell receptor interactions, resulting in inappropriate T-cell activation and subsequent polyclonal B-cell activation, autoantibody production and increased IgE synthesis (Pelletier *et al.*, 1985, 1986). The model of chronic local graft-*versus*-host reaction of Gleichmann and coworkers can be analysed within the same molecular framework (Hurtenbach *et al.*, 1987). However, in these two models, direct evidence for interaction of the toxic molecule with MHC class-II antigens, T-cell receptors or antigenic peptides is still awaited.

ANTIGEN PROCESSING

In order to be recognized by T lymphocytes, most antigens require processing so that immunogenic epitopes can be revealed and bound to MHC molecules. The interaction between processed peptides and MHC molecules has begun to be defined at the molecular level; however, much less is known about how these peptides are generated from foreign or self antigens and where they interact with the MHC molecule. There are at least three pathways of antigen processing, and each may be further subdivided into separate compartments (Long, 1988). First, exogenous antigens may be taken up by antigen-presenting cells through endocytosis and associated with newly synthesized class-II MHC molecules in endosomes. This pathway requires pH-dependent fusion and is sensitive to lysosomotropic agents (e.g., chloroquine). Second, antigenic molecules synthesized by any cell may be associated with MHC class-I antigens (Braciale *et al.*, 1987), possibly after degradation in the endoplasmic reticulum. Finally, cytoplasmic antigens (e.g., viral proteins in a virus-infected cell) are also processed and presented by class-I HLA antigen (Townsend, 1987), possibly by the ubiquitin-mediated protein degradation pathway. It is generally assumed that antigens processed by the exogenous pathway are recognized only by class-II restricted T cells (helper/inducer or cytotoxic), whereas endogenous processing of the same antigen leads to recognition by class-I restricted T cells (Germain, 1986). The two pathways may generate different peptides from the same antigen.

B-CELL DIFFERENTIATION

B-Cell receptors or antibody molecules are made of symmetrical pairs of light (L) and heavy (H) chains encoded by different sets of genes. The chromosomal location of these genes and their approximative numbers are listed in Table 1. Each gene is not functional in

Table 1. Human immunoglobulin genes

Chain	Chromosome	Segment	Genes			
			V	D	J	C
Heavy	14	14q32	1000(?)	4-50(?)	6	9
κ	2	2p12	100-200	0	4	1
λ	22	22q11		0	?	~10

its germinal configuration. A somatic rearrangement occurring during early B-cell differentiation between D-J_H then V_H-D-J_H segments for H genes, V-J for κ or λ genes, is necessary before the gene can be expressed (Alt, 1986; Gefter & Marrack, 1986). Added to the fact that each recognition unit (paratope) is made up of two independent H and L chains, the use of several gene segments to code for a single polypeptide accounts for the great structural diversity of antibody molecules (up to 10^9 different molecular species or even more). Germ line diversity is further enhanced by the very high rate of somatic mutations that may occur in V_H genes.

B Lymphocytes differentiate from lymphoid stem cells (or from haem-atopoietic pluripotent stem cells) in the fetal liver then in the bone marrow. This first stage of differentiation is under the control of interleukins (IL)-7 and -4 and other mediators produced within the microenvironment of the bone marrow. Orderly gene rearrangement and expression leads to a mature B cell expressing surface IgM and IgD bearing the same L chain (κ or λ) and the same V_H domain. During this first (central) stage of differentiation, B cells express a set of surface molecules, initially recognized by monoclonal antibodies and designated as CD (cluster of differentiation). Examples of such molecules are shown in Table 2. Most of them represent cell membrane receptors, which have a major function in cellular interactions, in the triggering and regulation of B-cell activation and differentiation (Zola, 1987).

The second stage of B-cell differentiation occurs in peripheral lymphoid organs. It is triggered by nonspecific mitogens (e.g., lymphokines, bacterial products) or by antigens and thus permits adaptation of the immune system to environmental stimuli (Melchers & Anderson, 1984; Jelinek & Lipsky, 1987). The endpoint of this peripheral B-cell differentiation is either a memory B cell or a plasma cell. The latter has a short half-life. Thus, all of the regulation of the antibody response affects activation, clonal expansion and terminal differentiation of B cells but not the rate of immunoglobulin secretion by plasma cells. Most of the regulation involves T cells *via* cognate T-B interaction and/or release of lymphokines such as IL-2, IL-4, IL-5 and IL-6. Accessory cells (e.g., monocytes, macrophages, dendritic cells) also contribute to this regulation by secreting mediators such as IL-1 and IL-6, which provide B-cell activation signals, or the prostaglandin E_2, which exerts suppressive effects.

A single B cell or B-cell clone may subsequently produce antibodies of different classes or subclasses by switching the heavy chain constant gene. Switching is regulated by interleukins and by isotypic networks involving antigen-antibody complexes and Fc receptors on various cell types (Revillard, 1985a,b). Class and subclass regulation depends on the chemical structure of the antigen and on its route of introduction.

Table 2. Main differentiation stages of the B-cell lineage

Characteristic[a]	Early pre-B	Pre-B	Immature B	Mature B	Activated B	Plasma cells
DNA recombinations	D-J_H	V_H-D-J_H	V_κ-J_κ V_λ-J_λ			
Intracytoplasmic Ig	0	μ	0	0	IgM	IgM/IgG/IgA/IgE
Surface Ig	0	0	IgM	IgM + IgD	IgM	0
HLA Class II (DR, DP, DQ)	-/+	+	+	+	+ +	+ /-
CD9 (p24)	0	+	+	+		0
CD10 (cALLA)	+	+	0	0	0	0
CD19 (p95)	+	+	+	+	+/-	
CD20 (p35)	0	+	+	+	+/-	+
CD21 (p140)	0	0	+	+	0	0
CD22 (gp130, 140)	0	-/+	+	+	+/-	+
CD23 (p45)	0	0	0	0	+	
CD24 (p42)	0	0	+	+	+	-
CDw40 (p50)	0	0	+	+	0	0

[a]Ig, immunoglobulin; p24, protein or glycoprotein of 24 kD.

T-CELL DIFFERENTIATION

Two types of specific antigen receptors, or Ti molecules, are expressed on distinct subsets of T cells. Each receptor consists of a heterodimer composed of two polypeptide chains (α and β, or γ and δ) linked by an interchain disulfide bond. The molecular structure of the Ti receptor is therefore similar to that of the Fab fragment of immunoglobulins (Williams, 1984; Royer & Reinherz, 1987; Claverie et al., 1989).

These polypeptides contain a number of sequences. Starting at the amino terminal, there is an L sequence (a hydrophobic signal peptide containing 20 amino acid residues) which is absent in the mature protein, a V sequence (or V + D in β and δ chains) including an interchain disulfide bond, a J sequence of about 15 residues, a C sequence of about 140 residues, a transmembrane hydrophobic sequence of about 20 amino acids, and a short intracytoplasmic tail about five amino acids long.

Each sequence is coded for by a different exon. Table 3 summarizes current knowledge on the numbers and chromosomal locations of T-cell receptor genes. A series of gene rearrangements, leading to a functional gene product, takes place during intrathymic cell differentiation. The recombination events are essentially identical to those involved in immunoglobulin gene rearrangements (Born et al., 1985). T-Cell receptor diversity arises as a result of multiple V and J gene segments (germ-line diversity and combination diversity) and junctional diversity (possible addition of nucleotides during D-J and V-D joining, and three different potential reading frames for translation of the Dβ sequence). Terminal deoxyribonucleotidyl transferase, present in immature cells, also plays a role in junctional diversity. Another factor that contributes to diversity is the heterodimeric structure of the Ti molecule. In contrast to the situation in B cells, somatic mutation does not seem to occur in α, β or γ genes. It should be kept in mind that many recombination events generate nonfunctional genes.

By analysing the specificity of monoclonal antibodies directed against human leukocytes, and monoclonal cell lines derived from leukaemia or lymphoma cells, groups of antibodies that recognize the same antigen have been classified as CD. The antigens defined in this way have been characterized, and the molecular structure and gene sequence of some of them, along with their biological functions, have been elucidated (Möller, 1983). Examples of the main T-cell differentiation antigens are given in Table 4. Some markers are present on all mature T cells (e.g., CD2, CD3, CD5), and others are displayed only at certain stages of differentiation (e.g., CD1) or on different subpopulations of T cells (e.g., CD4, CD8).

The CD3 molecule (Kanellopoulos et al., 1983) is made up of three peptide chains, γ, δ and ε (two others, ζ and p21, have been identified in mice). It is closely associated with the Ti receptor and plays a role in transducing the signal produced by antigen-Ti receptor interaction. This activates tyrosine kinase (protein phosphorylation) and phospholipase C

Table 3. Human T cell receptor genes

Gene	α	β	γ	δ
Chromosome	14	7	7	14
Segment	14q11 to 12	7q35	7p15	14q11 to 12
V genes	~100 (>58)	>76	8 (+7ψ)[a]	?~ 10
D genes	, 0	2	0	2
J genes	46 (~100)	13	5	3
C genes	1	2	2	1
Ti molecule	α β		γ δ	
Association with CD3	+		+	
Association with CD4 or CD8	+		_b	

[a]ψ refers to peudogenes.
[b]Some γδ receptors are associated with CD8.

Table 4. Main differentiation antigens of human T cells

Antigen	Apparent molecular mass (kDa)	Distribution	Remarks
CD1a	49	Thymocytes (and Langherhans' cells)	Expression associated with TE-3 antigen of the epithelial thymic cortex
CD1b	45		
CD1c	43		
CD2	50	Thymocytes and T lymphocytes	Adhere to lymphocyte function-association antigen-3
CD3	20,25,26	Mature T cells	Associated with Ti (α β or γ δ)
CD4	60	Stage II and III thymocytes and 2/3 of mature T cells	Adhere to HLA-DR
CD5	67	T Cells and immature B-cell subsets	
CD6	120	T Cells	
CD7	40	T-Cell subsets	IgM receptor
CD8	32	Stage II and III thymoytes and 1/3 of mature T cells	Adhere to HLA-A, B, C
CD25	55	Activated T cells	p55 light chain of interleukin-2 receptor
CD28	44	Cytotoxic T-cell subsets	(p44, 9 3 antibody)
CDw29	135	T-Cell subsets	4B4 antibody

(diacyl-glycerol synthesis), and opens ionic channels. Anti-CD3 antibodies activate T cells, as do certain anti-Ti antibodies (Royer & Reinherz, 1987).

The process of T-cell differentiation has been described by analysing the sequential expression of differentiation markersand by studying Ti receptor gene rearrangements. In the eighth week of development, at the stage when pre-T cells leave the fetal liver and settle in the thymus, CD7 antigens, a T200 (CD44) molecule and a CD2 antigen can be detected. This is the phenotype that corresponds to stage-I thymocytes as well as certain severe combined immune deficiencies. In the tenth week of development, CD4 and CD8 antigens are expressed, followed by CD3 and CD6 (twelfth week). During this period, γ genes (or γ and δ), β genes (D-J then V-D-J junctions), and finally α genes rearrange in sequential order. Another scheme of differentiation is coupled to this ontogeny. This sequential development is established after the fifteenth week and maintained after birth, and the stages of differentiation may be topographically related to a maturation gradient, originating in the outer cortex and ending in the medulla. Analyses of the phenotypic expression and T-cell receptor gene rearrangements occurring in lymphoma and leukaemia cells reveal that the diseased cells roughly correspond to discrete intrathymic differentiation stages. The data obtained from studies of monoclonal proliferation, along with the data on normal ontogeny, are summarized in Table 5. As this scheme is still very rough, modifications will probably need to be added as we gather more data.

Most thymocytes die in the thymus. This phenomenon has not been elucidated, and several explanations have been proposed. The first suggests that the probability of a nonfunctional rearrangement, which is inherent in the structure of Ti receptor genes, is high for γ, intermediate for β, and low for α. The second deals with intrathymic education, a mechanism of positive selection of T cells based on the capacity of the α and/or β receptor chains to interact with the polymorphic determinants of class-I or class-II HLA gene products.

Table 5. Main intrathymic differentiation stages of T cells

Stages	Pre-T	Thymocyte stage I	Thymocyte stage 2	Thymocyte stage III	Mature T lymphocyte
CD1	-	-	+	-	-
CD2	-	+	+	+	+
CD3	-	-	-	+	+
CD4/CD8	-	-	+/+	+/- or -/+	+/- or -/+
DNA rearrangement					
γ genes	-/+	+	+	+	+
β genes	-	-	+	+	+
α genes	-	-	-/+	+	+
mRNA					
γ	–	+	+/–	–	–
β	–	–	+	+	+
α	–	–	–	+	+

Thymocytes begin migrating towards the peripheral lymphoid organs (spleen) in the thirteenth week and continue to do so afterwards. In the twentieth week of gestation, mature T cells infiltrate the bone marrow (4-6% of CD8$^+$ cells). T-Cell activation occurs in peripheral lymphoid tissues (spleen, lymph nodes, mucosae-associated lymphoid tissues) as a result of interaction with an antigen-presenting cell (e.g., B lymphocyte, monocyte/macrophage, Langerhans' cells from the epidermis, dendritic cells in the thymus-dependent areas of lymphoid organs). Progression through the cell cycle, maturation and differentiation of T cells is controlled by a set of interleukins (mostly IL-2, IL-4 and interferon γ) and cytokines (IL-1, IL-6 and tumour necrosis factor-α). After clonal expansion of antigen-specific T cells, which interact either with HLA class-II molecules (CD4$^+$ T cells) or HLA class I (CD8$^+$ T cells), terminal differentiation leads to small circulating T lymphocytes endowed with cytotoxic capacity (cytotoxic T cells) or with the capacity to produce various lymphokines upon activation. The latter population contributes to immune regulation (T helper/inducer cells) or to effector mechanisms such as delayed hypersensitivity by secretion of lymphokines.

In summary, both B-cell and T-cell differentiation pathways are characterized by a central antigen-independent stage and a peripheral step which requires activation and concerns a limited number of clones. However, major differences exist between these two lineages. B-Cell differentiation gives rise to short-lived cells and operates throughout the organism's life span; somatic mutations are quite frequent. In contrast, intrathymic T-cell differentiation decreases after puberty and leads to long-lived cells with little or no somatic mutation. Hence, ageing of the immune system is characterized by a relative T-cell defect, which contrasts with elevated immunoglobulin production rate, decreased response to novel antigens and increased incidence of autoantibodies.

Finally, it should be emphasized that immune and neuroendocrine systems are closely interwoven at multiple levels of regulation. Most cells involved in specific and nonspecific immunity express receptors for steroids, peptidic hormones, neuropeptides and catecholamines. These mediators modulate the immune response by acting at various stages of cellular activation or differentiation. They can act at a distance from their production site, like hormones, but most act at the site of their release by neurones, which form pseudo synapses at the point of contact with lymphoid cells. Conversely, interleukins may act on the central nervous system and the hypothalamo-adrenal axis, and activated lymphocytes were shown to produce propiomelanocortin, a precursor of endorphins and adreno-corticotropic hormone.

CONCLUSION

This brief survey of the immune system shows that toxic compounds in the environment may interfere at multiple levels with the host's immunity. The prediction of immunotoxicity from in-vitro or animal studies may be an impossible goal if one excepts to be able to detect gross immunosuppression. Most biological sciences, including physiology, pharmacology and toxicology, deal with rather simple mechanisms which are shared by several animal species and are assumed to be identical among most individuals of a given species. Immunology, however, is concerned with the molecular and cellular basis of the polymorphism of individual reactions. Nearly all members of a community are exposed to the same load of airborne allergens (e.g., house dust, pollens), yet no more than a few per cent of them will suffer from conjunctivitis, rhinitis, asthma or allergic eczema. Industrial pollutants, which by themselves have no demonstrable direct effect on the immune system according to currently available tests, may increase the incidence of allergic reactions among exposed individuals. Adverse drug reactions, which range from benign cutaneous rashes to life-threatening Lyell syndrome, hepatitis or cytopenia, are very rare, and they involve either antigen-specific immune reactions or other types of nonimmunological hypersensitivity. The multiple effects of radiology contrast products on the complement and other inflammatory or immune reactions provide no clue to explain the severe or fatal hypersensitivity reactions that occur once among 30-100 000 injections. The same remarks apply to most drugs that induce autoantibodies in rare individuals.

The prediction of immunotoxic effects must take into account recent developments in understanding molecular interactions between antigenic peptides, MHC molecules and T-cell receptors. So far, most of these interactions have been analysed at the cellular level after administration of the toxic substance *in vivo* (e.g., popliteal lymph node assay, T-cell activation *ex vivo*). It is conceivable that in the near future most efforts will be devoted to the development of in-vitro procedures for investigating molecular interactions between toxic molecules and B- or T-cell receptors, HLA antigens and processed peptides, or the effect of toxic agents on antigen processing. The greatest challenge is the assessment of the effect of long-term exposure to environmental toxins on the incidence of altered immune responses (e.g., allergy, autoimmunity, susceptibility to infections or lymphomas and leukaemias). This approach has proved to be extremely rewarding when applied to long-term side-effects of immunosuppressive treatments (Nicolas *et al.*, 1988; Penn, 1988).

REFERENCES

Alt, F.W. (1986) Antibody diversity. New mechanism. *Nature*, **322**: 772-773

Amit, A.G., Mariuzza, R.A., Phillips, S.E.V. & Poljak, R.J. (1986) Three-dimensional structure of an antigen-antibody complex at 2.8Å resolution. *Science*, **233**: 747-753

Bjorkman, P.J., Saper, M.A., Samraoui, B., Bennett, W.S., Strominger, J.L. & Wiley, D.C. (1987) Structure of the human class I histocompatibility antigen, HLA-A2. *Nature*, **329**: 506-518

Bona, C. (1987) *Regulatory Idiotypes* (*Modern Concepts in Immunology*, Vol. 11), New York, J. Wiley

Born, W., Yague, J., Palmer, E., Kappler, J. & Marrak, P. (1985) Rearrangement of T cell receptor β chain genes during T cell development. *Proc. natl Acad. Sci. USA*, **82**: 2925-2929

Braciale, T.J., Braciale, V.L., Winkler, M., Stroynowski, I., Hood, L., Sambrook, J. & Gething, M.J. (1987) On the role of the transmembrane anchor sequence of influenza hemagglutinin in target cell recognition by class I MHC-restricted, hemagglutinin-specific cytolytic T lymphocytes. *J. exp. Med.*, **166**: 678-692

Brown, J.H., Jardetsky, T., Saper, M.A., Samraoui, B., Bjorkman, P.J. & Wiley, D.C. (1988) A hypothetical model of the foreign antigen binding site of class II histocompatibility molecules. *Nature*, **332**: 845-850

Claverie, J.M., Prochnika-Chalufour, A. & Bougueleret, L. (1989) Implications of a Fab-like structure for the T cell receptor. *Immunol. Today*, **10**: 10-14

Colman, P.M., Laver, W.G., Varghese, J.N., Baker, A.T., Tulloch, P.A., Air, G.M. & Webster, R.G. (1987) Three-dimensional structure of a complex of antibody with influenza virus neuraminidase. *Nature*, **326**: 358-363

Gefter, M. & Marrack, P. (1986) Development and modification of the lymphocyte repertoire. *Nature*, **321**: 116-118

Germain, R.N. (1986) The ins and outs of antigen processing and presentation. *Nature*, **322**: 687-689

Hurtenbach, U., Gleichmann, H., Nagata, N. & Gleichmann, E. (1987) Immunity to D-penicillamine: genetic, cellular and chemical requirements for induction of popliteal lymph node enlargement in the mouse. *J. Immunol.*, **139**: 411-416

Jelinek, D F. & Lipsky, P.E. (1987) Regulation of B lymphocyte activation, proliferation and differentiation. *Adv. Immunol.*, **40**: 1-59

Jerne, N.K. (1974) Towards a network theory of the immune system. *Ann. Immunol. (Paris)*, **125C**: 373-389

Jerne, N.K. (1984) Idiotypic networks and other preconceived ideas. *Immunol. Rev.*, **79**: 5-24

Kanellopoulos, J.M., Wigglesworth, N.M., Owen, M.J. & Crumpton, M.J. (1983) Biosynthesis and molecular nature of the T3 antigen of human T lymphocytes. *EMBO J.*, **2**: 1807-1814

Kunkel, H., Mannik, M. & Williams, R.C. (1963) Individual antigenic specificity of isolated antibodies. *Science*, **140**: 1218-1219

Long, 0. (1988) Processing requirements for presentation of antigens to T lymphocytes. *Current Opin. Immunol.*, **1**: 98-102

Melchers, F. & Anderson, J. (1984) B Cell activation: three steps and their variations. *Cell*, **37**: 715-720

Möller, G. (1983) Functional T cell subsets defined by monoclonal antibodies. *Immunol. Rev.*, **74**: 5-168

Nicolas, J.F., Cozon, G. & Revillard, J.P. (1988) Some viral infections and related disorders associated with long-term immunosuppressive treatments. *J. Autoimmun.*, **1**: 558-574

Oudin, J. & Michel, M. (1963) [A new form of allotyping γ globulins from rabbit serum apparently linked to the function and specificity of antibodies.] (in French) *C.R. Acad. Sci. (Paris)*, **257**: 805-808

Parham, P., Lomen, C.E., Lawlor, D.A., Ways, J.P., Holmes, N., Coppin, H.L., Salter, R.D., Wan, A.M. & Ennis, P.D. (1988) Nature of polymorphism in HLA-A, -B, and -C molecules. *Proc. natl Acad. Sci. USA*, **85**: 4005-4009

Pelletier, L., Pasquier, R., Hirsch, F., Sapin, C. & Druet, P. (1985) In vivo self-reactivity of mononuclear cells to T cells and macrophages exposed to HgCl$_2$. *Eur. J. Immunol.*, **15**: 460-465

Pelletier, L., Pasquier, R., Hirsch, F., Sapin, C. & Druet, P. (1986) Autoreactive T cells in mercury-induced autoimmune disease: in vitro demonstration. *J. Immunol.*, **137**: 2548-2554

Penn, 1. (1988) Cancer is a long-term hazard of immunosuppressive therapy. *J. Autoimmun.*, **1**: 545-558

Revillard, J P. (1985a) Isotype regulation: IgE. *Int. Rev. Immunol.*, **2**: 1-115

Revillard, J.P. (1985b) Isotype regulation: IgG and IgA. *Int. Rev. Immunol.*, **2**: 116-120

Royer, H.D. & Reinherz, E.L. (1987) T Lymphocytes: ontogeny, function, and relevance to clinical disorders. *New Engl. J. Med.*, **317**: 1136-1142

Sheriff, S., Silverton, E.W., Padlan, E.A., Cohen, G.H., Smith-Gill, S.J., Finzel, B.C. & Davies, D.R. (1987) Three-dimensional structure of an antibody-antigen complex. *Proc. natl Acad. Sci. USA*, **84**, 8075-8079

Townsend, A.R.M. (1987) Recognition of influenza virus proteins by cytotoxic T lymphocytes. *Immunol. Res.*, **6**: 80-100

Williams, A.F. (1984) The T-lymphocyte antigen receptor - elusive no more. *Nature*, **308**: 108-109

Zola, H. (1987) The surface antigens of human B lymphocytes. *Immunol. Today*, **8**: 308-315

CONCEPTS AND DEFINITIONS IN IMMUNOTOXICOLOGY

J.H. Exon

Department of Veterinary Science, University of Idaho
Moscow, Idaho 83843, USA

ABSTRACT

The scientific field of immunotoxicology has developed as a subdiscipline of toxicology. Although this area of study has become established, it is still a young science and faced with developmental problems. Definitions and concepts must be redefined to attain more understanding and agreement among scientists working in this and related fields. Few doubt the potential health significance of chemical- and drug-induced immune dysfunction, but opinions differ on how best to assess and interpret these effects. Certainly, we can measure a variety of immune responses and detect immunopathological alterations in lymphoid organs and changes in functional immunity. Complicating interpretations of these effects are concepts of 'immune reserve', or capacity for compensation, among different compartments of the immune system. Other considerations include predisposing factors of age, malnutrition, stress and genetic susceptibility. This important science is nevertheless progressing on the basis of sound experimental approaches, careful evaluation of data and genuine concern for public health through safe use of chemicals.

INTRODUCTION

Immunotoxicology can be defined as the scientific study of adverse effects resulting from occupational, inadvertant or therapeutic exposure to drugs, environmental chemicals and biological material on the immune system of living organisms. The fact that chemicals and non-immunotherapeutic drugs could alter the immune responses of the host and decrease resistance to pathogens was first shown by studies in the 1960s, later reviewed by several authors (Vos, 1977; Dean et al., 1982). During the 1970s and early 1980s, the number of immunotoxicological studies reported in the literature increased, and international attention to the field began to grow (Haber & Pfiter, 1982; Gibson et al., 1983; Berlin et al., 1987). A large boost in the awareness of the public and of regulatory agencies of the discipline resulted from epidemiological evidence that acquired immunodeficiency syndrome (AIDS) was associated with chronic drug abuse. The science of immunotoxicology is now a relatively well established and accepted subdiscipline of toxicology but is still a young science.

The consequences of exposure to immunotoxic chemical and drugs can be several. The immune system may be either suppressed or enhanced or may react against the chemical or drug or one of its metabolites. Immunosuppression may result in decreased resistance to opportunistic pathogens (e.g., viral, fungal, bacterial) or increased susceptibility to oncogenesis. Immuno-enhancement could increase the risk of autoimmune reactions. Immune responses to the xenobiotic *per se* could result in allergic reactions such as hypersensitivity-type responses. In fact, all of these sequelae have been documented in either laboratory animals or humans. There is substantial evidence that patients receiving immunosuppressive chemotherapy or radiation treatment are much more susceptible to opportunistic infections and usually have a higher incidence of certain cancers (Allen, 1976; Penn, 1985). Studies on irradiated laboratory animals also show the importance of the

Immunotoxicity of Metals and Immunotoxicology, Edited by
A. D. Dayan *et al.,* Plenum Press, New York, 1990

immune system in protection against skin cancer. In addition, genetically immunodeficient animals and humans also have a higher incidence of infections and certain cancers (Touraine, 1987).

Certain drugs and other chemicals have also been linked to the induction of autoimmune reactions and diseases. Examples are trichloroethylene-induced scleroderma (Saihan *et al.*, 1978; Lockey *et al.*, 1987) and a similar syndrome in vinyl chloride-exposed workers (Haustein & Ziegler, 1985). There is also a relationship between exposure to the drug procainamide and development of systemic lupus erythematosus (Koffler, 1980). In several examples of animal models, autoimmune diseases can be induced by a xenobiotic (Talal, 1987). In most instances, some genetic predisposition is required for induction of autoimmune responses.

Hypersensitivity reactions to xenobiotics in occupational and environmental settings are quite common (reviewed by Luster & Dean, 1982). The very nature of immediate hypersensitivity responses, i.e., antigen-IgE binding, indicates the potential for adverse immune-mediated interactions with a variety of chemicals and drugs. Xenobiotics can also induce contact sensitivity and immune complex formation as well as protein-chemical interactions and hapten formation.

It appears, then, that immune dysregulation induced by xenobiotics could present serious health effects. Although no widespread episode of immune-related diseases has been documented as a result of exposure to xenobiotics, certain compounds have been shown to alter immune function in humans (2,3,7,8-tetrachlorodibenzo-*para*-dioxin, polychlorinated biphenyls, polybrominated biphenyls and Spanish oil syndrome; Kamuller *et al.*, 1984; Bekesi *et al.*, 1985; Lee & Chang, 1985). What is not known, however, is the degree to which quality of life is compromised by subtle immune dysfunction caused by exposure to immunotoxic chemicals in the work place and the environment. This would not necessarily result in death or severe disablement but is more likely to manifest in higher incidences of common infectious diseases or spontaneous cancer.

ASSESSMENT OF IMMUNOTOXICITY

There are currently two very distinct concepts about the best methods for screening chemicals for immunotoxicity. Some argue that potential immunotoxic compounds can be detected by methods currently used in standard toxicological screening tests, such as changes in histopathology or weights of lymphoid organs, haematological parameters (i.e., differential cell counts, white blood cell counts, morphology), serochemistry (i.e., total immunoglobulin) and enumeration of immune cell populations (i.e., T and B cells).

Most immunotoxicologists argue that standard toxicological profiles are inadequate for screening immunotoxicants because they do not measure functional parameters of the immune system. In other words, a count of the number of white blood or B cells does not indicate an altered capacity for the function of these cells. Also, there is evidence that some toxicants may selectively target the immune system at doses below those that produce other evidence of toxic damage in other tissues. There is also some evidence that immune dysfunction can occur in the absence of any clinical sign or histopathological change in lymphoid organs. Conversely, morphological changes may occur without changes in immune system function.

It is also a consensus of immunotoxicologists that no single assay for immune system function is adequate to detect the majority of immunotoxic compounds. It appears that some immunotoxicants are quite selective in the segment of the immune system they affect. A given chemical may alter antibody production by affecting B lymphocytes, with no apparent effect on specific cell-mediated responses by T lymphocytes. Therefore, a panel of assays is required in immunotoxicity testing, composed of functional assays for each major type of immune response or population of cells. Typically, such a panel includes assays for humoral immunity (i.e., antibody production by B cells), specific cell-mediated immunity (mediated by T lymphocytes) and nonspecific cell-mediated immunity (mediated by natural killer cells or macrophages). The panel includes pathotoxicity profiles, including histopathology and weights of major lymphoid organs (thymus and spleen), haematological parameters (red blood cell, white blood cell and differential cell counts) and enumeration of specific cell populations (B and T cells). Also included in the test scheme are host resistance assays (e.g., bacterial, viral, parasitic, fungal, tumour).

These assays are generally performed in some sort of tier-testing scheme. Tier-1 assays are chosen as a screening process to identify potential immunotoxicants. Compounds that have effects in one or more of the tier-1 assays would then require further testing for immunotoxic properties by a panel of tier-2 assays. The tier-2 assays are chosen to identify more definitively the types of immune responses altered, the cell populations affected, the reversibility of effect and relevance of the effect to host resistance to an appropriate model. For example, if tier-1 assays indicate a reduced capacity to produce a specific antibody to an injected antigen, as measured by antibody levels in the serum, tier-2 assays may be performed to examine if the numbers of antibody-producing cells are diminished, if B cells are impaired to undergo division, if the response is T cell-dependent or T cell-independent and if the host is more susceptible to an infectious agent that is sensitive to B cell-mediated responses. Alternatively, if tier-1 studies indicate a defect in T cell-mediated responses, tier-2 assays would be directed more toward examination of T-cell functions. Therefore, the tier-2 assay panel should have some flexibility of design to adapt to results of tier-1 screening results.

Several tier-type approaches to immunotoxicological testing have been proposed. Luster *et al.* (1988) published the results of an extensive study sponsored by the US National Toxicology Program. Several laboratories participated in an intra- and interlaboratory validation study of a battery of assays in B6C3F1 mice, in which assays were tested for sensitivity, reproducibility and predictive value to host resistance models. A panel of assays was recommended for use in tier-1 and tier-2 immunotoxicity testing studies (Table 1). Vos and Van Loveren (1987) and Exon *et al.* (1986) published similar, but less extensively validated, tier-1 and tier-2 assay panels for immunotoxicity testing in rats (Tables 2 and 3). Also, the US Environmental Protection Agency has published recommended guidelines for immunotoxicity testing of biochemical pest control agents and are in the process of formulating similar testing schemes for other pesticides (Sjobad, 1988). An extensive study to validate use of the rat for immunotoxicity testing, organized by the International Collaborative Study for Immunotoxicology, is currently under way, involving approximately 20 laboratories throughout the world. Part of this study is designed to compare conventional and 'enhanced' pathotoxicological responses in a battery of assays to assess functional parameters of immunity. These studies, if properly conducted and controlled, could provide valuable insight into exactly what procedures are adequate in screening for immunotoxic chemicals.

ASSAYS FOR IMMUNOTOXICITY

Numerous assays are available to measure different immunological endpoints in the major arms of the immune system. The criteria for choosing an assay for use in immunotoxicological testing are several. Of most importance is that the endpoint be correlated to the ability of the host to defend itself against a pathogen or tumorigenesis. Other important considerations are reproducibility, sensitivity, economy, automation and relevance to extrapolation to immune responses in humans.

The assays used most commonly to assess humoral immune responses are the plaque-forming cell assay and the enzyme-linked immunosorbent assay and their variations. Both appear to be sensitive for detecting altered antibody production, and each can be modified to measure different types of antibody responses to T cell-dependent or -independent antigens, and primary and secondary antibody responses. The plaque-forming cell assay is easy to perform and very economical in that specialized instruments are not required for quantification, and reagents are relatively inexpensive. Disadvantages to this assay may be that only one source of antibody (i.e., spleen) is measured, and only the number of antibody forming cells in that organ is assessed, not the amount of antibody they produce. Also, this assay is somewhat labour-intensive and does not lend itself well to large numbers of samples. The enzyme-linked immunosorbent assay, on the other hand,

Table 1. Panel for detecting immune alterations following exposure of rodents to chemicals or drugs[a]

Parameter	Procedure
Screen (tier I)	
Immunopathology	Haematology - complete blood count and differential cell count
	Weights - body, spleen, thymus, kidney, liver
	Cellularity - spleen
	Histology - spleen, thymus, lymph node
Humoral-mediated immunity	Enumeration of IgM antibody plaque-forming cells to T-dependent antigen; lipopolysaccharide mitogen response
Cell-mediated immunity	Lymphocyte blastogenesis to mitogens (concanavalin A) and mixed leukocyte response against allogeneic leukocytes
Nonspecific immunity	Natural killer cell activity
Comprehensive (tier II)	
Immunopathology	Quantification of splenic B- and T-cell numbers
Humoral-mediated immunity	Enumeration of IgG antibody plaque-forming cells to T-dependent antigen
Cell-mediated immunity	Cytotoxic T lymphocyte cytolysis; delayed hypersensitivity response
Nonspecific immunity	Macrophage function; quantification of resident peritoneal cells and phagocytic ability (basal and activated by macrophage activating factor)
Host resistance challenge models (endpoints)[b]	Syngeneic tumour cells
	PYB6 sarcoma (tumour incidence)
	B16F10 melanoma (lung burden)
	Bacterial models
	Listeria monocytogenes (mortality)
	Streptococcus species (mortality)
	Viral models
	Influenza (mortality)
	Parasite models
	Plasmodium yoelii (parasitaemia)

[a] The testing panel was developed using B6C3F1 female mice; from Luster *et al.* (1988).
[b] For any particular chemical tested, only two or three host resistance models are selected for examination.

Table 2. Methods for detecting immunotoxic alterations in the Wistar rat (currently being evaluated at the National Institute of Public Health and Environmental Protection, Bilthoven, The Netherlands)[a]

Parameter	Procedure
Tier 1	
Immunopathology	Routine haematology; serum IgM and IgG; lymphoid organ weights (spleen, thymus, lymph nodes) and histology; bone-marrow cellularity
Tier-2 panel	
Cell-mediated immunity	Sensitization to T-cell dependent antigens (e.g., ovalbumin, tuberculin, *Listeria*) and skin test challenge; lymphoproliferative responses to specific antigens (*Listeria*); mitogen responses
Humoral immunity	Serum titration of IgM, IgG, IgA, IgE responses to T-dependent antigens (ovalbumin, tetanus toxoid, *Trichinella spiralis*) with enzyme-linked immunosorbent assay; T cell-independent IgM response to lipopolysaccharide; mitogen response to lipopolysaccharide
Macrophage function	In-vitro phagocytosis and killing of *Listeria monocytogenes* by adherent spleen and peritoneal cells; cytolysis of YAC-1 lymphoma cells by adherent spleen and peritoneal cells
Natural killer cell function	Cytolysis of YAC-1 lymphoma cells by non-adherent spleen and peritoneal cells
Host resistance	*Trichinella spiralis* challenge (muscle larval counts and worm expulsion); *Listeria monocytogenes* hypersensitivity

[a] From Vos and Van Loveren (1987).

Table 3. Tier-I multiple immunoassay model for assessing immunotoxicity in Sprague-Dawley rats[a]

Parameter	Procedure
Humoral immunity	Enzyme-linked immunosorbent assay to keyhole limpet haemocyanin antigen (IgG)
T Cell-mediated immunity	Delayed-type hypersensitivity reaction to keyhole limpet haemocyanin antigen
Natural immunity	Natural killer cell cytotoxicity to tumour cells Macrophage production of prostaglandin E_2
Immunopathology	Thymus-spleen weights and histopathology Spleen and macrophage cell numbers Haematology (complete and differential blood counts)

[a]From Exon *et al.* (1986).

measures serum antibody from all sources in the body and therefore may be more indicative of overall humoral immunity. It is also automated to handle large numbers of samples and does not require killing the animal, since only a serum sample is needed. Disadvantages to this assay are that the reagents are more expensive than for the plaque-forming cell assay and some investment in instrumentation is needed (e.g., a reader) in order to quantify accurately. Although there are pros and cons to each assay, both are acceptable methods of assessing humour immunity, and investigators choose between them mainly on the basis of preference.

Another assay commonly used to assess B-cell function is lymphoblastogenesis to selected mitogens or antigens. Lymphocyte proliferation in response to mitogens is not a definitive measure of functional immunity and too often does not correlate well with responses *in vivo*. This may be because mitogens do not bind to antigen receptors, but rather to mitogen receptors, to induce proliferation. Also, many compounds, including some metals, have innate mitogenic properties. This is, however, an assay commonly used in human immunology, generally as a support assay, however, rather than as the sole assay for humoral immunity.

The assays used most commonly to measure specific T cell-mediated immune responses include the delayed-type hypersensitivity reaction, the mixed lymphocyte reaction (MLR) and cytotoxic T-cell lympholysis. These assays measure the functions of different types of T-cell subpopulations. The cytotoxic T-cell lympholysis response involves T cells that are responsible for allograft rejection and require recognition of class-I major histocompatibility antigens. The T cells involved in DTH reactions and in the MLR are of a different phenotype and recognize class-II major histocompatibility antigens and mediate graft-*versus*-host reactions. Some consider the MLR to be the in-vitro correlate of the DTH. Any one of these three assays is acceptable for measuring T-cell function, but the DTH reaction and the MLR are most commonly used in immunotoxicity studies. Some researchers prefer the DTH assay because it is carried out entirely *in vivo*, although the MLR assay seems to correlate well with T cell-sensitive host-resistance assays in mice (Luster *et al.*, 1988).

The assay used most commonly to measure nonspecific cell-mediated immunity is natural killer cell cytolysis of tumour cells. Natural killer cells are believed to be one of the first lines of defence against developing tumour cells or some virally infected cells. Also, natural killer function has been shown to correlate with some tumour host resistance models in mice. Therefore, these assays are usually included in a screen for immunotoxicity in tier 1. The other major cell population involved in natural immunity (i.e., non-major histocompatibility complex-dependent) is macrophages. Many investigators, however, have found macrophages quite resistant to chemically induced modulation *in vivo*. Consequently, a number of macrophage assays have been attempted, but there is no consensus that any one is really adequate for immunotoxicity testing.

BIOMARKERS IN IMMUNOTOXICOLOGY

The US National Academy of Sciences, through the National Research Council Board of Environmental Studies and Toxicology, has recently formed a Committee on Biological Markers, with a subcommittee on Biological Markers of the Immune System composed of statisticians, immunologists and immunotoxicologists. The charge of the committee is to identify biological markers of immunotoxicity that can be used in regulatory decision-making. The biomarkers are divided into three types - exposure, effect and susceptibility. An exposure biomarker is defined as 'an exogenous substance or its metabolite(s) or the product of an interaction between a xenobiotic and some target molecule that is measured in a compartment within an organism.' An effect biomarker is defined as 'a measurable biochemical, physiological, or other alteration within that organism that, depending on the magnitude, can be recognized as an established or potential health impairment or disease.' A susceptibility biomarker is defined as 'an indicator of inherent or acquired limitation of an organism's ability to respond to the challenge of exposure to a specific xenobiotic.' These immunobiomarkers will be examined for use in species extrapolation and as indicators of exposure and impaired health. The committee will also make recommendations as to appropriate animal models for assessing immunotoxicity and future research needs in this field. One of these research needs was to establish a national registry for retrospective analysis of immune defects. The first workshop of the committee was held on 8 February 1988; recommendations are expected by late 1989.

One area the committee will address is validation of animal models, immunoassays and testing approaches. The concept of 'validation' of these parameters has not previously been well understood. The US National Toxicology Program multi-laboratory immunotoxicology studies in the mouse seem to provide an acceptable method of validation (Luster *et al.*, 1988). In these studies, all laboratories used the same animal strains, assays and reagents and tested the same chemicals by the same exposure regimens. These studies lend a degree of 'validity' to immunotoxicity studies in the B6C3F1 mouse and in the assays employed. Areas of validation that need improvement are demonstrated consistency across species (e.g., rodent to human) and ability to predict toxicant-induced human disease. At the 1989 meeting of the Society of Toxicology in Atlanta, Georgia, USA, convincing evidence for validation of immunoassays in rat models was presented. It was evident that the process of developing assays in different species did not require a 'reinvention of the wheel', but rather could be based on previous work and assays in other species. Thus, the mouse model developed by Luster *et al.* (1988) provides what I believe is a sound method for approaching the concept of validation. As previously mentioned, a similar international validation study is under way on the rat model.

INTERPRETATION OF IMMUNOTOXICOLOGICAL DATA

The science of immunotoxicology has evolved to the point of sophistication that regulatory agencies are beginning to ask how the data can be used in risk assessment and regulation of chemicals and drugs. A concept (question) that continually surfaces in this regard is that of 'immune reserve capacity' or 'immune resilience.' This was a major topic at a recent (1988) workshop of the US National Institutes of Environmental Health on risk assessment in immunotoxicology. The question raised was at what point we classify a compound as immunotoxic and on what criteria; how much can the immune system be altered before serious health effects ensue? As with most other systems in the body, the immune system is capable of compensatory responses, but to what degree this occurs is largely unknown. In the strictest sense, any xenobiotic that significantly alters immune responses must be considered a potential risk, especially when predisposing factors are present, such as senescence, stress, malnutrition and any other idiosyncratic condition that may result in concomitant immune suppression or enhancement. Even though a 50% suppression of antibody production in a healthy individual may not manifest in clinical signs of illness, the individual is still compromised and may show effects under different environmental or health conditions. This almost necessitates treating each immunotoxicant on a case-by-case basis, taking into account the population exposed, the conditions of exposure, uses of the chemical/drug and other pertinent factors. This approach is not significantly different from that applied to other types of toxicants. In other words, some judgement should be made on the basis of risk-benefit analysis.

Another question of interpretation that has arisen is what types of immunotoxic effects are most relevant. Should only compounds that can be demonstrated to alter host resistance or cause hypersensitivity responses be regulated or used in risk assessment, or must any functional change also be considered relevant? Again, it seems that any change should be considered potentially detrimental to health. A statement recently prepared by the Immunotoxicology Specialty Section of Regulatory Affairs and Legislative Assistance Committee of the Society of Toxicology in the USA echoes this conclusion. It states, 'Any xenobiotic which significantly increases or decreases immune function is considered an immunotoxicant.' The statement also indicates that this does not imply clinical effects, but merely potential risk. These concepts of risk assessment of immunotoxicological data are just beginning to be formulated and should spawn considerable discussion and controversy in the coming months. At this point, it is really unknown how much damage the immune system can sustain without a real compromise in the health of the host; however, it is in the nature of tolerance setting to stay on the safe side. Therefore, it can be expected that immunotoxicity data will be treated conservatively.

REFERENCES

Allen, J.C. (1976) Infection complicating neoplastic disease and cytotoxic therapy. In: Allen, J.C., ed., *Infection and the Compromised Host*, Baltimore, Williams and Wilkins, pp. 151-171

Bekesi, G.J., Roboz, J., Fischbein, A., Roboz, J.F., Solomon, S. & Graves, J. (1985) Immunological, biochemical and clinical consequences of exposure to polybrominated biphenyls. In: Dean, J.H., Luster, M.I., Munson A.E. & Amos, H., eds, *Immunotoxicology and Immunopharmacology*, New York, Raven Press, pp. 393-406

Berlin, A., Dean, J., Draper, M.H., Smith, E.M.B. & Spreafico, F., eds (1987) *Immunotoxicology. Proceedings of the International Seminar on the Immunological System as a Target for Toxic Damage*, Dordrecht, Martinus Nijhoff

Dean, J.H., Luster, M.I., Boorman, G.A. & Lauer, L.D. (1982) Procedures available to examine the immunotoxicity of chemicals and drugs. *Pharmacol. Rev.*, **34**: 137-148

Exon, J.H., Koller, L.D., Talcott, P.A., O'Reilly, C.A. & Henningsen, G.M. (1986) Immuno-toxicity testing: an economical multiple-assay approach. *Fundam. appl. Toxicol.*, **7**: 387-397

Gibson, G.G., Hubbard, R. & Parke, D.V. (1983) *Immunotoxicology, Proceedings of the First International Symposium on Immunotoxicology*, New York, Academic Press

Haber, E. & Pfiter, E.A. (1982) Immunologic aspects of toxicology, a workshop. *Regul. Pharmacol. Toxicol.*, **2**: 247-256

Haustein, U.F. & Ziegler, V. (1985) Environmentally induced systemic sclerosis-like disorders. *Int. J. Dermatol.*, **24**: 147-256

Kammuller, M.E., Penninks, A.H. & Seinen, W. (1984) Spanish toxic oil syndrome is a chemically induced GVHD-like epidemic. *Lancet*, i: 1174-1175

Koffler, J. (1980) Systemic lupus erythematosus. *Sci. Am.*, **July**, 52-64

Lee, T.P. & Chang, K.J. (1985) Health effects of polychlorinated biphenyls. In: Dean, J.H., Luster, M.I., Munson A.E. & Amos, H., eds, *Immunotoxicology and Immunopharmacology*, New York, Raven Press, pp. 415-422

Lockey, J.F., Kelly, C.R., Cannon, C.W., Colby, T.V., Aldridge, V. & Livingston, G.K. (1987) Progressive systemic sclerosis associated with exposure to trichloroethylene. *J. occup. Med.*, **29**: 493-496

Luster, M.I. & Dean, J.H. (1982) Immunological hypersensitivity resulting from environmental or occupational exposure to chemicals. A state-of-the-art workshop summary. *Fundam. appl. Toxicol.*, **2**: 327-330

Luster, M.I., Munson, A.E., Thomas, P.T., Hosapple, M.P., Fanters, J.D., White, K.L., Lauer, L.D., Germolc, D.R., Rosenthal, G.J. & Dean, J.H. (1988) Methods evaluation: development of a testing battery to assess chemical-induced immunotoxicity: National Toxicology Program guidelines for immunotoxicity evaluation in mice. *Fundam. appl. Toxicol.*, **10**: 2-19

Penn, I. (1985) Neoplastic consequences of immunosuppression. In: Dean, J.H., Luster, M.I., Munson, A.E. & Amos, H., eds, *Immunotoxicology and Immunopharmacology*, New York, Raven Press, pp. 79-90

Saihan, E. M., Burton, J. L. & Heaton, K.W. (1978) A new syndrome with pigmentation, scleroderma, gynaecomastia, Raynaud's phenomenon and peripheral neuropathy. *Br. J. Dermatol.*, **99**: 437-440

Sjoblad, R.D. (1988) Potential future requirement for immunotoxicology testing of pesticides. *Toxicol. ind. Health*, **4**: 391-394

Talal, N. (1987) Autoimmunity. In: Mehlman, M.A., ed., *Advances in Modern Environmental Toxicology*, Vol. 13, *Environmental Chemical Exposures and Immune System Integrity*, Princeton, NJ, Princeton Scientific, pp. 167-180

Touraine, J. (1987) Primary immunodeficiencies. In: Berlin, A., Dean, J., Draper, M.H., Smith E.M.B. & Spreafico, F., eds, *Immunotoxicology*, Boston, Martinus Nijhoff, pp. 61-68

Vos, J.G. (1977) Immune suppression as related to toxicology. *CRC crit. Rev. Toxicol.*, **5**: 67-101

Vos, J.G. & Van Loveren, H. (1987) Immunotoxicity testing in the rat. In: Mehlman, M.A., ed., *Advances in Modern Environmental Toxicology*, Vol. 13, *Environmental Chemical Exposures and Immune System Integrity*, Princeton, NJ, Princeton Scientific, pp. 147-159

IMMUNOGENETICS

K.I. Welsh

Molecular Immunogenetics, Guy's Hospital, GT18, London SE1 9RT, UK

ABSTRACT

The associations between genetic markers and immune reactions caused by exposure to metals are not strong. Those related to direct hypersensitivity are not proven, but immune reactions in which auto-immune processes are involved are associated with specific genetic markers, and one of these is used clinically in certain centres.

HYPERSENSITIVITY AND AUTOIMMUNITY

The types of hypersensitivity reactions (I, II, III and IV) described by Coombs and Gell (1975) have stood the test of time and are described fully elsewhere in this volume. All that is necessary in addition, for a consideration of the immunogenetics of the responses induced by metals, is to expand the distinction between reaction to self as opposed to reaction to an outside insult.

The immune system can be activated in two distinct ways. In the first, a specific response is formed directly to the agent or to the product(s) that the agent produces. The various types of hypersensitivity responses can and do occur during this type of response, and I therefore refer to it as the direct hypersensitivity-type response (DHTR). In the second, a response to self is generated as a result of the environmental insult. This autoimmune process (autoimmune hypersensitivity-type response, AHTR) can occur by one of two main mechanisms, in one of which it loses specificity, while in the other, it retains it. In the first group, the agent causes the exposure in host tissue of epitopes that are normally 'hidden' to the immune system. This type of response is not a hypersensitivity response, since it is a natural reaction to a new determinant and occurs due to the lack of any active suppressive mechanism. It is possible that two or more factors can lead to exposure of the same 'hidden' determinant. This group of AHTR is not covered in the classic definitions of hypersensitivity. In the second group, the normal type of autoimmune process associated with hypersensitivity reactions, the environmental agent or its product forms an epitope which resembles a self epitope. The response to the agent may override the natural suppression and lead directly or indirectly to an autoimmune reaction.

These two groups of autoimmune reactions are quite distinct. In the first, a number of different insults can expose the same epitope; hence, specificity of the induction can degenerate, but specificity as regards target structure remains. This situation is thought to pertain in Kawasaki's disease, in which abnormal up-regulation of endothelial cells by an external agent induces an IgM response to an epitope found only on activated cells. Deactivation of the cell, i.e., a return to the resting state, removes the 'hidden' determinant, and the disease regresses. The same or a different endothelial activator can up-regulate the target antigen at a later date, causing relapse. In the second group of autoimmune responses, the environmental agent directly resembles or reacts to produce a product which resembles a host antigen.

The DHTR, in which a specific response can be formed to the agent or its product with host tissue, is much better described than the AHTR. The cell-mediated hypersensitivity

Immunotoxicity of Metals and Immunotoxicology, Edited by
A. D. Dayan *et al.*, Plenum Press, New York, 1990

reactions caused by nickel, chromium and cobalt are examples of DHTR. The toxicity induced by the gold chelates used in the treatment of rheumatoid arthiritis is an example of an AHTR - almost certainly a group-1 AHTR.

In general terms, DHTR are not under tight immunogenetic control, as demonstrated by accumulated evidence that particular polymorphisms in genes which control the immune response occur in equal proportions in affected and unaffected individuals. A possible flaw is that the statement implies that all possible polymorphisms have been investigated. Table 1 shows that they have not. In contrast, AHTR are often under very tight genetic control in both animals and humans.

AREAS OF THE HUMAN GENOME IMPORTANT TO IMMUNOGENETICS

The important areas are: (i) the major histocompatability complex (MHC) region on chromosome 6; (ii) the immunoglobin region on chromosome 14; and (iii) the T-cell receptor areas on chromosomes 9 and 14.

The MHC region on chromosome 6 is equivalent in size to the total contained in the *Escherichia coli* chromosome. Further, it is the most polymorphic area of the genome, so that only identical twins have an identical MHC.

The immunoglobulin regions are limited in their polymorphism but can rearrange to produce tens of thousands of new sequences. Within these hypervariable regions are relatively constant portions which partially determine the ability to rearrange. These regions define so-called gene families, and certain antibodies can be formed only in individuals who have a particular gene family present in their genome. For example, the majority of rheumatoid factors utilize a particular variable light gene family.

The T-cell receptor areas mimic the immunoglobulin areas in broad terms, with particular gene families occasionally being associated with particular disorders.

Immunoglobulin and T-cell genomic regions of circulating B and T cells are thus multiclonal, and even identical twins differ, since these areas of the genome rearrange to combat internal or external insults to the immune system.

An excellent and interesting introduction to these topics is provided by the book *Natural History of the Major Histocompatibility Complex* written by Jan Klein (1986).

METALS, HYPERSENSITIVITY REACTIONS AND IMMUNOGENETIC DISPOSITIONS

Nickel

Analysis of published data from studies in Europe on 183 patients with allergy to nickel have shown no association with MHC class-I antigens (Liden *et al.*, 1978; Dumont-Frutyier *et al.*, 1980; Kapoor-Pillarisette *et al.*, 1981; Liden *et al.*, 1981). In an additional, Finnish study (Silvennoinen-Kassinen *et al.*, 1979), both MHC class-II and class-I antigens

Table 1. Associations between immune genes and responses to metals

Metal	Immune gene association[a]			Hypersensitivity reaction	
	MHC	Ig	TCR	Direct	Autoimmune
Nickel	-	ND	?	+	-
Chromium	-	ND	ND	+	-
Cobalt	-	ND	ND	+	+
Gold	+	ND	ND	+	+
Mercury	+	ND	ND	+	+
Potassium	+	ND	ND	-	+
Silicon	+/-	ND	ND	-	+

[a]MHC, major histocompatibility complex; Ig, immunoglobulin gene family or polymorphism association; TCR, T-cell receptor gene family or polymorphism association; ND, not determined.

were studied; again, no association was observed. Studies of families and of twins confirm the absence of association between the MHC and the hypersensitivity response to nickel. The same may not be true for the T-cell receptor area, because cloned T cells obtained from such individuals could be oligoclonal (Kapsenberg *et al.*, 1987). In a study of such clones from eight patients, five responded to nickel only when it was applied to skin antigen-presenting cells (Langerhans cells) and three responded to nickel applied to peripheral blood antigen-presenting cells.

Chromium

As for nickel, several studies have been carried out within Europe, but no correlation has been seen between any particular MHC allotype and the allergic reaction observed (Liden *et al.*, 1978; Roupe *et al.*, 1979; Kapoor-Pillarisette *et al.*, 1981; Liden *et al.*, 1981).

Cobalt

Specific antibodies to cobalt have been detected in cases of hard-metal asthma induced by this metal: specific IgE antibodies to cobalt-HSA were observed (Shirakawa *et al.*, 1988).

Mercury

Mercury salts can induce both DHTR- and AHTR-type reactions. They also differ from most other metal compounds in that they can induce type-IV hypersensitivity reactions (cell-mediated DHTR). Early work on DHTR type IV in guinea-pigs suggested a very strong genetic control (Polak *et al.*, 1968). To my knowledge, this work has not been confirmed, but much of the early work of this group has been proven to be accurate, and I suggest that the observation will be correct. In recent years, animal models of glomerular nephritis and of scleroderma have been developed by giving rats mercury compounds.

Potassium

Polak *et al.* (1968) observed that potassium dichromate induced type-IV hypersensitivity reactions in a particular guinea-pig strain. We suspect that the reaction can be further classified as a group-1 AHTR.

Gold

Two forms of gold chelate therapy are used to alleviate the symptoms of rheumatoid arthritis. Both induce side-effects, but intramuscular gold, the most effective therapy, induces side-effects that are related to the immunogenetic make-up of the patient. Proteinuria develops in 1-10% of patients treated intramuscularly with gold, but the nephropathy is not related to dose or to gold concentrations in the blood or urine and may commence at any time following the first week of therapy. The renal lesion is described more fully in other papers in this volume, but it is important to state that gold is not associated with the lesion and that the lesion is histologically identical to that seen in idiopathic membranous nephropathy. Further, the work of our own group and others (Woolley *et al.*, 1980) has shown that both conditions are strongly associated with possession of the same specific MHC allotypes. The particular haplotype involved is A1, B8, C4AQ0, DR3, which is known to be associated with a range of autoimmune disorders, including myasthenia gravis and systemic lupus erythematosus.

This evidence indicates that gold induces an AHTR as a result of the DHTR that it is known to generate. Certain centres use HLA typing to decide which individuals should be given intramuscular gold.

Silicon

A subset of individuals get systemic sclerosis-like problems following cosmetic surgery with silicon implants or after exposure to silica dust. These two forms of induced scleroderma are considered briefly because, although they have no reported association with the MHC, genetic factors have been established for idiopathic and vinyl chloride-induced scleroderma (Black *et al.*, 1983; Kondo *et al.*, 1985a). One may speculate that an underlying, genetically determined, constitutional diathesis predisposes to systemic sclerosis, and silica may precipitate the disease in those predisposed by genetic background through its effect on the immune system. Altered drug metabolism may also be important, and a recent study has indicated that some white South African gold miners with a scleroderma-like illness have an altered step in the tryptophan metabolic pathway, which is more marked than that recorded in the idiopathic disease.

A further subset of individuals suffer silicosis after exposure to silica dust. One study of the association with the MHC has been carried out on patients exposed to French gold, tungsten and uranium and to some in porcelain industries. There was no strong association, but the incidence of B7 was low (6.7% in patients, 20% in controls). There was weak evidence of a higher incidence of B8 in those with pulmonary tuberculosis (Gualde *et al.*, 1977). No study of class-II antigens was carried out.

The post-mammoplasty scleroderma-like syndrome is well known, particularly to the Japanese (Kondo *et al.*, 1985b), who have used various substances, including both paraffin and silicon, for breast augmentation. Since paraffin is a solvent, these results accord with what is known for other solvent-induced diseases, but we suspect that the major culprit is silicon, which has a myofibroblast proliferating effect thought to be due to the liberation of silica. The type of scleroderma reported ranged from morphoea to diffuse cutaneous with oesophageal and pulmonary involvement. Unfortunately, no genetic analysis has been carried out on post-mammoplasty scleroderma.

It would seem very unlikely (partly because a range of environmental agents can lead to similar scleroderma-like diseases) that the process responsible is an AHTR rather than any direct response to the agents. We would expect the same to be true for silicosis. The main problem in these diseases, however, is overproduction of collagen, and immune factors are, at best, secondary.

REFERENCES

Black, C.M., Welsh, K.I., Walker, A.E., Bernstein, R.M., Catoggio, L.J., McGregor, A.R. & Lloyd Jones, J.K (1983) Genetic susceptibility to scleroderma-like syndrome induced by vinyl chloride. *Lancet*, **i**: 53-55

Coombs, R.R.A & Gell, P.G.H. (1975) Classification of allergic reactions responsible for clinical hypersensitivity and disease. In: Gell, P.G.H., Coombs, R.R.A. & Lachmann, P.J., eds, *Clinical Aspects of Immunology*, 3rd ed., Oxford, Blackwell, p. 671

Dumont-Frutyier, M., Van Neste, D., De Bruyere, M., Tenstedt, D. & Lachpelle, J.M. (1980) Nickel contact sensitivity in women and HLA antigens. *Arch. dermatol. Res.*, **269**: 205-208

Gualde, N., De Leobardy, J., Serizay, B. & Malinvaud, G. (1977) HL-A and silicosis. *Am. Rev. respir. Dis.*, **116**: 334-336

Kapoor-Pillarisette, A., Mowbray, J.F., Brostoff, J. & Coronin, E.A. (1981) HLA dependence of sensitivity to nickel and chromium. *Tissue Antigens*, **17**: 261-264

Kapsenberg, M.L., Res, P., Bos, J.D., Schootemijer, A., Teunissen, M.B.M. & Van Schooten, W. (1987) Nickel-specific T cell clones derived from allergic nickel-contact dermatitis lesions in man: heterogeneity based on requirement of dendritic antigen presenting cell subsets. *Eur. J. Immunol.*, **17**: 861-866

Klein, J. (1986) *Natural History of the Major Histocompatibility Complex*

Kondo, H., Kumagai, Y. & Shiokawa, Y. (1985a) Scleroderma following cosmetic surgery ('adjuvant disease'): a review of nine cases reported in Japan. In: Black, C.M. & Myers, A.R., eds, *Systemic Sclerosis (Scleroderma)*, New York, Gower, pp. 97-102

Kondo, H., Yoshii, M., Kashiwazaki, S. & Kashiwagi, N. (1985b) Histocompatibility antigens in progressive systemic sclerosis. In: Black, C.M. & Myers, A.R., eds, *Systemic Sclerosis (Scleroderma)*, New York, Gower, pp. 97-102

Liden, S., Beckman, L., Cedergren, B., Goransson, K. & Nyqist, H. (1978) HLA antigens in contact dermatitis. *Acta dermatovenereol.*, **79** (Suppl.): 54-56

Liden, S., Beckman, L., Cedergren, B., Groyh, O., Goransson, K. & Wahlby, L. (1981) Lack of association between contact dermatitis and HLA antigens of the A & B series. *Acta dermatovenereol.*, **61**: 155-157

Polak, L., Barnes, J.M. & Turk, J.L. (1968) The genetic control of contact sensitisation to inorganic metal compounds in guinea pigs. *Immunology*, **14**: 702

Roupe, G., Rydberg, L. & Swanbeck, G. (1979) HLA antigens and contact hypersensitivity. *J. invest. Dermatol.*, **72**: 131-132

Shirakawa, T., Kusaka, Y., Fujimara, N., Goto, S. & Morimoto, K. (1988) The existence of specific antibodies to cobalt in hard metal asthma. *Clin. Allergy*, **18**: 451-460

Silvennoinen-Kassinen, S., Tiilikainen, A. & Karvonen, J. (1979) No significant association between HLA and nickel contact sensitivity. *Tissue Antigens*, **14**: 459-461

Woolley, P.H., Griffin, A.J., Panayi, G.S., Batchelor, J.R., Welsh, K.I. & Gibson, T.G. (1980) HLA-DR antigens and toxicity to sodium aurothiomalate and D-penicillamine in rheumatoid arthritis. *New Engl. J. Med.*, **303**: 300-302

DOSE-EFFECTS AND DOSE-RESPONSES IN IMMUNOTOXICOLOGY: PROBLEMS AND CONCEPTUAL CONSIDERATIONS

S. Nicklin & K. Miller

British Industrial Biological Research Association
Carshalton, Surrey SM5 4DS, UK

ABSTRACT

While traditional pathological approaches have implicated various lymphoid organs as possible targets for toxic insult, it is only relatively recently that the complexity and far-reaching consequences associated with local and systemic immunotoxic interactions have been fully appreciated. Whereas it is perfectly possible to examine the effects of a given agent on lymphoid weight, for example, some form of antigen challenge must be implemented if one wishes to address the effect of a particular dose of chemical upon immune reactivity; indeed, it is this requirement for antigen challenge that actually separates conventional toxicology from immunotoxicology. Although difficult to assess using conventional methods, recent advances in molecular biology have provided new techniques for the detection and precise evaluation of immunotoxic events and processes. These novel approaches to the study of toxicity have not only increased our understanding of the immune mechanism, they offer for the first time a rapid and effective means of exploring the intricacies of dose-effect:dose-response relationships at the level of the target cell.

INTRODUCTION

The dose-response relationship remains a central concept in a range of scientific disciplines, including pharmacology, drug metabolism and toxicology. In its simplest form, the relationship is most often presented graphically, usually as an S-shaped, exponential or hyperbolic curve with dose on the x-axis and the measured effects or response on the y-axis (Fig. 1 presents a typical hypothetical curve, a variation on the common theme previously devised by Hatch, 1968, and modified more recently by Emil Pfitzer, 1976, among others).

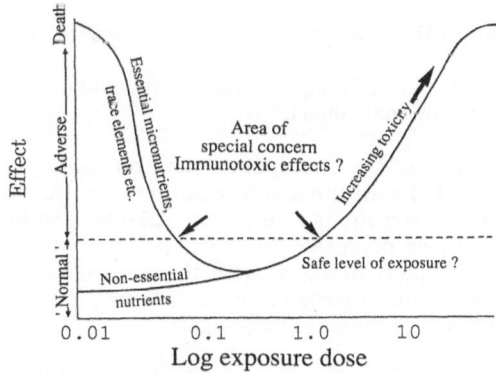

Fig. 1. Schematic representation of the dose-effect:dose-response relationship

Immunotoxicity of Metals and Immunotoxicology, Edited by
A. D. Dayan *et al.,* Plenum Press, New York, 1990

Although first appraisals reveal a delightfully simple picture, it takes but a moment's consideration to appreciate how many external factors can influence the nature of the curve. In reality, a complete graphical summarization of the dose-effect:dose-response relationship requires a family of curves yielding a much more detailed three-dimensional profile.

Definitions

Whereas it is common practice to use the words 'effect' and 'response' almost synonymously in everyday language, traditional toxicology has evolved and retained special and separate applications for the terms:

A dose-effect relationship is said to exist if the change in an administered dose of a xenobiotic causes a quantifiable alteration in the specific biological effect observed. A reduction in circulating $CD8^+$ T cells, increased production of interleukin-2 (IL-2) and decreased antigen-specific IgA secretion at mucosal membranes would all be considered effects rather than responses as far as toxicologists are concerned. Most notably, however, the effects must be quantifiable and graded with respect to dose. For example, a compound that affects CD25 expression on T cells may have no effect on the basal level expression at one dose, whereas twice the dose may produce a 20-fold increase in expression, and four times the dose a maximal effect, but with no further effect observed above that level.

When the observed effect cannot be measured but represents an all-or-none effect, a dose-response relationship is said to exist if the percentage of the population presenting an effect depends on the dose of agent received. Death is clearly the ultimate all-or-none effect. When using death as a 'biological' indicator, therefore, it is necessary to consider a population given a specific dose and measure the percentage of that population showing the specific effect. Thus, the LD_{50} value may be described as the dose that causes a 50% response in a population tested for the lethal effect.

The distinction between quantal and graded effects, however, is not necessarily always absolute, and from the point of view of the immune system dose-effect relationships must be considered at a number of levels. In a strictly biological sense, individual lymphocytes may function on a quantal basis, but when a large number of cells reacts to a drug or a virus, then the summation of the individual responses may result in a measurable response that is observed as a graded effect; conversely, many graded effects can be expressed as a percentage of the control or maximal effect.

In order to utilize dose-response effects in any predictive fashion in toxicological studies, three main assumptions must be satisfied:

(1) Dose and effect must be causally related.
(2) The effect must be related to the dose administered, i.e.,
   (i) There is a specific receptor(s) with which the agent interacts to produce the effect.
   (ii) The magnitude of the effect is related to the concentration of the agent at the reactive site.
   (iii) The concentration of the agent at the site is dependent upon the magnitude of the exposure dose.
(3) One must have both a quantifiable method of measuring and a precise means of expressing the nature of the toxic effect.

Although a great variety of toxic endpoints may be used, the ideal criterion is that which is most closely associated with the insult resulting from the particular exposure. Until recently, such early or direct assessments were unassailable, and investigators were obliged to moniter secondary effects or processes as markers or indicators of more distant toxic events. As will be discussed later, however, with the increasing applicability of molecular biological techniques, assessment of early events is now very much within reach, especially in respect to early immunotoxic processes (see below).

Knowing what to measure is, of course, central to establishing dose-effect or dose-response relationships; but what does one measure? Such information is usually available only after some form of toxicological screening exercise, often dependent on other markers and measures of toxicity. Traditionally, such studies might start with some form of lethality testing, or, more recently, studies designed to establish a maximal tolerated dose. This form of testing, when used in conjuction with conventional histopathology, provides initial information on the events leading to the lethal effect and the apparent target organ or organs involved and may even suggest a possible mechanism.

When we attempt to apply the same rules to immunotoxicity studies, however, the climate changes somewhat; we not only enter a different 'ball park', we have to play a different game with a different set of rules. Previous reference points alter; the immune system is not a static concept, it is an intergrated, interdependent system capable of reacting to changing circumstances. In addition, we must consider not only the effects of the toxic agent upon and within the system as a whole, we must also consider the effects and constraints imposed by antigen. Antigenic challenge is inseparable from immune reactivity; it occurs continuously, and, by definition, drives the immune mechanism. Without antigen, there is no immune response and the concept of immunotoxicity becomes meaningless. Thus, antigen not only adds another dimension to the dose-effect or dose-response relationship, the requirement of antigen actually separates conventional toxicity from immunotoxicity (Fig. 2). Whereas it is perfectly possible to examine the effect of an agent upon lymphoid organ weight, for example, some form of antigen challenge must be considered if one wishes to address the effect of the agent upon immune reactivity.

The purpose of this paper is to highlight some of the difficulties associated with the generation and interpretation of dose-effect and dose-response data for immunotoxic compounds. It does not attempt to create a single model of the effect or response relationship *per se* but rather sets out to define the nature of the problem so that the limitations as well as the utility of our present knowledge relating to immunotoxic processes may be better appreciated and communicated to non-immunotoxicologists (see Fig. 3). As alluded to above, we are, at the onset of this excercise, faced with a number of conceptual problems arising from the nature of the immune response itself, as the immune system, unlike the conventional target organ, is a highly integrated mechanism in which minor 'nontoxic' effects at the level of regulatory cells may have dramatic, even life-threatening consequences for the organism as a whole. At the same time, a measure of the redundancy within the immune system can protect the host, so that overtly toxic effects in one effector system may be compensated for by enhanced reactivity in parallel pathways. The concept of redundancy and the processes for compensatory reactivity can cloud both the nature and sequence of events in toxicological studies, making it difficult to resolve immunotoxic target cell or organ-specific effects with any degree of certainty. Nevertheless, accumulating evidence based on human and experimental animal studies now links exposure to a variety of drugs and chemical agents with various immunotoxic processes, including the induction of aberrant or inappropriate responses to self-determinants, resulting in autoimmune disease, or an exaggerated respose to antigen leading to hypersensitization. In addition, the direct or indirect suppression of effector functions of the immune response may leave the host more susceptible to infectious agents and may in the long run produce an increased risk for cancer following the loss of immune surveillance.

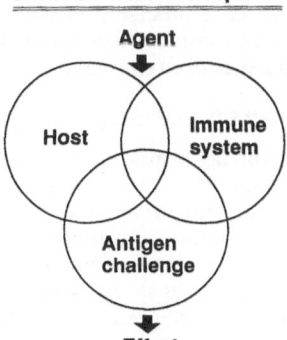

Fig. 2. Schematic representation of the link between host, antigen challenge and the immune system

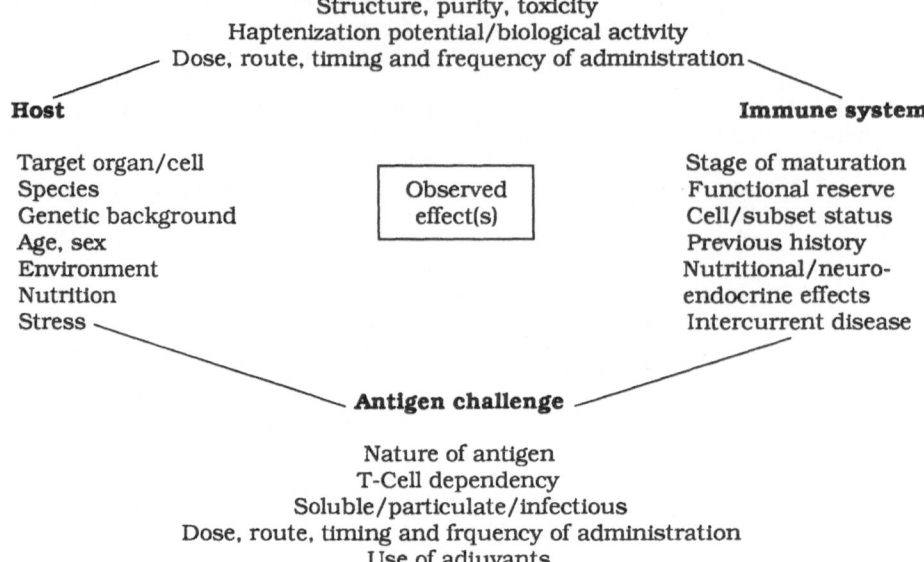

Test compound

Structure, purity, toxicity
Haptenization potential/biological activity
Dose, route, timing and frequency of administration

Host

Target organ/cell
Species
Genetic background
Age, sex
Environment
Nutrition
Stress

Observed
effect(s)

Immune system

Stage of maturation
Functional reserve
Cell/subset status
Previous history
Nutritional/neuro-
endocrine effects
Intercurrent disease

Antigen challenge

Nature of antigen
T-Cell dependency
Soluble/particulate/infectious
Dose, route, timing and frquency of administration
Use of adjuvants

Fig. 3. Factors influencing the immune dose-effect or dose-response relationship

It is clearly not feasible within the confines of a short text to review fully all of the possible interactions that may occur between xenobiotics and the mammalian immune system. In the following subsections, we consider the effects of several model compounds upon the lymphoid tissues and the immune response of various experimental animals. It must, however, be stated that in many instances the immunotoxic element of the discussion stems by necessity from investigations in which the primary objectives of the studies presented relates to the experimental analysis of normal immune function rather than to immunotoxic events *per se*. Clearly, the practice of appropriating results of assays designed to test one particular hypothesis to support a secondary premise must be questioned and the implications tempered accordingly. It must be further noted that many of the assay systems that have been designed and used by experimental investigators over the years have been optimized (even customized) for a set of precisely defined experimental circumstances; thus, many test methods and experimental regimens depend on species- and often strain-specific responses. Many reactions are age-dependent, and, because of the progressive nature of immune reactions, certain aspects of a particular response can be examined only within the confines of a precisely limited time-frame. It is anticipated that other papers will provide additional examples of other effects and correlations as they relate to specific chemicals, species and exposure regimens.

CYCLOPHOSPHAMIDE AND RELATED COMPOUNDS

Cyclophosphamide (CY) is a nitrogen mustard derivative that has found clinical use in both the treatment of various autoallergic immune disorders and in alleviating the problems of graft rejection associated with human organ and tissue transplantation. The drug has found particular favour with experimental immunologists, since it has a high selectivity for lymphoid tissues, yet it is surprisingly sparing of haemopoiesis and, depending on dose and time of administration, can be used to dissect discrete aspects of the immune response. Thus, CY treatment has been shown to depress antibody production, inhibit various cell-mediated responses, including allograft rejection and the graft-*versus*-host reaction, when given both prior to and following challenge, but to enhance delayed-type hypersensitivity responses if given prior to sensitization.

In rodents, a single dose of CY within the LD_{10} dose range (300 mg/kg for mice) produced thymic cortex involution and cell depletion in the B-cell zone of the spleen and lymph nodes within two to three days; T-cell areas within these organs remained relatively intact, demonstrating that immature thymocytes and B cells are preferential cell targets at this dose level (Turk & Poulter, 1972). This dose also produced profound lymphopenia, but there was no marked alteration in the haematocrit, endorsing the relative selectivity of the drug for the lymphoid tissues. Indeed, the ratio between the dose of drug that caused a 50% reduction in haematocrit as opposed to a 50% reduction in plaque-forming cells is in the region of 10:1 in the mouse.

These results are in accordance with those of earlier experiments which had indicated that CY was a potential immunosuppressive drug for thymus-dependent antigens (Stender et al., 1963; Berenbaum & Brown, 1964; Santos & Owens, 1966). However, suppression of humoral immune responses by CY is not only dose-dependent, the dose-response curve being in general steep and exponential, it is more significantly influenced by other factors, most notably the timing of drug administration relative to the time of antigen challenge. In fact, although reduction of humoral responses can be obtained with administration before and after antigen, maximal depression is seen with treatment at the time of, or shortly after, antigen challenge. This finding is clearly consistent with the supposition that CY acts on dividing cells. Prolongation of the interval between drug administration and challenge results in a progressively lower effect and/or in the requirement for higher doses. The effect is, however, transient, and, in mice given a single dose of 150 mg/kg, complete functional recovery from the effects of CY is usually observed within six to seven days.

As one might expect, CY also suppresses antibody response against thymus-independent antigens, and a direct comparison between the immunosuppressive activities of various drugs on antipolysaccharide responses revealed that a single injection of CY was distinctly superior to the alkylating agents melphalan or chlorambucil and even to daily injection of 6-mercaptopurine, azathioprine or A-methopterin (Howard & Hale, 1978).

The relative susceptibility of B and T lymphocytes to CY *in vivo* remains somewhat controversial. The original observation in chicken (Lerman & Weidanz, 1970) that CY was selectively toxic for B cells was later confirmed in guinea-pigs utilizing morphological criteria (Turk & Poulter, 1972). These experiments implied that B cells were affected to a much greater extent then were T cells, in agreement with earlier findings that CY induced a more substantial inhibition of the antibody responses than of allograft rejection (Berenbaum & Brown, 1964). In contrast, neither B cells nor T helper cells from the spleen of CY-treated mice responded to antigen following transfer to naive recipients (Bach, 1975).

The antigen used and the immunoglobin class evaluated can also significantly influence the picture of CY-induced immunosuppression. In guinea-pigs pretreated with the drug and challenged with different antigens, it was shown that agglutinating antibody production was more easily inhibited than reaginic antibody production, which, depending on the particular antigen used, may be reduced, not affected or even increased (Turk & Parker, 1982). Similarly, in mice, CY pretreatment was found to increase IgE, while reducing the IgG response to the same antigen (Chiorazzi et al., 1976); this response was attributed to the different sensitivities to the drug among different B-cell isotype precursors of antibody forming cells and of their helper and regulatory T cells. In the light of the available evidence, the cellular basis of the inhibition by CY of humoral responses now appears to involve inhibition of both T and B cells. The sensitivity of the latter is supported by the histopathological demonstration of B-cell area depletion following drug administration and its capacity to inhibit the response to T-independent antigens. An effect on T helper cells is indicated by the observation that both B and T helper cells from CY-treated donors are nonresponsive when transferred to syngeneic, irradiated hosts (Bach, 1975).

Turning now to the effects of CY on cell-mediated responses, relatively large doses of CY (200 mg/kg) have been shown to suppress those lymphocyte functions that are mediated exclusively by T cells, e.g., graft-*versus*-host reaction and delayed-type hypersensitivity (DTH; Turk & Parker, 1982). In contrast, in a contact-sensitizing system with dinitrofluorobenzene in guinea-pigs, it was shown that 200 mg/kg CY enhanced rather than suppressed the subsequent skin reaction if the drug was administered prior to the sensitizing antigen (Turk *et al.*, 1972). This observation has been confirmed in a number of alternative models and is now used routinely as a method to promote induction of DTH to certain antigens. Further work has established that even small doses of CY (20-30 mg/kg), which do not suppress antibody synthesis, still dramatically enhanced a DTH reaction, provided the drug was administered prior to the sensitizing agent (Askenase *et al.*, 1975; Gill & Liew, 1978). The general consensus of opinion is that this potentiation of the DTH response is due to the elimination of T suppressor (Ts) cells by CY. A similar inhibitory effect of CY, also apparently targeting Ts cells, was reported by L'Age-Stehr and Diamantstein (1978), who demonstrated that autoreactive T-cell clones became transiently demonstrable in mice pretreated with CY and injected subsequently with lipopolysaccharide. Their interpretation of this phenomenon was that CY-resistant precursors of autoreactive T lymphocytes were stimulated by neodeterminants expressed on B lymphoblasts recruited into the CY-damaged spleen during a temporary absence of CY-sensitive Ts cells.

Nevertheless, it is apparent from the literature that Ts cells are not uniformly sensitive to CY. For example, the precursors of Ts cells induced by an injection of picryl sulfonic acid were found to be resistant to CY (Zembala & Asherson, 1976). Those induced by tumour allografts were equally resistant (Bonavida, 1977). Further studies by Shand (1978) indicated that murine-specific T cells that are destined to become suppressors following activation with concanavalin A are also fully resistant to CY. It therefore appears that only certain Ts-cell precursors are sensitive to CY.

Evidence in support of this concept is provided by studies of Spreafico *et al.* (1982), who used a passive transfer method to investigate the differential sensitivity of DTH and antibody regulating Ts cells. In these studies, CY effectively inhibited Ts-DTH activity at doses as low as 20 mg/kg, with 100 mg/kg totally abrogating Ts-cell activity for eight to nine days. In contrast, antibody suppressing T (Ts-Ab) cells were inhibited only by higher levels of CY (200 mg/kg). It is clearly tempting to speculate that Ts-Ab precursors may be a more slowly replicating and therefore less sensitive population than Ts-DTH cells; however, our lack of knowledge with respect to the structure and function of the networks within which these cells act, and their mode of communication with their respective effector cells, makes such a naive conclusion immediately open to criticism. Indeed, in respect of the latter aspect of cell-cell communication, CY has been demonstrated to inhibit the production and release of a number of antigen-specific suppressive cytokines, a finding in accordance with earlier work indicating that macrophage migration inhibition factor produced by lymphocytes was suppressed following treatment with this drug (Winkelstein, 1979).

In guinea-pigs, the antineoplastic drug bleomycin has also been shown to enhance DTH to dinitrofluorobenzene. In these studies, the drug was given as a single dose of 125 mg/kg on the day of, or up to three days after, sensitization. When administered two or three days after sensitization, bleomycin increased T-cell proliferation in the lymph nodes draining the skin site. This suggested to the investigators (Parker & Turk, 1984) that it may trigger IL-2 production. This capacity was confirmed when bleomycin was co-incubated with spleen cells from Lewis rats or Balb/c mice in the presence of a suboptimal dose of concanavalin A. Significant stimulation of IL-2 production occurred with as little as 1 ng/ml; the effect peaked at 10-100 ng, and toxicity became evident with doses in excess of 1 µg/ml.

Bleomycin has been examined for its ability to alter IL-1 production by peritoneal exudate macrophages; however, the effect on IL-1 was less significant than that on IL-2. The authors argued that it was unlikely that the increased production of IL-2 occurred as a direct result of an effect on IL-1 production, even though there was some alteration in the release of this monokine (Hamied *et al.*, 1986). Adriamycin had a similar effect to bleomycin down to a dose of 1 ng/ml; 4-hydroperoxycyclophosphamide and mafosfamide, on the other hand, markedly inhibited IL-2 release but had no effect on the release of IL-1 (Hamied *et al.* 1987).

Finally, an analysis of natural killer activity in murine systems revealed that a single dose of 150 mg/kg CY produced a marked reduction in splenic natural killer activity; the effect was transient, and full recovery was seen in seven to eight days (Mantovani et al., 1987). Data are confusing and incomplete, however, with regard to other nonspecific immune reactions. In mice, injection of 150 mg/kg CY has been reported to reduce the cytotoxic capacity of lymph node mononuclear cells, as judged in terms of both antibody-dependent cell-mediated cytotoxicity activity and mitogen-induced cytolytic activity (Winkelstein et al., 1979). In guinea-pigs, however, neither antibody- nor mitogen-dependent cytotoxicity of blood mononuclear cells and alveolar macrophages was influenced by a single injection of 200 mg/kg CY, whereas repeated daily administration of CY caused significant impairment of these effector functions (Hunninghake & Fauci, 1977). CY has also been demonstrated to decrease circulating monocytes in a number of different species (Mantovani et al., 1980). Impaired degradation of antigen-antibody complexes and phagocytosis of bacteria by peritoneal macrophages has also been described, but other workers have not observed a reduction in the capacity of macrophages to clear colloids from the circulation even after higher doses; increased phagocytosis by murine macrophages has also been reported following long-term treatment (see Spreafico et al., 1982). Similarly, CY did not interfere with the expression of tumoricidal activity of normal murine peritoneal macrophages (Mantovani et al., 1978,1980), and enhanced anti-tumour potential has been reported (Stoychkov et al., 1979) in the regenerating spleen after CY treatment. Thus, whereas mature macrophages appear to be relatively resistant, large and/or repeated doses of CY may adversely affect macrophage-dependent immune functions, presumably by blocking the maturation of macrophages at the level of the bone marrow. Clearly, further data are required in this area before firm conclusions can be drawn regarding the effects of CY on better defined macrophage populations and functions.

The immunosuppressive effects of CY are clearly most divergent. From the early evidence that the drug possessed an inherent selectivity for B cells, it soon became clear that certain Ts-cell subsets are even more affected by this compound. The reason for their sensitivity is not immediately apparent, but it is suggested that since CY-induced effects in B cells are reversible it is possible that the regulatory suppressor cells lack necessary enzyme-mediated DNA repair mechanisms. It is equally possible that, unlike the B-cell memory, there is little or no reserve of suppressor cell precursors that can be recruited into the general circulation. The latter situation could therefore be considered an example of what may occur in systems lacking inbuilt redundancy. Whatever the final mechanism is, this aspect of drug-induced immunoregulation clearly warrants further, more detailed exploration.

EFFECTS OF CARRAGEENAN

Carrageenan is the generic name given to high-molecular-weight (> 100 000 D) sulfated polygalactans derived from certain species of red algae. They are used extensively in the food industry as thickening, gelling or protein-suspending agents. Initially, all grades of carrageenan were considered safe and were permitted for use as regulated food additives; however, subsequent reports implicated degraded forms of carrageenan (< 20 000 D) in the induction of ulcers and metaplastic chages in the intestinal tract of a number of species of experimental animal (Sharratt et al., 1971; Fabian et al., 1973). Herbivores such as guinea-pigs and rabbits were shown to be particularly sensitive. In guinea-pigs, the ulcerogenic capacity of the carrageenan was related to the ability of intestinal macrophages to endocytose the material, and it was suggested that, following uptake, carrageenan caused lysosomal enzyme release and macrophage necrosis, prior to local tissue damage and ulceration (Abraham et al., 1974). Although some of the initial findings were contested (Sharratt et al., 1971), the US Food and Drug Administration ruled that food-grade carrageenans have an average molecular weight exceeding 100 000 D.

Subsequent studies using food-grade carrageenans in a variety of species, including man, have failed to demonstrate any adverse effect within the gastrointestinal tract. The consensus of scientific opinion remains, therefore, that, whereas degraded carrageenan may produce inflammatory lesions within the gastrointestinal tract of certain herbivores, omnivores are resistant.

Nevertheless, although native carrageenans are not ulcerogenic, trace amounts of this molecule has been shown to cross the intestinal barrier. Sharratt et al. (1971) reported that when native carrageenan 'labelled' with ferric iron was administered orally to guinea-pigs, particulate Pearls'-positive material could be demonstrated within lamina propria cells and in the subepithelial macrophages of the caecum. Likewise, using the carrageenan-specific Alcian blue staining technique, we have demonstrated the presence of carrageenan in the villus and lamina propria macrophages of rats given 0.5% carrageenan in their drinking-water (Nicklin & Miller, 1984). More recently, we confirmed and extended these observations using ^{3}H-labelled carrageenan and demonstrated the uptake of very low concentrations of radioactive label. Absorption occurred via the Peyer's patches and caecal lymph node, the lymphatic drainage from these organs leading to subsequent accumulation of radioactivity within the mesenteric lymph node (Baker, 1986; Nicklin et al., 1988). Uptake occurred in the absence of inflammatory or pathological changes and seemed consistent with the concept that the specialized cells present within the Peyer's patches and caecal lymph node take carrageenan from within the intestinal lumen and provide transport to the mesenteric lymph node, presumably for presentation to the immune system.

While there is no evidence to suggest that human intestinal uptake poses any toxic hazard, carrageenans are physiologically active molecules and, following their systemic administration, have been demonstrated to influence a number of biological systems, including blood clotting, the complement system, the inflammatory process and various aspects of the immune response (see Di Rosa, 1972 and Thomson & Fowler, 1981, for reviews).

If introduced into a suitable site, such as the planar surface of a rat's paw, the pleural cavity or a subcutaneous air bubble, carrageenan (0.05 ml of a 1% solution in saline) will induce an inflammatory response. In this response, oedema is followed by the migration of cells, mostly poly-morphonuclear leukocytes, and at some sites the eventual formation of a granuloma (Di Rosa, 1982). Other studies have demonstrated that systemic administration is associated with increased allograft survival. Rios and Simmons (1972) reported that histo-incompatible skin grafts had extended survival on mice treated intraperitoneally with carrageenan, unless the mice were also treated with poly-2-vinylpyridine N-oxide, a lysosome stabilizing agent. The authors concluded that the immunosuppression, as evidenced by loss of host-versus-graft responses, was mediated by macrophage cytotoxicity.

In vivo, administration of carrageenan at 40-160 mg/kg as four single injections during the week prior to challenge has been associated with a reduction in primary cytotoxic lymphocyte responses to allogeneic cells and, conversely, an augmentation of the secondary cytotoxic lymphocyte response (Sakemi et al., 1980). This differential effect was considered to be attributable to differences in the macrophage requirement of lymphocytes in maturation or sensitization processes. The augmentation of the secondary responses could also be due to macrophage injury caused by carrageenan, resulting in prolonged retention of injected allogeneic cells in the host and persistent antigenic stimulation of T cells (Yung & Cudkowicz, 1977). Treatment of guinea-pigs with carrageenan has also led to inhibition of both the induction and elicitation of DTH reactions (Bice et al., 1971).

In the study described above, bovine serum albumin-sensitive guinea-pigs received 40, 80 or 160 mg/kg carrageenan intraperitoneally for five days prior to challenge. In a parallel study, guinea-pigs received 40 or 80 mg/kg carrageenan intraperitoneally at 72, 48 and 24 h before immunization with human γ globulin, on the day of immunization and 24 h after immunization. In the presensitized group, the erythema and oedema associated with the Arthus reaction produced following challenge with bovine serum albumin were not affected at the 40 mg/kg dose level, but a marked decrease was apparent in the 80- and 100-mg/kg treatment groups. In the highest dose group, all animals became emaciated, with the development of ascites, and three out of ten died within two weeks. Autopsy revealed abundant serosanguinous ascites fluid with a sterile mucoid peritoneal exudate and nodular liver and spleen. The marked inhibition of Arthus and 24-h skin reactions observed in these animals may therefore be attributed to direct toxic effects of carrageenan at this dose rather than to a specific immunosuppressive effect. Animals treated with carrageenan during the sensitization phase were similarily affected. The Arthus reaction in guinea-pigs treated with

40 mg/kg was within the control range, whereas in animals treated at 80 mg/kg it was totally suppressed.

In other studies in which carrageenan and antigen were administered together, the carrageenan acted as an adjuvant and was shown to be as effective as Freund's complete adjuvant in potentiating the DTH response to lysozyme (Mizushima et al., 1974). In these studies, however, carrageenan was administered as a single dose, at 10 mg/kg, admixed with antigen. As mentioned above, the timing and dose of agent with respect to antigen are crucial in directing the outcome of the response measured.

In the main, however, there is general agreement that animals administered carrgeenan via the intraperitoneal route have a significantly reduced capacity to mount primary antibody responses against T cell-dependent antigens (see Thomson & Fowler, 1981). Antibody responses to T cell-dependent antigens are either unaffected (Wong & Herscowitz, 1979) or suppressed (Chaouat & Howard, 1976).

More importantly, Bash and Vago (1980) and Cochran and Baxter (1984) demonstrated that oral administration of carrageenan (5 and 50 mg/kg on five days per week for four weeks) to rats also resulted in a dose-dependent suppression of lymphocyte responsiveness to phytohaemagglutinin and concanavalin A in vitro . The latter results, in particular, are in accordance with those of more recent studies performed at our institute, which also demonstrated that intestinal persorption of small quantities of orally administered food-grade carrageenan at 5 mg/kg per day for 90-228 days was associated with depressed systemic humoral immunity against a heterologous T cell-dependent antigen (Nickin & Miller, 1984; Baker, 1986; Nicklin et al., 1988). Since T-cell responses, as judged by a popliteal lymph node assay for graft-versus-host reactivity, remained unchanged during these studies (Nicklin & Miller, 1984), it was postulated that altered humoral immunity was the result of modified antigen processing by macrophages rather than a direct effect on lymphocytes. This view is supported by the results of studies which demonstrated that carrageenans depressed some responses (Rumjanek & Brent, 1978; Pugh-Humphreys & Thomson, 1979) but enhanced others (Richou et al., 1968; Turner & Higginbotham, 1979), including the initiation of de-novo reaginic antibody production against proteins (Nicklin et al., 1985) and associated haptens (Nicklin & Miller, 1985).

These studies led to the suggestion that macrophages exposed to carrageenan may modify immune responses by the timed release of specific immunoregulatory products. Evidence in support of this possibility came from in-vitro studies which demonstrated that carrageenan-treated macrophages could, depending on conditions and time of administration, release either stimulatory or inhibitory factors. The former was shown to be the immunostimulatory agent IL-1 (Baker, 1986). This is particularly noteworthy, since IL-1 has been shown to be released from macrophages by other adjuvants (Oppenheim & Gerry, 1983). The inhibitory factor, which was shown to be produced at an early stage following exposure to non-toxic doses of carrageenan, is believed to be a prostaglandin because of its mode of action and short biological half-life.

Prostaglandins have been shown to inhibit effectively a range of in-vitro immune responses, including humoral antibody production (Webb & Nowowiejski, 1977), mitogen-induced lymphocyte transformation (Rao et al., 1979), lymphocyte-mediated cytolysis (Henney et al., 1972) and the production of leukocyte (Lomnitzer et al., 1976) and macrophage migration inhibition factor (Gordon et al., 1976). Further evidence that directly implicates prostaglandins as inhibitory immunoregulatory molecules is derived from the ability of inhibitors of prostaglandin synthesis to enhance antibody production (Webb & Nowowiejski, 1977) and mitogenic responses (Vosixa & Thies, 1979). Bash and Cochran (1980) also reported that a suppressor factor produced by incubating rat spleen cells with carrageenan was inhibited by indomethacin, a prostaglandin synthetase inhibitor. In reviewing these studies, it is possible to put forward explanations for certain aspects of the immunoregulatory properties of carrageenan. It would appear that the adjuvant properties of carrageenan stem from its ability both to act as a protein carrier and to elicit enhanced IL-1 release by antigen-presenting macrophages. Indeed, recent in-vitro studies using molecular biological tools have confirmed at the level of gene expression the ability of high-molecular-weight carrageenan to enhance IL-1 transcription (Fig. 4). This, in turn, would induce preferential amplification of T helper cells, which, if triggered at an appropriate time, would result in an enhanced immune response, including the elicitation of reaginic antibody production.

The immunodepressive effects observed when carrageenan is given orally or systemically prior to antigen are more difficult to explain but could involve carrageenan-induced IL-1-dependent expansion of a Ts-cell population, the release of inhibitory prostaglandin molecules and direct macrophage toxicity. These effects are, of course, not necessarily mutually exclusive, and in view of the previous observations it seems likely that the final outcome on the immune system must be influenced by both the dose of carrageenan administered and the conditions of exposure.

DIOCTYLTIN DICHLORIDE

Effects of organotin compounds on the immune system are described in detail in the paper by Penniks *et al.* in this volume. Within the constraints of this paper, however, it is worth emphasizing that di-*n*-octyltin dichloride is of particular interest in that its effects on the T cell-dependent pathways of the rat immune system are not mediated by a stress-induced increase in steroid hormones but occurs in the absence of other pathological changes and at dose levels that do not interfere with the growth of the animals (Miller & Scott, 1985; Vos *et al.*, 1985). This chemical may therefore be an ideal candidate for investigating dose-response relationships, as well as the mechanism whereby immunoselective effects are exerted on both proliferating thymocytes and a specific subpopulation of T lymphocytes (Miller *et al.*, 1986). Recent investigations at our institute, using the gene probing and dot blot hybridization techniques described above, have demonstrated that treatment with di-*n*-octyltin dichloride produces a rapid decrease in IL-2

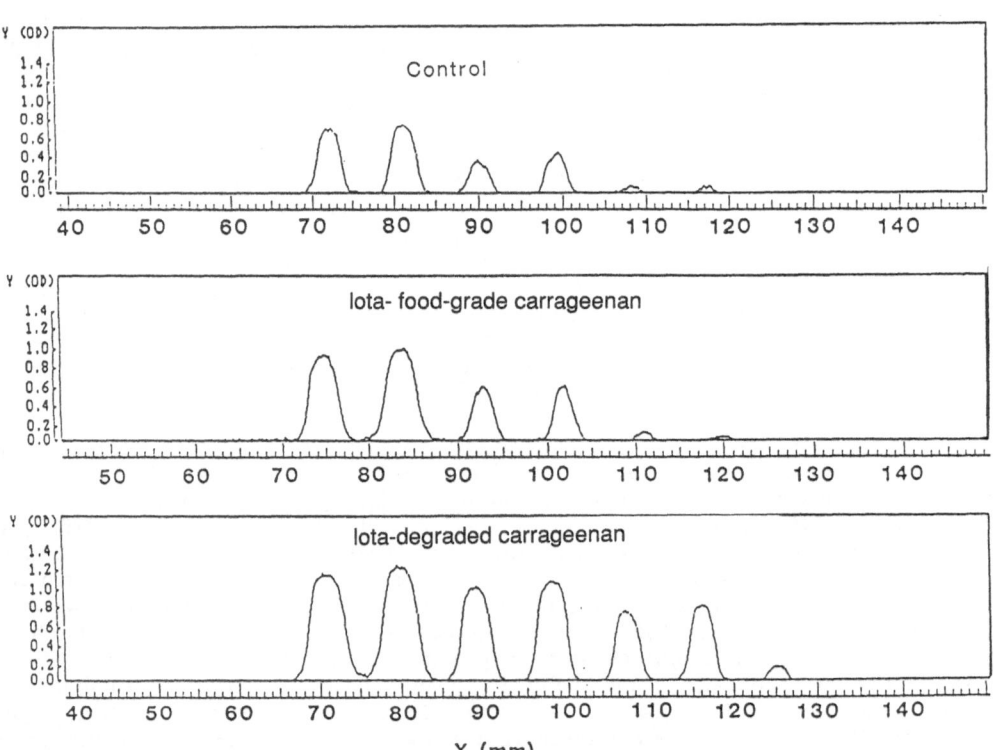

Fig. 4. Effects of carrageenan treatment on interleukin-1 gene expression in rat peritoneal macrophages; scanning densitometry of cytoplasmic mRNA dot blots

expression in the thymocyte population (Volsen *et al.*, 1989). This cytokine is thought to be produced by medullary thymocytes and is essential for sustaining thymocyte proliferation within the organ. The effects were time- and dose-dependent, occurred within 24 h and appeared to correlate with a significant reduction in the expression of a phenotypic marker positive for the MRC OX18 monoclonal antibody (a phenotype expressed on some medullary thymocytes as well as peripheral T cells). This effect was specific for the IL-2 regulatory gene, as the expression of the actin gene (a 'house-keeping' gene used to control for toxic effects) was unaffected by the treatment. It is possible, therefore, to explain some of the immuno-modulatory events associated with exposure to organotin compounds in terms of a treatment-related down-regulation of IL-2 or the expression of IL-2 receptors on sensitive cell populations.

This finding is in marked contrast to the effects of the immunosuppressive agent, azathioprine. A gene-probing investigation of thymocyte cell populations after 28-day oral administration to rats demonstrated that the immunosuppressive effects of azathioprine were due entirely to its general cytotoxic effects on proliferating cells and not to any direct effect on the immune system (Fig. 5). At levels of 2 mg/kg, at which no significant effect was seen with respect to thymic weight and cellularity, gene expression of *both* IL-2 and actin was markedly reduced; at 10 mg/kg, marked thymic involution had occurred and the remaining thymocyte population was obviously azathioprine-resistant.

CONCLUDING REMARKS AND COMMENTS

There is now a wealth of experimental evidence that the mammalian immune system can be damaged and immune reactivity subsequently altered following exposure to a wide and diverse range of drugs and environmental chemicals. There are also accumulating data to support the hypothesis that susceptible populations may be expected to suffer adverse immunological effects following accidental or occupational exposure to immunotoxic agents. As discussed above, such effects may be manifested in a number of ways; these include a loss or reduction in immune surveillance leading to heightened susceptibility to infections and increased risks of developing some forms of cancer, or loss of control within the system leading to autoimmune disease processes and/or hypersensitive reaction(s) to the agent itself. These and other basic principles underlying immunotoxic effects are adequately covered in other papers.

Progress in dose-effect, dose-response and risk analysis, as they relate to immunotoxic chemicals, has so far been relatively slow. This is due in part to the inherent complexity of the immune system and the diverse range of interconnected effects that may be altered. Perhaps more importantly, the lack of appropriate and effective screening assays for investigating dose-effect and dose-response relationships has held up progress in this field. Better procedures for assessing lymphoid histopathology are currently being reviewed and

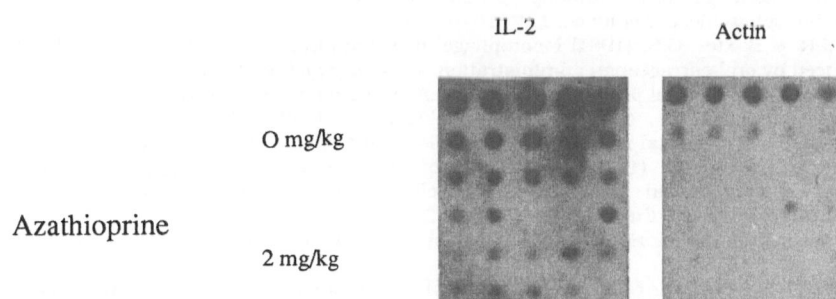

Fig. 5. Effect of azathioprine treatment on interleukin-2 (IL-2) and α-actin gene expression in rat thymocytes; mRNA expression in thymocytes isolated from rats following 28-day oral exposure to azathioprine

validated in a number of laboratories, with a view to their possible inclusion within the existing framework of acute/subacute and chronic toxicity testing and safety evaluations, as presently established for routine regulatory purposes. Agents that are deemed to be potentially immunotoxic may then be subjected to more specialized immunological screening procedures, as dictated by the nature of the lesion detected. Another approach is the use of molecular biological techniques to screen for the effects of the expression of immunoregulatory genes (Meredith *et al.*, 1989). The analysis of mRNA in defined immune cell populations may offer a simple, sensitive, specific scientific method for assessing the immunodulatory potential of compounds. An in-vitro screening strategy has been developed at our institute under the auspices of the Biotechnology Action Programme of the Commission of the European Communities, which could easily be extended to material derived from immune cells *in vivo*. These assays are based on the finding that the development of immune responses depends on precise intercellular communication involving a series of soluble polypeptide mediators, which include interleukins, cytokines, growth factors and their respective receptors on the cell surface. Clearly, before one can explore the feasibility and utility of the conventional dose-effect and dose-response relationships, it will be necessary to build up an adequate data base specifically relating the immunomodulating potential of a particular chemical with its more conventional toxicity profile - a daunting prospect but an exercise that clearly warrants further consideration.

REFERENCES

Abraham, R., Fabian, R.J., Goldberg, L. & Coulston, F. (1974) Role of lysosomes in carrageenan-induced caecal ulceration. *Gastroenterology*, **67**: 1169-1181

Askenase, P.W., Hayslen, B.J. & Gershon, R.K. (1975) Augmentation of delayed type hypersensitivity by doses of cyclophosphamide which do not affect antibody responses. *J. exp. Med.*, **141**: 697-702

Bach, J.F. (1975) The mode of action of immunosuppressive agents. In: Neuberger, A. & Tatum, E.L., eds, *Frontiers of Biology*, Vol. 41, Amsterdam, Elsevier, pp. 67-141

Baker, K.C. (1986) *The absorption from the gut and immunomodulatory effects of the sulphated polygalactan food additive carrageenan: studies in the inbred rat*, PhD Thesis, University of Reading, UK

Bash, J.A. & Cochran, F.R. (1977) Carrageenan-induced suppression of T lymphocyte proliferation in the rat: *in vitro* production of a suppressor factor by peritoneal macrophages. *J. reticuloendothel. Soc.*, **28**: 203-215

Bash, J.A. & Vago, J.R. (1980) Carrageenan-induced suppression of T lymphocyte proliferation in the rat: *in vivo* suppression induced by oral administration. *J. reticuloendothel. Soc.*, **28**: 213-221

Berenbaum, M.C. & Brown, I.N. (1965) Dose-response relationships for agents inhibiting the immune response. *Immunology*, **7**: 65-71

Bice, D., Schwartz, H.J., Lake, W.W. & Salvaggio, J. (1971) The effect of carrageenan on the establishment of delayed hypersensitivity. *Int. Arch. Allergy*, **41**: 628-636

Bonavida, B. (1977) Antigen-induced cyclophosphamide-resistant suppressor T cells inhibit the *in vitro* generation of cytotoxic cells from one-way mixed leukocyte reactions. *J. Immunol.*, **119**: 1530-1533

Chaouat, G. & Howard, J.G. (1976) Influence of reticuloendothelial blockage on the induction of tolerance and immunity by polysaccharides. *Immunology*, **30**: 221-227

Chiorazzi, N., Fox, D.A. & Katz, D.H. (1976) Hapten-specific IgE antibody responses in mice: selective enhancement of IgE antibody production by low doses of X-irradiation and by cyclophosphamide. *J. Immunol.*, **117**: 1629-1637

Cochran, F.R. & Baxter, C.S. (1984) Macrophage mediated suppression of T-lymphocyte proliferation induced by oral carrageenan administration. *Immunology*, **53**: 291-297

Di Rosa, M. (1972) Biological properties of carrageenan. *J. Pharmacol.*, **24**: 89-102

Fabian, R.J., Abraham, R., Coulston, F. & Goldberg, L. (1973) Carrageenan-induced squamous metaplasia of the rectal mucosa in the rat. *Gastroenterology*, **65**: 265-272

Gill, H.K. & Liew, F.Y. (1978) Regulation of delayed type hypersensitivity. III. Effect of cyclophosphamide on the suppressor cells for delayed type hypersensitivity to sheep erythrocytes in mice. *Eur. J. Immunol.*, **8**: 172-176

Gordon, D., Bray, M.A. & Morley, J. (1976) Control of lymphokine secretion by prostaglandins. *Nature*, **262**: 159-166

Hamied, T.A., Parker, D. & Turk, J.L. (1986) Potentiation of release of IL-2 by bleomycin. *Immunopharmacology*, **12**: 127-134

Hamied, T.A., Parker, D. & Turk, J.L. (1987) Effects of adriamycin, 4-hydroperoxycyclophosphamide and AstaZ 7557 (non Mafosfamide) on the release of IL-2 and IL-1 *in vitro*. *Int. J. Immunopharmacol.*, **9**: 355-361

Hatch, T.F. (1968) The dose-effect, dose-response relationship. *Arch. environ. Health*, **16**: 571-584

Henney, C.S., Bourne, H.R. & Lichtenstein, L.M. (1972) The role of cyclic 3'5'-adenosine monophosphate in the specific cytolytic activity of lymphocytes. *J. Immunol.*, **8**: 1526-1535

Howard, J.G. & Hale, C. (1978) Drug-promoted B cell tolerance induction: a selective activity of cyclophosphomide dependent suppression on the tolerogenicity of thymus-independent antigens. *Eur. J. Immunol.*, **8**: 492-496

Hunninghake, G.W. & Fauci, A.S. (1977) Immunological reactivity of the lung. IV. Effect of cyclophosphamide on alveolar macrophage cytotoxic effector function. *Clin. exp. Immunol.*, **27**: 555-559

L'Age-Stehr, J. & Diamantstein, T. (1978) Induction of autoreactive T lymphocytes and their suppressor cells by cyclophosphamide. *Nature*, **271**: 663-665

Lerman, S.P. & Weidanz, W.P. (1970) The effect of cyclophosphamide on the ontogeny of the humoral immune response in chickens. *J. Immunol.*, **105**: 614-617

Lomnitzer, R., Rabson, A.R. & Koornhof, H.J. (1976) The effects of cyclic AMP on leucocyte inhibition factor (LIF), production and inhibition of leucocyte migration. *Clin. exp. Immunol.*, **24**: 42-50

Mantovani, A., Luini, W., Peri, G., Vecchi, A. & Spreafico, F. (1978) Effect of chemotherapeutic agents on natural cell mediated cytotoxicity in mice. *J. natl. Cancer Inst.*, **61**: 1255-1261

Mantovani, A., Luini, W., Peri, G., Vecchi, A. & Spreafico, F. (1980) Effect of chemotherapeutic agents on natural and BCG-stimulated macrophage mediated cytotoxicity in mice. *Int. J. Immunopharmacol.*, **2**: 333-339

Meredith, C., Scott, M.P. & Miller, K. (1989) Immunotoxicology screening *in vitro*: modulation of expression of immunoregulatory genes. *Human Toxicol.*, **8**: 411-412

Miller, K. & Scott, M.P. (1985) Immunological consequences of dioctyltin dichloride (DOTC)-induced thymic injury. *Toxicol. appl. Pharmacol.*, **78**: 395-401

Miller, K., Scott, M.P., Hutchinson, A.P. & Nicklin, S. (1986) Suppression of thymocyte proliferation *in vitro* by a dioctyltin dichloride-induced serum factor. *Int. J. Pharmacol.*, **8**: 237-241

Mizushima, Y., Murata, J. & Horiuchi, Y. (1974) Use of carrageenan as an adjuvant of delayed hypersensitivity. *Int. Arch. Allergy appl. Immunol.*, **47**: 532-542

Nicklin, S. & Miller, K. (1984) Effect of orally administered food-grade carrageenans on antibody-mediated and cell-mediated immunity in the inbred rat. *Food chem. Toxicol.*, **22**: 615-621

Nicklin, S. & Miller, K. (1985) Induction of a transient reaginic antibody response to tartrazine in the rat. *Int. Arch. Allergy appl. Immunol.*, **76**: 185-187

Nicklin, S., Atkinson, H. & Miller, K. (1985) Carrageenan induced reaginic antibody production in the rat. Characterisation and kinetics of the response. *Int. J. Immunopharmacol.*, **7**: 677-685

Nicklin, S., Baker, K.C. & Miller, K. (1988) Intestinal uptake of carrageenan: distribution and effects on humoral immune competence. *Adv. exp. Med. Biol.*, **237**: 813-832

Oppenheim, J.J. & Gerry, I. (1983) Interleukin 1 is more than an interleukin. In: Inglis, J.R., ed., *T-Lymphocytes Today*, Amsterdam, Eslevier, pp. 265-279

Parker, D. & Turk, J.L. (1984) Potentiation of T-lymphocyte function by bleomycin. *Immunopharmacology*, **7**: 109-113

Pfitzer, E.A. (1976) General concepts and definitions for dose-response and dose-effect relationships of toxic metals. In: Nordberg, G.F., ed., *Effects and dose-response Relationships of Toxic Metals*, Amsterdam, Elsevier, pp. 140-146

Pugh-Humphreys, R.G.P. & Thomson, A.W. (1979) An ultrastructural study of mononuclear phagocytes from iota carrageenan-injected mice. *Cytobios*, **16**: 241-252

Rao, K.M.K., Schwartz, S.A. & Good, R.A. (1979) Modulation of the mitogenic response of lymphocytes from young and aged individuals by prostaglandins and indomethacin. *Cell Immunol.*, **48**: 155-167

Richou, R., Lallouette, P. & Legger, H. (1968) [Carrageenan, an adjuvant and stimulant substance.] (in French) *C.R. Acad. Sci. (D) (Paris)*, **267**: 257-263

Rios, A. & Simmons, R.L. (1972) Poly-2-vinylpyridine-N-oxide reverses the immunosuppressive effects of silica and carrageenan. *Transplantation*, **13**: 343-432

Rumjanek, V.M. & Brent, L. (1978) Immunosuppressive activity of carrageenan for cell-mediated responses in the mouse. *Transplantation*, **26**: 113-118

Sakemi, T., Kuroiwa, A & Nomoto, K. (1980) Effect of carrageenan on the induction of cell-mediated cytotoxic responses *in vivo*. *Immunology*, **41**: 297-302

Santos, G.W. & Owens, A.H. (1966) 19s and 7s antibody production in cyclophosphamide or methotrexate-treated rats. *Nature*, **209**: 622-624

Shand, F.L. (1978) The capacity of microsomally-activated cyclophosphamide to induce immunosuppression *in vitro*. *Immunology*, **35**: 1017-1025

Sharratt, M., Grasso, P., Carpanini, F. & Gangolli, S.D. (1971) Carrageenan ulceration and ulcerative colitis. *Gastroenterology*, **61**: 410-418

Spreafico, F., Tagliabue, A. & Vecchi, A. (1982) Chemical immunodeppressants. In: Sirois, P. & Rola-Pleszcznski, M., eds, *Immunopharmacology*, Amsterdam, Elsevier, pp. 315-348

Stender, H.S., Strauch, D., Winter, H. & Textor, W. (1963) The effect of cyclophosphamide on antibody formation with fractional and massive dosage. *Arzneimittel-Forsch.*, **13**: 1031-1034

Stoychkov, J.N., Schultz, R.M., Chigoros, M.A., Pavlidis, N.A. & Goldin, A. (1979) Effects of adriamycin and cyclosphosphamide treatment on induction of macrophage cytotoxic function in mice. *Cancer Res.*, **39**: 3014-3017

Thomson, A.W. & Fowler, E.F. (1981) Carrageenan. A review of its effects on the immune system. *Agents Actions*, **1**: 265-273

Turk, J.L. & Parker, D. (1982) Effect of cyclosphosphamide on immunological control mechanisms. *Immunol. Rev.*, **65**: 99-113

Turk, J.L. & Poulter, L.W. (1972) Selective depletion by cyclosphosphamide. *Clin. exp. Immunol.*, **10**: 285-296

Turk, J.L., Parker, D. & Poulter, L.W. (1972) Functional aspects of the selective depletion of lymphoid tissue by cyclosphosphamide. *Immunology*, **23**: 493-501

Turner, E.V. & Higginbotham, R.D. (1979) Effects of intravenous carrageenan on immune responses and on the reticuloendothelial system. *J. reticuloendothel. Soc.*, **26**: 763-773

Volsen, S.G., Barrass, N., Scott, M.P. & Miller, K. (1989) Cellular and molecular effects of di-n-octyltin dichloride on the rat thymus. *Int. J. Immunopharmacol.*, **6**: 703-715

Vos, J.G., Erajnc, E.I. & Wester, P.M. (1985) Immunotoxicity of bis (tri-n-butyltin) oxide. In: Dean, J., Luster, M., Munson, A.E. & Amos, H., eds, *Immunotoxicology and Immunopharmacology*, New York, Raven Press, pp. 327-339

Vosixa, G. & Thies, J. (1979) Effects of indomethacin on blastogenesis of lymphocytes from cancer patients, differentiation of patient types. *J. clin. Immunol. Immunopharmacol.*, **13**: 30-42

Webb, D.R. & Nowowiejski, I. (1977) The role of prostaglandins in the control of the primary IgA immune response to SRBC. *Cell Immunol.*, **33**: 1-11

Winkelstein, A. (1979) The effects of azathiorpine and 6-MP on immunity. *J. Immunopharmacol.*, **1**: 429-454

Winkelstein, A., Brizzi, J.A. & Kift, B.L. (1979) Mechanisms of immunosuppression: effects of cyclophosphamide on lymphocytes and macrophanges. *J. Immunopharmacol.*, **1**: 139-156

Wong, M. & Herscowitz, H.B. (1979) Immune activation by T-independent antigen. Lack of effect of macrophage depletion on the immune response to TNP-LPS, PVP and dextran. *Immunology*, **37**: 765-775

Yung, Y.P. & Cudkowicz, G. (1977) Abrogation of resistance to foreign bone marrow grafts by carrageenans. *J. Immunol.*, **119**: 1310-1315

Zembala, M. & Asherson, G.L. (1976) The effect of cyclophosphamide and irradiation on cells which suppress contact sensitivity in the mouse. *Clin. exp. Immunol.*, **23**: 554-561

RECOGNITION OF METALS BY PROTEINS

R.J.P. Williams

Inorganic Chemistry Laboratory, University of Oxford
Oxford OX1 3QR, UK

ABSTRACT

This paper describes the way in which metal ions of different classes interact with proteins of different kinds. The metal ions are divided into those which usually interact weakly through oxygen-centre donors, e.g., calcium, and those which interact with nitrogen or sulfur donors, e.g., mercury. The proteins are divided into those which do not fold except when bound to a metal ion and those with a more permanent fold. The combinations of metal with protein are then relatively specific in their chemistry but the physical shape of the metal/protein complex is highly specific. This specificity allows ready recognition of different metal ions by the immune system.

INTRODUCTION: METAL IONS AND THE IMMUNE SYSTEM

The immune system can be classified into levels of activity as far as the effect of metal ions is concerned. Here, I am no expert, but it would seem worthwhile to separate the following:

(i) the generation of antigenic sites by metal ions; and
(ii) the interference by metal ions in recognition steps at the molecular (antibody) and cellular levels.

Antigenicity

We know now that metal ions can control the shapes of proteins so that a well-established protein could be adjusted by an unusual metal ion to generate antigenicity. Whether or not this would just be a clearance mechanism for the metal ion, it could also result in a sustained attack on a self-protein. Which of the possibilities dominates seems to me to depend on whether the metal ion-induced conformation had always been present but in very low amounts, implying that response is dose-related. However, once switched on, the immune system remains super-sensitive.

Antibodies

I cannot see an easy mechanism for metal ions to affect antibodies directly, although antibodies will bind metal ions.

Cellular response

Here, I chart unknown waters. The striking effects of some metal ions in cellular growth patterns, both as poisons and useful drugs, suggests that at the level of cell growth and division metal ions and their complexes would be damaging to selected organs.

Finally we must try to pinpoint where the whole immune system is dependent on metals as opposed to where it may be sensitive to metal ions which damage a pathway that is not dependent on metal ions. We need to consider different parts of the immune response.

Immunotoxicity of Metals and Immunotoxicology, Edited by
A. D. Dayan *et al.,* Plenum Press, New York, 1990

The immune system has different modes of action. If we put to one side the antigen-antibody response as being largely independent of particular metal ions, since there is no role for metal ions in antibodies or the complement system (except for calcium-dependent effects), we are left with the immune response based on neutrophils. Here, there is no metal-ion requirement for dioxygen activation but one for superoxide removal - the superoxide dismutases. It is suspected that the inadequate clearance of superoxide could be a major cause of inflammation, but such topics are best left to other contributors to this volume. In such discussions, I would make one plea: the definition of metal ion function has to be referred to a location in a biological system not only at the level of the organ but particularly its cellular location. Figure 1 is an attempt to give some ideas about the locations and functions of metal ions in cells.

METAL IONS AND PROTEINS: GENERAL CONSIDERATIONS

I take it that my task in this volume is to highlight the ways in which different metal ions behave in their reactions with proteins, so that one can begin to understand chemically how metal ions could affect the parts of the immune system listed above. I go back, therefore, to first principles. I shall not discuss cell killing by chemical attack on DNA, as occurs with alkylating agents and with drugs such as *cis*-platinum. The topics under review are covered in the proceedings of the Dahlem conference (Nriagu, 1984), in which there are extensive references.

I shall discuss the problem of metal toxicity and its relation to the immune system in the following terms. (I assume that free metals are of little concern generally, although this may not be true of elements such as lithium and rubidium, the free ions of which carry current.):

    (i) the combining ability of metal ions;
    (ii) the nature of proteins as metal ion partners; and
    (iii) metal toxicity and exchange.

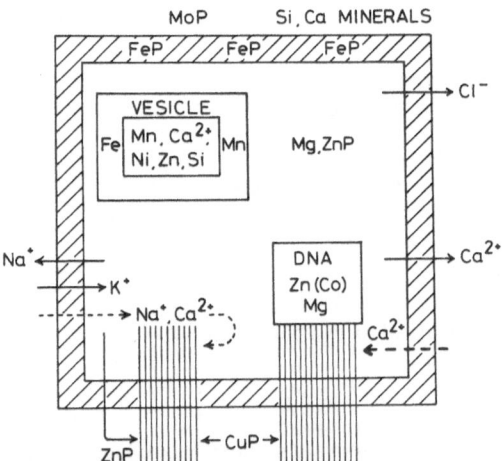

Fig. 1. Location of metal ion functions in cells. The metals are shown to occur in compartments to greater and lesser extents. For example, Ca²⁺ and CuP (P=proteins) are usually in extracellular fluids; Fe is often in membranes; K usually occurs at high levels in intracellular fluids. Some metal ions have special features, such as the ability to assist energy capture (Mg, Cu, Fe, Mn); a role in contractile devices (Ca); and a role in synthesis and destruction of filaments (Zn, Cu in collagen reactions).

COMBINING ABILITY OF METAL IONS

Metal ions in themselves are spherical and range in radius from about 0.05-0.2 nm. The first parameter of selectivity is then size. They also vary in electron affinity, i.e., Lewis acid strength. The size and electron affinity are dependent on charge. These three parameters can be used to explain the classification of metal ions into hard and soft or 'a' and 'b', which relates to the way in which they bind selectively to nonmetals. Figure 2 shows a plot of z/r (z the charge and r the ion radius) for divalent ions against I_2 which is the ionization potential from the M atomic state to the M^{2+} ion. Changing the sign of the I_2 gives the electron affinity, or roughly the Lewis acid strength of the ion. Those metal ions that lie higher in the plot are more 'a'-class (hard) than the lower, i.e., 'b'-class (soft) metal ions. If we take a series such as $Ca^{2+} < Mn^{2+} < Fe^{2+} < Co^{2+} < Ni^{2+} < Cu^{2+} > Zn^{2+}$ (the Irving-Williams series), Cu^{2+} is the softest cation. The distinction is revealed in chemistry, when we observe that soft cations prefer soft anions or neutral donors. Approximatively, the list with regard to donor centre softness is: $F^- < Cl^- < Br^- < I^-$ and $O < N < S$. Thus, we find (and expect from the rules) that Ca^{2+} will be bound to O-donor ligands but Cu^{2+} may be bound with either N or S donors. All such descriptions of the properties of metal ions are independent of shape.

Shape arises from the capacity of the metal ion to polarize in a complex. Energetically, some metal ions prefer one geometric arrangement of ligands and others prefer a very different arrangement. Some of the geometric arrangements that arise in coordination chemistry are given in Table 1. The problem can be treated at different levels of sophistication - e.g., by ligand field theory.

When we consider shape around a metal ion, we must consider the size of the ion first, since any radial field effect due to the electron affinity is limited in direction by covalency; then we can consider the so-called polarizability. Size is the important property for most

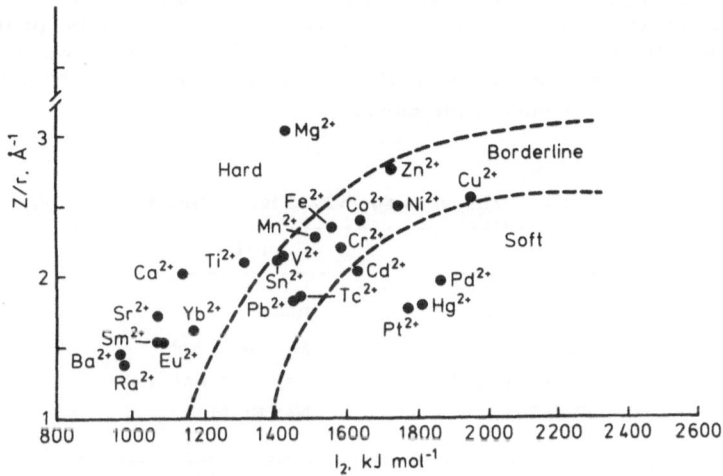

Fig. 2. Plot of z, charge, over r, ion radius against I_2, the ionization potential of the metal (M) atom to the ion M^{2+} for divalent ions

Table 1. Shapes of metal ion complexes

Shape	Example of complex
Linear	$Ag(NH_3)_2^{2+}$, $HgCl_2$
Planar (tetragonal)	$[Cu(NH_3)_4]^{2+}$, $[PtCl_4]^{2-}$
Tetrahedral	$[AuCl_4]^-$, $[HgI_4]^{2-}$
Octahedral	$[Co(NH_3)_6]^{3+}$, $[AlF_6]^{3-}$

hard ions such as Na^+, K^+, Mg^{2+} and Ca^{2+}. For a very small positive ion, the best packing of large nonmetal donors gives a tetrahedral form; next in size yields an octahedral form, and for still larger ions there is no preferred packing: those with 7-, 8- and 9-coordination are of similar stability. Roughly, ions with a radius of less than 0.06 nm are tetrahedral, ions with a radius between 0.06 and 0.09 nm are octahedral, and ions above this size are of ill-defined geometry. These are rules of packing for electrostatic association. Table 2 groups the ions accordingly. Covalent effects due to unoccupied orbitals of the ion come into play increasingly for ions toward the end of the first transition series and for all 'b'-class elements thereafter. Thus, Hg^{2+} forms two colinear bonds, Pt^{2+} forms four square (coplanar) bonds, and so on. The polarizability term is the effect of the field of ligands on the core electrons of the positive ion. For example, the core of Cu^{2+}, d^9, gives rise to square coplanar complexes. In many such cases, there is an additive influence of covalence after polarizability has been considered on the basis of symmetry, making it difficult to have a clear-cut separation of effects.

When a metal ion enters a biological system, it is partitioned among a wide variety of the small and large molecules. I shall not concern myself with combinations with DNA and RNA nor with polysaccharides for the most part. The reaction with small molecules leads to the formation of complexes in which the shape of the combined complex molecule is often decided by the metal ion. In the case of large molecules, e.g., proteins, the fold energy of the protein may or may not dictate the geometry around the metal ion. In other words, the metal ion makes demands, and the protein fold demands may be in conflict. The resolution of this conflict depends on the strength of the protein fold and the strength of the geometric demand of the metal.

PROTEIN FOLDING

The dogma that the protein sequence determines the fold of a protein is but a partial truth. Several protein do not fold (Table 3), some have several folds of approximately the same energy, and a majority perhaps have a fixed fold. Even within the last group, we must be careful to define 'fixed' as a description of a fold which shows one major backbone but many side-chain conformations. In view of the diversity of protein folds, we can address the principles of recognition of metal ions by proteins only by considering extreme examples. We start with recognition by random coil proteins.

Table 2. Shapes of some hard ion hydrates

Shape	Examples
Tetrahedral	Be^{2+}
Octahedral	Mg^{2+}, Al^{3+}, Sc^{3+}
8/9 Coordinate	Ca^{2+}, Sr^{2+}, Ba^{2+}, Ln^{3+}
Ill-defined	Na^+, K^+, Rb^+

Table 3. Folds of proteins

Unfolded	Loosely folded	Strongly folded
Metallothionein (Cd)	Calmodulin (Ca)	Phospholipase A2 (Ca)
Apocytochrome c (haem)	Ferric uptake regu-	Apoplastocyanin (Cu)
Osteocalcin (Ca)	latory protein (Fe)	Superoxide dismutase (Zn,Cu)
Tooth phosphoproteins		Carboxypeptidase (Zn)
Resilin		

Recognition by random coils

The basic reaction here is as follows:

$$\text{Random polymer} + \text{metal ion} \rightarrow \text{folded protein}$$

Let us take metallothionein as an example. Nuclear magnetic resonance (NMR) studies show that this protein has no fold in solution. On addition of heavy metal ions, such as copper, cadmium, zinc or mercury, it folds to a relatively well defined form in which the metal ions (all soft or rather soft) are bound by thiolates in two clusters of three and four metal ions. The reaction is extremely cooperative. The fact that the fold occurs only with metal ion cooperation means that the folded form is different for each metal ion. Thus, once a metal, A, is bound in a metallothionein molecule, it can be handled specifically. For example, zinc metallothionein is largely a storage form of zinc and remains in the cytoplasm, but copper metallothionein is rejected from cells. Copper is toxic inside cells and is more greatly used outside cells.

An example of a similar recognition of a metal complex (not a metal ion) is the uptake of iron porphyrins into cytochrome c. Apocytochrome c, as shown by NMR studies, is a random coil protein. In the presence of porphyrins - even metal-free porphyrin - it folds; although this fold is not yet very stable, the protein has already taken on a fold dictated by Van der Waals' interactions. In the presence of iron protoporphyrin, the fold is similar, but now two bonds are formed from His-18 and Met-80 to the iron. In this situation, the two allyl groups of protoporphyrin IX are very close to two thiolates, Cys-14 and Cys-17 of cytochrome c. Oxygen from the air now aids oxidative addition, which is assisted catalytically by the iron:

$$-SH + CH_2 = CH \; -C \rightarrow \; CH_3 \; - \underset{\underset{S}{|}}{CH} \; -C.$$

The fold is now very tight, as NMR and X-ray crystallographic studies show.

Here again, the fold is defined by the reaction of a rather soft metal ion with two soft bases. We return to cytochrome c, as we can use it to analyse surface recognition of a protein fold dictated by a metal ion or a metal ion complex.

A final example of this type of recognition is provided by a hard metal ion reacting with hard bases, e.g., calcium reacting with O-atom donors. The case is that of osteocalcin. The protein itself is poorly folded. The reaction with three or four calcium ions gives a folded form in which calcium is bound mainly by the carboxylate groups of Glu, Asp or Gla. This protein-metal ion complex recognizes bone crystallites.

Most of the observations described above are based on NMR studies of proteins. Note that once the metal ion or complex is taken up by the proteins in this way it is no longer represented by a small surface but can be detected through the surface of the large protein in which it is trapped. This represents a chance for the recognition of specific metal ions by antibodies (see below).

Almost rigid proteins for recognition of metal ions

Numerous large proteins have very stable folds based on a unique backbone construction. An example is lysozyme. In Table 3 we gave examples of metalloproteins that do not alter shape to any marked degree when their metal ion is removed. All of these proteins are heavily cross-linked between remote parts of the chain by either H-bonds, typically a β-sheet, or by chemical bridges such as -S-S- bridges. Such cross-linking is a major constraint, so that the fold controls the geometry around any metal ion that is taken up. This constrained metal site has been called an entatic state. Metals replace one another on the sites of these proteins isomorphously, so that the metal protein is recognized as a protein no matter which metal ion is involved. Such proteins are not particularly valuable in the control of toxicity, but their sites are obviously at risk from contamination since replacement depends only on the thermodynamics of metal ion binding.

Good examples of these principles are provided by carboxypeptidase and carbonic anhydrase - both zinc proteins. It has been shown that many metal ions can enter these sites, e.g., Cu, Ni, Co, Mn, Cd, Hg, Pb. The metal ions accept the geometry provided by the site to a first approximation. It would appear that most enzymes and simple electron transfer proteins are based on this principle of relative rigidity. An example of a hard metal centre is provided by phospholipase A2, the calcium-binding protein. Carrier proteins may be much more flexible, as we shall see.

As an aside, we must observe that the surfaces of these proteins do not have motionless recognition patterns. Recognition is of a particular conformation of the side-chains, but the side-chains themselves have considerable motion. Our studies by NMR of sequential antigenic sites show that they usually occur on loops, and the loop itself has considerable mobility. The best examples are cytochrome c and acyl phosphatase. Similar observations have been made on other proteins using X-ray crystallographic B-factors to discern mobility. However, the mobile surfaces are virtually independent of the metal ion incorporated, unlike the first group of random coil apo-proteins and unlike the next group of proteins described.

Intermediate strength of fold

Some proteins are folded but have a variety of significantly different shapes with similar energy. When such proteins combine with a metal ion, they change shape somewhat. Indeed, they change average shape with temperature change. A good example is calmodulin, with which we can contrast phospholipase A2, a member of the rigidly folded class of protein. When calmodulin binds to calcium, there is a considerable change in the atoms which coordinate to the calcium, i.e., side-chains of carboxylate amino acids in contrast to the negligible movement of the carbonyls of the main chain of phospholipase A2, which are its donors to calcium. The changes to the calmodulin amino acids on binding calcium affect the small β-structure at the heart of the calcium site, and its adjustment causes a larger change in helices and loops elsewhere in the protein, so that calcium calmodulin is recognized by target proteins that do not recognize apocalmodulin. Although other cations compete for the calcium site, the conformational change for each is relatively specific. Thus, clearly, calmodulin can be a recognition site for the presence of calcium. Now, although magnesium binds to the same site as calcium, its effect on the protein fold is different. Once again, the metal ion can be recognized specifically by the shape it gives to a large protein molecule. We see that recognition principles are similar for soft and hard metal ions but they have selective chemical centres.

Controlled incorporation

Metal ions can be incorporated almost irreversibly into small cyclic molecules by catalysed transfer reaction sequences. The sequences are of the kind:

$$M_1 + L_1 \rightleftarrows M_1L_1 + L_2 \rightarrow M_1L_2;$$

compare $\qquad\qquad M_2 + L_1 \rightleftarrows M_2L_1 + L_2 \rightarrow$ no reaction.

The first step is based on the principle outlined above that the ligand, or protein L_1, can select metal ions to some degree to give an ML_1 complex. This selectivity could be quite strong or relatively weak and is based on the hard acid/hard base and soft acid/soft base selectivity (Fig. 2). The second step has greatly enhanced selectivity, since it is based both on these properties and the recognition by L_2 of the individual shape of ML_1 complexes. Now each ML_1 complex has its own shape (see above), so that M_1 may enter L_2 almost specifically. Examples are given in Table 4. The complexes such as M_1L_2 that are formed can then be folded into selected proteins. The immune system could select different M, by its reaction with either ML_1 or ML_2 (more selective) or ML_2 in a protein, when the selectivity may be further enhanced.

Table 4. Highly selective uptake of metal ions

Metal ion	Small complex	Protein (example)
Iron	Protoporphyrin	Cytochrome c
Cobalt	Corrin (vitamin B_{12})	Carrier protein
Nickel	F-430	Hydrogenases
Magnesium	Chlorophyll	Reaction centre
Molybdenum	Molybdenum factor	Xanthine oxidase
Iron/Molybdenum	Iron/molybdenum/cobalt	Nitrogenase
Zinc	—	Carbonic anhydrase
Copper	—	Plastocyanin
Calcium	—	Calmodulin
Manganese	—	O_2-release system

METAL TOXICITY AND EXCHANGE

It would appear that biological systems have adopted their intake of metal ions within narrow limits for optimal function and that generally this is based on the availability of metal ions. Thus, toxicity can arise from the intake of 'too much' of any element. The definition of 'too much' depends heavily on the element. For mercuric ions, it is a very low concentration, but for sodium a much greater tolerance exists. Again, speciation of the metal ion is important in the intake. Clearly toxic conditions exist through change in the environment, e.g., of pH, or through the genetic nature of the organism, i.e., reduced tolerance. The toxic effects of, say, aluminium on organisms are very much dependent on pH and the age - very young or very old - of the population. Teratogenic effects are displayed in the growing organism by, e.g., lithium.

Now, the toxicity to the immune system must depend on the time of residence of the toxic ion. Throughout the above discussion, the metal ion has been treated as if it were in a static chemical container. In fact, biological systems are flow systems. It is not likely that the immune system will be affected greatly by an invasion of the body that is very short lived or that passes from one organ to another rapidly, unless the invasion is continuous. We should carefully distinguish an uptake that will remain or accumulate in the body from one that is transient. We must look at rates of exchange of metal ions from metal complexes and proteins as well as strengths of binding.

RATES OF EXCHANGE OF METAL IONS

Table 5 lists some generalities that can be made in this context. It is hard to retain locally ions such as Li, Na, K, Mg, Ca, Sr, Ba and lanthanides, except in bone. When used medicinally, these elements can be given in quite high doses and continuously and do not appear to affect the immune system greatly. They are hard ions. For another group of very hard ions, the situation is much less clear. These are Be^{2+} and Al^{3+} (common) and ions such as Ti^{4+}. They can be retained for long periods. The next group has a mixed character and lies appropriately between hard and soft metal ions. They include Cr, Mn, Fe, Co, Ni, Cu, Zn and Ga. In some oxidation states they exchange easily, and most easily from oxygen-donor complexes; in others they exchange very slowly. Small amounts may be retained for long periods. Finally, there are the very soft metals, the heavier transition metals, including Cd, Hg, Ag, Au, Tl, Sn and Pb. Once combined, they remain in the body for long periods.

Table 5. Rates of exchange of metal ions

Metal ion[a]	Exchange rate
Na, K, (Mg), Ca, (Mn)	Fast
(Zn), (Mn), (Fe), Ln	Intermediate
Co, Ni, Cu, Hg, Pt, (Zn), (Mn), (Fe), (Mg)	Slow

[a]Metal ions given in parentheses occur in two or more groups.

Noticeably, it is the latter groups of elements that most affect the immune system. Why? At the same time, we notice that the series of elements - hard, intermediate and soft - represents the series of abundance of the elements in the body. One factor could well be that the immune system is not normally exposed to elements in the last category. In other words, the whole body, and not just the immune system, does not know how to handle the soft elements.

CONCLUSION

It appears from the above that the immune system, which is highly idiosynchratic, could generate anti-metal proteins specifically in individuals. Metal ions could also affect components of the immune system in a general way. The less common the element is to biological systems and the more it falls into class 'b', the stronger its effect.

REFERENCE

Nriagu, J.O., ed. (1984) *Changing Metal Cycles and Human Health*, Berlin (West), Springer

HYPERSENSITIVITY

HYPERSENSITIVITY : CLINICAL ASPECTS

G. Kazantzis

London School of Hygiene and Tropical Medicine
London WC1E 7HT, UK

ABSTRACT

Immune status must be taken into account in any consideration of factors that influence the toxicity of metals. Commonly occurring phenomena are described that result from increased cellular reactivity to nickel, chromium, cobalt, beryllium, zirconium, mercury, gold and platinum, and an attempt is made to classify these phenomena into the four main categories of hypersensitivity reaction. The clinical effects can be varied, giving rise to conjunctivitis, rhinitis, asthma, urticaria, contact dermatitis, proteinuria, nephrotic syndrome, thrombocytopenia and other blood dyscrasias. Of these effects, cutaneous hypersensitivity is the most common, affecting both the general population and occupationally exposed groups. Metal compounds used in therapeutics have also been responsible for hypersensitivity reactions. A brief account is given of the principal diagnostic procedures used in eliciting evidence of a hypersensitive state.

INTRODUCTION

Hypersensitivity is a state in which an exaggerated and adverse response follows exposure to a particular foreign substance, the heightened sensitivity being the result of immunological 'memory' of previous contact with that substance. The mechanisms underlying these inappropriate reactions are those normally employed by the body in combating infection. Awareness of certain forms of hypersensitivity reaction, in particular the allergies, has for long preceded our knowledge of impaired immunological responses, in large part because of their often dramatic clinical presentation and by identifying outcome with an immediately previous exposure, as for example the potentially fatal response to a bee sting from angioneurotic oedema in sensitized individuals, the asthmatic response to a variety of inhaled and ingested allergens and the skin rashes which develop in sensitized individuals following exposure to a wide range of materials including foods, plants, and jewellery.

Hypersensitivity reactions cover a broad range of disease, the commonly recognized allergies representing no more than 'the tip of the iceberg'. The reactions may be classified into four main types, dependent on the ways in which immune components behave abnormally, although a disease process may involve more than one category. Examples of the types of hypersensitivity reaction as classified by Coombs and Gell (1975) are shown in Table 1, to illustrate the broad range of diseases to which they give rise. Metals are involved in each of the four types of hypersensitivity reaction, but in particular in cell-mediated hypersensitivity (Kazantzis, 1978).

Immunotoxicity of Metals and Immunotoxicology, Edited by
A. D. Dayan *et al.*, Plenum Press, New York, 1990

Table 1. Types of hypersensitivity reaction

Type	Basic mechanism	Examples of disease state
Type I Immediate or anaphylactic	IgE, mast cells and basophils	Anaphylaxis Asthma Conjunctivitis Rhinitis Hay fever
Type II Cytotoxic, antibody dependent	IgM, IgG Complement activation Lysis	Transfusion reactions Drug-induced: - haemolytic anaemia - agranulocytosis - thrombocytopenia Autoimmune haemolytic anaemia Goodpasture's syndrome
Type III Immune complex	IgA, IgM, IgG Complement activation	Extrinsic allergic alveolitis Serum sickness Systemic lupus erythema- tosus Glomerulonephritis (some forms)
Type IV Delayed-type hypersensitivity	Delayed hypersensitivity T Lymphocytes	Mantoux reaction Graft rejection Contact dermatitis

CATEGORIES OF IMMUNE RESPONSE

Type I - Anaphylactic or immediate hypersensitivity

Antigen reacts with specific IgE antibody bound to the surface of mast cells, leading to the release of vasoactive amines, including histamine, leukotrienes and platelet activating factor, together with eosinophil and neutrophil chemotactic factors. Hay fever and extrinsic asthma are the commonest clinical disorders, and anaphylactic reactions are also brought about in this way. The tendency to produce high levels of IgE is an important contributory factor, a strong familial predisposition being evident. Hypersensitivity can be transferred from a sensitized to a normal subject by means of serum which contains the humoral antibody.

Type II - Antibody-dependent cytotoxic hypersensitivity

The humoral antibody, which is an IgG or IgM immunoglobulin, reacts with antigen bound to the cell surface and fixes complement to produce cell death. This is one of the mechanisms by which invading organisms are destroyed, but cytotoxic hypersensitivity also gives rise to transfusion reactions, to haemolytic disease in the newborn and to drug-induced haemolytic anaemia, agranulocytosis and thrombocytopenia. A similar mechanism may give rise to autoimmune reactions, good examples being autoimmune haemolytic anaemia, idiopathic thrombocytopenic purpura and Goodpasture's syndrome.

Type III - Immune complex-mediated hypersensitivity

The antibody combines with soluble antigen, and the complex deposits in tissues, fixing complement and giving rise to a polymorphonuclear inflammatory response. Localization of preformed, circulating immune complexes depends on their size, charge and concentration, the nature of the antigen and the local concentration of complement. Where circulating antibody levels are high, the complexes are precipitated close to the site of origin of the antigen. In the skin, this is characterized by the Arthus reaction, consisting of erythema and oedema with polymorph infiltration, while in the lung various forms of extrinsic allergic alveolitis result. With a relative antigen excess, soluble antigen-antibody complexes are formed which may be deposited on the glomerular basement membrane, in joints, skin or choroid plexus. In the glomerular basement membrane, these complexes build up as 'lumpy' granules staining for antigen, immunoglobin and C3 complement by immunofluorescence, and appear as amorphous masses on electron microscopy. A second mechanism for injury in the kidney is glomerular fixation of antibody directed against the glomerular basement membrane, giving rise to a smooth linear deposition of antibody in a continuous distribution along the glomerular basement membrane.

Type IV - Cell-mediated hypersensitivity

This form of hypersensitivity is encountered in the contact dermatitis resulting from sensitization to a variety of chemicals, tissue damage following bacterial, viral, parasitic and fungal infections and in the rejection of transplanted tissues. Essentially, the reaction is initiated by delayed hypersensitivity T cells which react with antigens to which they have been previously specifically sensitized to release lymphokines. Lymphokines are soluble mediators which attract and activate macrophages and polymorphs, which in turn liberate lysosomal enzymes that cause local tissue damage. Erythema and induration develop some 24-72 h after exposure to the antigen; the lesion is typified by the Mantoux reaction. The time may be contrasted with the 15-30 min required for an anaphylactic reaction to develop, and 4-8 h for Arthus reactions.

METALS THAT GIVE RISE TO HYPERSENSITIVITY REACTIONS

A metal requires complexing with protein, nucleic acid or a polysaccharide to develop antigenic properties, which involves the formation of covalent bonds to form a hapten-carrier conjugate. Clinical observation has shown an individual predisposition to a hypersensitivy reaction following exposure to a potential allergen. Experimental animal studies provide some evidence that the ability to become sensitized is genetically controlled. For example, of two inbred strains of guinea-pig, 80% of one strain could be sensitized to mercuric chloride but not to potassium dichromate, while the second strain could not be sensitized to mercury but over 70% could be sensitized to the other metal compound (Polak et al., 1968).

Certain metals, in particular mercury and gold, give rise to autoimmune reactions in susceptible subjects. Animal models of metal-induced autoimmunity have been developed, and these aspects are presented and discussed in this symposium by Pelletier et al. and by Panayi. Those metals observed in humans to give rise to hypersensitivity reactions are shown in Table 2.

Nickel

Epidemiological studies of contact dermatitis have shown nickel to be the commonest skin sensitizer at a population level, as it is very widely distributed in the environment, as a

Table 2. Metals observed to give rise in humans to hypersensitivity reactions

Type I	Platinum
	Chromium
	Cobalt
	Nickel
Type II	Gold
Type III	Mercury
	Gold
Type IV	Nickel
	Chromium
	Cobalt
	Beryllium
	Gold
	Mercury
	Zirconium

constituent of jewellery, buttons, clips, coins, various alloys and in glass. Even abrasive cleaning of kitchenware has been shown to release nickel in washing-up water and to give rise to hypersensitivity reactions.

Nickel dermatitis usually presents as an itching, papular erythema on the neck, thighs or elsewhere on the body where contact is made with a nickel alloy, and in workers more often on the hands, where in its chronic stage it presents as a papulovesicular dermatitis with a tendency to lichenification. On repeated exposure, the hypersensitive reaction can become increasingly severe, involving other parts of the body not in direct contact with the metal and including swelling of the eyelids.

Nickel dermatitis provides a good example of a type-IV delayed hypersensitivity reaction. Nickel has been shown to act as a specific stimulant in subjects with nickel hypersensitivity when examined by the lymphocyte transformation test. During the lymphocyte transformation process, lymphokines have been identified which temporarily inhibit the migration of macrophages. Leukocyte migration inhibition has been demonstrated in subjects with both positive and negative patch tests and a history of nickel dermatitis (Forman & Alexander, 1972).

Chromium

Chromium is the second most common skin sensitizer in the general population after nickel, and is the commonest in men, probably as a result of occupational exposure. Such exposures involve handling cement, the tanning of leather, chromium plating, printing, the handling of chrome colours, dyes, lubricating oils and greases. The hands are involved in the majority of cases but with spread to other parts of the body. Hexavalent chromium readily traverses cell membranes and then undergoes intracellular reduction to the trivalent state, forming a conjugate with proteins to act as the complete antigen. Circulating antibodies against trivalent but not against hexavalent chromium have been identified in sensitized animals (Novey et al., 1983).

Chromium may be involved in not only type-IV cell-mediated hypersensitivity, but also less commonly in immediate or type-I hypersensitivity reactions. Cases of asthma with an immediate or a delayed response have been observed following occupational exposure to chromic acid, dichromates, chromite ore, chrome pigments and to welding fume (Keskinen et al., 1980; Novey et al, 1983).

Cobalt

Cobalt hypersensitivity, also an example of a type-IV cell-mediated reaction, is often found in association with nickel and chromium sensitivity. Sensitization reactions have been observed in workers in the hard metal industry, in offset printers and in building workers handling paint and cement, and also following contact with cobalt in hair dyes and in patients with orthopaedic implants. Loosening of such implants has been shown to occur more frequently in patients with chromium or cobalt sensitivity (Benson et al., 1975). Cobalt dust has been implicated as an etiological agent in bronchial asthma and contact dermatitis in refinery workers.

Beryllium

Chronic berylliosis is a multisystem disorder affecting principally the lungs. The lesion is a noncaseating granuloma with giant-cell formation similar to that seen in sarcoidosis, with helper/inducer T cells and macrophages. A patch test developed in the 1950s was found to give rise to both dermal and pulmonary exacerbations of the disorder and was subsequently abandoned. Berylliosis has now been confirmed as a type-IV cell-mediated hypersensitivity disorder, the beryllium ion acting as a hapten; complexes in which the beryllium ion is unavailable are inactive (Krivanek & Reeves, 1972). Lymphocyte blast transformation and macrophage migration inhibition are now used as diagnostic tests for beryllium hypersensitivity. Alekseeva et al. (1974) postulated on the basis of clinical and experimental observations that the systemic lesions of chronic berylliosis were conditioned by an autoimmune process resulting from the abolition of natural tolerance to autologous proteins. The complex nature of the immunotoxic effects of beryllium has been considered by Reeves and Preuss (1985), and the immunological diagnosis is considered by the same authors in this volume.

Zirconium

Hypersensitivity reactions have been observed in persons exposed to zirconium, which is present in a number of deodorant preparations. A granulomatous reaction develops at the site of application, in particular where minor abrasions of the skin allow penetration of the antigen. The granolomas consists of aggregates of distinctive epithelioid and Langerhans giant cells. Patch and intradermal testing has produced a sarcoid-like granulomatous infiltrate.

Mercury

Mercury contrasts with the metals considered above in giving rise to both type-IV and type-III hypersensitivity reactions. Patch testing was begun following the observation in 1896 of an acute eczmatous reaction confined to sites treated with grey mercurial ointment. Severe allergic reactions have developed in sensitized subjects exposed to mercury vapour, one extreme form being the 'baboon syndrome'. Thiomersal and ammoniated mercury were found to be common skin sensitizers in a survey performed by the North American Contact Dermatitis Group (1973). A high incidence of contact dermatitis to mercury has been observed in Japan, where mercurochrome has been used widely as a topical disinfectant. Patch tests performed on subjects with amalgam fillings have provided evidence of sensitization to mercury (Finne *et al.*, 1982), and facial dermatitis has been reported in a few cases. Cutaneous hypersensitivity to mercury, as demonstrated by a standard patch test, has been investigated in dental students, who showed more positive reactions with longer exposure (White & Brandt, 1976). In a comparative study of medical and dental students, while none showed a positive patch test to mercury, there were significantly higher total lymphocyte and total T-cell counts, T helper/inducer cells and T suppressor/cytotoxic cells in the dental compared with the medical students (Eedy *et al.*, 1988). Both aryl and alkyl mercury seed dressings have been shown to be skin sensitizers, but there is no evidence for an immunological cross-reaction between organic and inorganic mercury compounds.

It has for long been known that workers exposed to metallic mercury vapour developed proteinuria, initially observed in the felt-hat industry. Less commonly, the proteinuria may progress to the nephrotic syndrome (Kazantzis *et al*, 1962). The nephrotic syndrome has also been observed in Africans using skin-lightening creams based on mercury, following treatment with organomercurial diuretics and with other mercury-containing medicaments (Fillastre *et al.*, 1988). Both minimal lesions and evidence of membranous glomerulonephritis have been observed, with widespread basement membrane thickening and partial fusion of epithelial cell foot processes under the electron microscope. Immunofluorescence has shown finely granular IgG, IgM and C3 complement deposits, indicative of a membranous glomerulonephritis probably with an immune complex pathogenesis (Lindqvist *et al.*, 1974). The possible consequences for general health following slow release of mercury from dental amalgam fillings is reviewed in this symposium by Friberg and Eneström.

Gold

Proteinuria develops in 1-10% of patients treated with organic gold compounds for rheumatoid arthritis, although in a proportion of these cases renal amyloid rather than gold-induced renal damage may be the cause. As with mercury, the nephrotic syndrome may develop in a proportion of these cases. The nephropathy is unrelated to other side-effects of gold, is not related to dose, may present at any time following commencement of therapy, although more often during the first six months, and is not related to gold concentrations in blood or urine. The lesion observed most often is a membranous glomerulonephritis (Fillastre *et al.*, 1988). Subepithelial electron-dense deposits and granular deposition of IgG, C3 and, less frequently, IgM on the capillary basement membrane have been demonstrated by immunofluorescence. The deposits are presumed to be immune complexes, but they have not been shown to contain gold, although gold has been identified elsewhere in the glomeruli (Palosuo *et al.*, 1976). The renal lesion appears to regress over a period of months or years following cessation of gold therapy. Thus, gold, as mercury, appears to be capable of inducing a type-III immune complex hypersensitivity reaction.

Gold has also been implicated in bone-marrow depression, including thrombocytopenia, and granulocytopenia. Lymphocyte blast transformation has been demonstrated with an organogold complex in patients with bone-marrow depression (Denman & Denman, 1968). Pulmonary eosinophilia, eosinophilic pneumonia and Loeffler's syndrome have been observed in association with chrysotherapy. Fibrosing alveolitis has also been observed both with and without eosinophilia, with positive and negative lymphocyte transformation, but the role of gold in these cases is difficult to assess. Allergic contact dermatitis has been reported in patients on chrysotherapy, preceded by eosinophilia and raised circulating IgE levels (Davis & Hughes, 1975). Metallic gold has also been reported, on rare occasions, to give rise to an allergic dermatitis, in particular involving areas subject to sweating, pressure and friction. Thus, gold appears, under appropriate circumstances, to give rise to types-II, -III or -IV hypersensitivity reactions.

Platinum

Hypersensitivity reactions have been observed following exposure to the complex salts of platinum, ammonium tetrachloroplatinate and hexachloro-platinate. In addition to conjunctivitis, rhinitis and asthma, urticaria and anaphylactic reactions have been reported. Platinum refinery workers have become sensitized following exposures ranging from a few months to many years. Immediate, late and dual bronchial constrictor reactions have been demonstrated in sensitized subjects exposed to dusts of complex salts of platinum in lactose (Pepys,1973). An Arthus reaction, indicative of the additional presence of precipitating antibody, has also been demonstrated, but IgG antibody has not been identified (Levene, 1971). The allergic response, as shown by skin tests, to various platinum halide complexes is confined to a small group of charged compounds containing reactive ligand groups, such as chlorine, and is related both to their charge and their overall reactivity towards protein. Neutral complexes and those containing more strongly bound ligands were found to be inactive (Cleare *et al*, 1976). Complex salts of platinum clearly give rise to type-I, immediate hyper-sensitivity.

Other metals

Hypersensitivity reactions have been implicated, but without confirmatory evidence for a number of metals. Thus, the role of copper in intrauterine contraceptive devices has been queried in giving rise to hypersensitivity reactions. Similarly, the role of nickel in stainless-steel components in indwelling catheters, molybdenum and vanadium in hip prostheses, and tin in preparations containing stannous chloride has been similarily queried, but without supporting evidence.

METAL HYPERSENSITIVITY - DIAGNOSTIC ASPECTS

Type-I hypersensitivity can be assessed by the response to intradermal challenge with the suspected allergen. The release of histamine and other mediators rapidly produces a wheal-and-flare reaction, maximal within 30 min and then subsiding. An immediate reaction may be followed by a late-phase reaction which may last for 24 h, characterized by an oedematous, dense cellular infiltrate. IgE antibodies can be demonstrated by testing the ability of the sensitized individual's serum to sensitize the skin of a normal subject or primate passively, the Prausnitz-Kustner reaction - but of course, this is not carried out in routine diagnostic practice. There is a good correlation between skin prick test response and the radioallergosorbent test for allergen-specific IgE. The skin prick test is employed routinely for screening workers exposed to soluble platinum complexes. Atopic subjects, as identified by a positive skin test prick using house dust or grass pollen, are not normally employed in the platinum industry. Screening for sensitization following employment is usually carried out at three-monthly intervals by a skin prick test with a complex platinum salt. A nasal reaction, with sneezing and nasal discharge, can also be elicited within minutes of a challenge with the platinum complex instilled into the nose. Similarily, an inhalation challenge may be performed with a platinum complex, sensitized subjects giving an immediate asthmatic reaction.

Inhalation bronchial provocation tests provide the most accurate means for identifying the responsible agent, and they enable previously unsuspected sensitizing substances to be identified. They do not, however, differentiate between asthma caused by nonspecific irritation and that due to a specific immunological reaction, which may be relevent in view of the heightened response of asthmatic subjects to nonspecific irritants.

Bronchial provocation testing is potentially hazardous and should be performed only under well-controlled conditions, preferably in hospital by experienced personnel. The initial challenge should be short and followed by regular estimation of ventilatory function for a period of 24 h, in case a late or nocturnal asthmatic reaction occurs. The concentration may be increased on subsequent days, but not beyond the level likely to be encountered in the workplace or environment. In the case of platinum, a dust can be created by tipping the complex, diluted with an inert material such as dried lactose, from one tray to another, to produce a concentration of the salt close to the occupational threshold limit value. A control exposure should be employed to ensure that the observed reaction is specific.

Type-IV cell-mediated hypersensitivity, giving rise to allergic contact dematitis, can be confirmed by patch testing. In this procedure, the agent, for example a nickel or a chromium salt, is applied to the skin surface on a carrier material with an occlusive dressing. It is usually applied to the back and the skin reaction assessed two and four days later, the covering adhesive tape having been removed some 2 h before reading. Care should be taken to avoid irritant materials, as false-positive results may arise from sensitivity to adhesive tape, to sweat gland occlusion or to increased irritability of the skin due to active eczema. False-negative reactions are not uncommon and may be due to inadequate skin penetration of the test material, to an inappropriate carrier that prevents release or to too low a concentration of the suspected allergen. A positive patch test presents with a palpable papular erythema, which may become vesicular. An internationally agreed standard battery of patch testing agents includes the metal compounds potassium dichromate, cobalt chloride and nickel sulfate.

The patch test was at one time employed for the diagnosis of chronic beryllium disease; however, it was found that the beryllium compounds used led to a flare up of chronic berylliosis in patients in a state of remission and noncaseating granuloma formation at the test site. Both false-positive and false-negative reactions were also encountered, and the test was abandoned as a diagnostic procedure. The immunological diagnosis of beryllium disease is considered in detail elsewhere in this volume (Reeves and Preuss). Suffice it to state here that, while the patch test, the macrophage migration inhibition test and the blood lymphocyte blast transformation test provide information on systemic beryllium hypersensitivity, the lymphocyte blast transformation test performed on bronchoalveolar lavage fluid is the current procedure of choice for the diagnosis of chronic beryllium disease involving the lungs.

A number of in-vitro tests have been devised for the detection and recognition of antigen. Tests may be based on cellular response, as for example on histamine release from mast cells, on inhibition of macrophage migration and on lymphocyte blast tranformation, but such tests are of limited value in the clinical situation. Antibody forming cells can be identified by the plaque-forming cell assay, which can be modified to identify cells that produce specific IgG or IgM antibodies. The direct antiglobulin or Coombs' test provides evidence of IgM or IgG antibody on the surface of red blood cells and is of value in assessing cases of drug-induced haemolytic anaemia.

The enzyme-linked immunosorbent assay and radioimmunoassay are sensitive laboratory techniques for the detection of antigens and antibodies. The radioimmunosorbent test and the radioallergosorbent test are modifications of the radioimmunoassay. The radioallergosorbent test is a useful and sensitive method for the quantification of IgE reaginic antibodies in serum in the diagnosis of type-I immediate hypersensitivity.

REFERENCES

Alekseeva, O.G., Vasil'eva, E.V. & Orlova, A.A. (1974) Abolition of natural tolerance and the influence of the chemical allergen beryllium on autoimmune processes. *Bull. World Health Organ.*, **51**: 51-58

Benson, M.K.D., Goodwin, P.G. & Brostoff, J. (1975) Metal sensitivity in patients with joint replacement anthroplastics. *Br. med. J.*, **iv**: 374-375

Cleare, M.J., Hughs, E.G., Jacoby, B. & Pepys, J. (1976) Immediate (Type I) allergic responses to platinum compounds. *Clin. Allergy*, **6**: 183-195

Coombs, R.R.A. & Gell, P.G.H. (1975) Classification of allergic reactions responsible for clinical hypersensitivity and disease. In: Gell, P.G.H., Coombs, R.R.A. & Lachmann, P.J., eds, *Clinical Aspects of Immunology*, 3rd ed., Oxford, Blackwell, pp. 761-781

Davis, P. & Hughes, G.R.V. (1975) A serial study of eosinophilia and raised IgE antibodies during gold therapy. *Ann. rheum. Dis.*, **34**: 203-204

Denman, J.E. & Denman, A.M. (1968) The lymphocyte transformation test and gold hypersensitivity. *Ann. rheum. Dis.*, **27**: 582-589

Eedy, D.J., Burrows, D., Clifford, T. & Fay, A. (1988) *Alterations in the Immunological Status of Dental Students*, Belfast, Society of Dental Research

Fillastre, J.P., Druet, P. & Mery, J.-P. (1988) Proteinuric nephropathies associated with drugs and substances of abuse. In: Cameron, J.S. & Glassock, R.J., eds, *The Nephrotic Syndrome*, New York, Marcel Dekker, pp. 697-744

Finne, K., Göransson, K. & Winckler, L. (1982) Oral lichen planus and contact allergy to mercury. *Int. J. oral Surg.*, **11**: 236-239

Forman, L. & Alexander, S. (1972) Nickel antibodies. *Br. J. Dermatol.*, **87**: 320-326

Kazantzis, G. (1978) The role of hypersensitivity and the immune response in influencing susceptibility to metal toxicity. *Environ. Health Perspect.*, **25**: 111-118

Kazantzis, G., Schiller, F.R., Asscher, A.W. & Drew, R.G. (1962) Albuminuria and the nephrotic syndrome following exposure to mercury and its compounds. *Q. J. Med.*, **31**: 403-407

Keskinen, H., Kalliomaki, P.L. & Alanko, K. (1980) Occupational asthma due to stainless steel welding fumes. *Clin. Allergy*, **10**: 151-159

Krivanek, N. & Reeves, A.L. (1972) The effect of chemical forms of beryllium on the production of the immunologic response. *Am. ind. Hyg. Assoc. J.*, **33**: 45-52

Levene, G.M. (1971) Platinum sensitivity. *Br. J. Dermatol.*, **85**: 590-593

Lindqvist, K.J., Makene, W.J., Shaba, J.K. & Nantulya, V. (1974) Immunofluorescence and electron microscopic studies of kidney biopsies from patients with nephrotic syndrome, possibly induced by skin lightening creams containing mercury. *East Afr. med. J.*, **51**: 168-169

North American Contact Dermatitis Group (1973) Epidemiology of contact dermatitis in North America, 1972. *Arch. Dermatol.*, **108**: 537-540

Novey, H.S., Habib, M. & Wells, L.D. (1983) Asthma and IgE antibodies induced by chromium and nickel salts. *J. Allergy clin. Immunol.*, **72**: 407-412

Palosuo, T., Provost, T.T. & Milgrom, F. (1976) Gold nephropathy. Serological data suggesting an immune complex disease. *Clin. exp. Immunol.*, **25**: 311-318

Pepys, J. (1973) Immunopathology of allergic lung disease. *Clin. Allergy*, **3**: 1-22

Polak, L., Barnes, J.M. & Turk, J.L. (1968) The genetic control of contact sensitization to inorganic metal compounds in guinea-pigs. *Immunology*, **14**: 707-711

Reeves, A.L. & Preuss, O.P. (1985) Immunotoxicity of beryllium. In: Dean, J.H., Luster, M.I., Munson, A.E. & Amos, H., eds, *Immunotoxicology and Immunopharmacology*, New York, Raven Press, pp. 441-455

White, R.R. & Brandt, R.L. (1976) Development of mercury hypersensitivity among dental students. *J. Am. dental Assoc.*, **92**: 1204-1207

ANIMAL MODELS FOR PREDICTING
HYPERSENSITIVITY REACTIONS
TO SMALL MOLECULES

P.A. Botham

ICI Central Toxicology Laboratory
Alderley Park, Macclesfield, SK10 4TJ UK

ABSTRACT

Hypersensitivity reactions to low-molecular-weight chemicals represent a significant health problem among both manufacturing and user populations. The most common clinical manifestations are rhinitis and asthma or dermatitis, but there have also been reports of anaphylaxis and autoimmunity. Animal models for predicting these effects are, with the notable exception of allergic contact dermatitis, poorly developed. Recent studies have shown, however, that it is possible to reproduce type-I (immediate-type) hypersensitivity reactions to chemicals in the guinea-pig, and work is now in progress to determine the utility of this type of model for assessing the potential of a material to cause respiratory allergy. Little progress has been made in the development of predictive tests for chemicals that may cause autoimmunity, although the mouse popliteal lymph node assay may provide some indication of the autoimmunogenic potential of certain types of drugs. Allergic contact dermatitis (a type-IV, delayed-type hypersensitivity reaction) can be predicted by means of many well-validated guinea-pig tests, several of which are accepted worldwide by regulatory authorities. Although these tests have proved to be very successful over the last 20-30 years, new tests are emerging, based on the mouse as an experimental model, which offer the possibility of more objective, immunologically based endpoints (thus reducing, for example, interpretive difficulties with coloured or irritant chemicals) and which are quicker and cheaper to perform.

INTRODUCTION

Clinical manifestations of hypersensitivity reactions to low-molecular-weight drugs and industrial chemicals, including rhinitis and asthma, urticaria, contact dermatitis and autoimmunity, are seen in both manufacturing and user populations. The overall frequency of these reactions is not known, although in the UK, the Health and Safety Executive has indicated that cases of occupational asthma and contact dermatitis (due to hypersensitivity reactions to chemicals) are associated with significant costs for employers in terms of sickness absence and compensation payments. For some individuals, a hypersensitivity response can mean a transient skin rash or a brief episode of sneezing, but for others it can mean a disabling autoimmune condition, asthma or dermatitis and, in a few cases, life-threatening conditions such as anaphylaxis.

Animal models for predicting the potential of a chemical to cause hypersensitivity in man are, with one exception (the prediction of allergic contact dermatitis), poorly developed. Consequently, the first indication that a material is capable of causing allergy or auto-immunity is often the reporting of symptoms by exposed individuals. This paper summarizes some recent work on the development of novel predictive animal tests for chemicals that could cause respiratory allergy or autoimmunity. In addition, the current status of animal

Immunotoxicity of Metals and Immunotoxicology, Edited by
A. D. Dayan *et al.,* Plenum Press, New York, 1990

testing for the potential of a chemical to cause allergic contact dermatitis is discussed, including several newly-developed mouse models which appear to offer the possibility of improved predictive capacity.

RESPIRATORY ALLERGY

Within the context of this review, the term 'respiratory allergy' is used synonymously with the conditions of chemically-induced rhinitis and asthma. In many (but by no means all) cases of respiratory allergy, it is possible to detect allergen (chemical)-specific IgE antibodies in the circulation by means of radioimmunoassay, or in the skin by means of a prick test (Chan-Yeung & Lam, 1986). The clinical history of such individuals often confirms that, after a period of exposure ranging from weeks to years, symptoms develop which usually occur either minutes or a few hours following re-exposure to the allergen. This pattern of symptoms, together with the finding of specific IgE antibodies, is highly suggestive of an immediate-type (or type-I) hypersensitivity mechanism; however, in some individuals, symptoms may have a delayed onset (up to 24 h after re-exposure), and the circulating antibodies are of the IgG class. It is possible that in these cases the disease is mediated through a type-III (immune-complex) hypersensitivity mechanism.

A wide variety of animal models for allergic asthma has been developed, primarily to aid in the development of therapeutic agents. The toxicological and preclinical aspects of model development have been the subject of considerable debate (e.g., Doe, 1983), but until recently there have been few practical advances.

Over the last ten years, Karol *et al.* have published a number of papers (reviewed by Karol *et al.*, 1985) describing guinea-pig models of respiratory allergy to low-molecular-weight materials. Their strategy has been to simulate the conditions present in an industrial environment. Thus:

1. animals are exposed *via* the inhalation route;
2. animals are unrestrained and unanaesthetized during sensitization and elicitation;
3. free (unconjugated) chemicals are used to sensitize the animals; and
4. the use of adjuvants is avoided.

The Karol protocol involves sensitization by inhalation of a chemical for 3 h/day for five consecutive days, followed two weeks later by a challenge with a chemical-protein conjugate, again administered by inhalation. Karol *et al.* were thus able to demonstrate that inhalation of toluene diisocyanate, a well-recognized respiratory allergen in man, induced a serological response (i.e., toluene diisocyanate-specific IgG1 and IgE antibodies; in the guinea-pig, both IgG1 and IgE can mediate type-I hypersensitivity reactions) and that, following a challenge, a proportion of the animals developed broncho-constriction, measured as an increase in respiratory rate.

We were able to confirm these observations (Botham *et al.*, 1988); however, both the antibody and pulmonary responses to toluene diisocyanate were critically dependent on the physicochemical properties of the hapten-protein conjugate used in the antibody assay or as the challenge antigen. In addition, we were unable to demonstrate pulmonary responses in animals that had been sensitized (as shown by the presence of antibodies) to two other known human respiratory sensitizers, trimellitic anhydride and a dichlorotriazine reactive dye. Our lack of understanding of the nature of the 'ideal' conjugate for the Karol procedure and the inconsistency of the pulmonary responses following challenge of sensitized guinea-pigs led us to consider an alternative protocol for inducing respiratory allergy to small molecules.

It has been assumed for many years that a chemical can cause pulmonary sensitization only when it exists as a vapour or as inhalable droplets or particles (Doe, 1983). It has been shown, however, that animals can develop homocytotropic antibodies (i.e., IgG1 and/or IgE) when chemicals are painted on their skin or injected intradermally (e.g., Thomas *et al.*, 1976; Karol *et al.*, 1981; Karol & Magreni, 1982). We have investigated whether respiratory allergy can be induced in the guinea-pig following intradermal injection of a chemical (Botham *et al.*, 1989). We have also studied whether intradermally sensitized animals can respond to a challenge of inhaled free chemical (rather than hapten-protein conjugate), in an attempt to improve the consistency of the pulmonary responses. The protocol employed is shown in Table 1.

The results of a typical study are shown in Table 2. Between 0.3 and 30 mg of trimellitic anhydride, injected into guinea-pigs in corn oil, resulted in the development of high-titre chemical-specific homocytotropic antibodies and, in the majority of animals, the subsequent elicitation of bronchoconstriction following inhalation challenge with free trimellitic anhydride. Similar results (not shown) were obtained using another human respiratory sensitizer, diphenylmethane diisocyanate.

Table 1. The intradermal injection protocol for the induction and elicitation of respiratory allergy to small molecules (Botham *et al.*, 1989)

Day		Treatment
1	Induction (sensitization)	Chemical injected intradermally (0.1 ml of a range of doses up to the maximum well-tolerated dose)
19		Blood sample taken for IgG1/IgE anti-hapten antibody assays
22	Elicitation (challenge)	Chemical administered by inhalation (15 min) (maximal non-irritant dose) Effect on respiratory rate determined

Table 2. Summary of serological and pulmonary responses in guinea-pigs injected intradermally with trimellitic anhydride (TMA)

Sensitizing dose of TMA (% w/v in corn oil)	Anti-TMA antibody titres (day 19) (serum dilution^{-1})[a]		Pulmonary responses[b] (day 22) to 30-60 mg^{-3} TMA		
	IgG1 (ELISA)	IgE (PCA)	O	M	S
0	0 (n = 8)	0 (n = 8)	8	0	0
0.3	51 200 (n = 1) 204 800 (n = 5)	0 (n = 1) 8 (n = 1) 32 (n = 2) 128 (n = 3)	2	0	5
1.0	51 200 (n = 1) 204 800 (n = 7)	8 (n = 5) 32 (n = 3)	3	2	3
3.0	12 800 (n = 2) 51 200 (n = 1) 204 800 (n = 4)	0 (n = 2) 2 (n = 1) 8 (n = 3) 128 (n = 1)	3	0	5
10.0	51 200 (n = 2) 204 800 (n = 6)	0 (n = 4) 8 (n = 2) 32 (n = 2)	4	1	2
30.0	12 800 (n = 3) 204 800 (n = 5)	0 (n = 4) 8 (n = 2) 32 (n = 1) 128 (n = 1)	3	2	3

[a]ELISA, enzyme-linked immunosorbent assay; PCA, plaque-forming cell assay.
[b]0, no response (changes in respiratory rate within 71-129% of the mean pre-challenge rate); M, moderate response (increase in respiratory rate to 130% or more of the mean pre-challenge rate); S, severe response (decrease in respiratory rate to 70% or less of the mean pre-challenge rate).

In marked contrast, 1-5 mg dinitrochlorobenzene, also injected intra-dermally in corn oil, resulted in only low-titre antibodies (maximal titre, 3200 compared with 204 800 with trimellitic anhydride) and a failure to elicit pulmonary responses following inhalation challenge with free dinitrochlorobenzene (see Table 3). The animals were, however, contact-sensitized by the single intradermal dose, as shown by the development of dermal responses to a topical challenge with dinitrochlorobenzene. This compound is a potent inducer of allergic contact dermatitis in man (Cronin, 1980), but respiratory symptoms have not been reported in exposed individuals.

These results suggest that our protocol can discriminate between low-molecular-weight respiratory sensitizers and non-sensitizers. Work is in progress to validate the method further, using a more extensive range of chemicals.

AUTOIMMUNITY

Autoimmunity is a possible side-effect associated with the administration of drugs such as procainamide, isoniazide, hydralazine, D-penicillamine and thiouracils. Clinically, the most common presentation is a systemic lupus erythematosus-like condition, which usually disappears after cessation of drug treatment. A strong genetic association is present; individuals who are 'slow acetylators' (i.e., less able to metabolize the drugs) are significantly more at risk of developing the condition. Autoimmune symptoms have also been associated with exposure to industrial chemicals, such as solvents, heavy metals (glomerulonephritis, for example) and asbestos; however, the causality of the relationship is, in these cases, much less clear than for drug-induced autoimmunity (reviewed by Trizio et al., 1988).

The relative infrequency of chemically induced autoimmunity, together with its complexity, including the genetic influences mentioned above, have contributed to making the development of predictive animal models unattractive. The only notable contribution has come from the group of Gleichmann et al, who have proposed that the potential of a chemical to induce autoimmunity can be detected by injecting the material subcutaneously into the hind footpad of a mouse. This results in increased cellular proliferation in the draining popliteal lymph node, as shown by weight increase or by uptake of tritiated thymidine. Using this protocol, positive responses have been seen with, for example, diphenylhydantoin and D-penicillamine and also with mercuric chloride (Gleichmann, 1981;

Table 3. Summary of serological, pulmonary and dermal responses in guinea-pigs injected intradermally with dinitrochlorobenzene (DNCB)

Sensitizing dose of DNCB (% w/v in corn oil)	Anti-DNCB antibody titres (day 19) (serum dilution[-1])[a]		Pulmonary responses[b] (day 22) to 10 mg[-3] DNCB			Dermal responses[c] (day 15) to 1% DNCB			
	IgG1 (ELISA)	IgE (PCA)	O	M	S	O	1	2	3
0	0 (n = 8)	0 (n = 8)	8	0	0	8	0	0	0
1.0	0 (n = 1) 50 (n = 2) 200 (n = 3) 400 (n = 1) 800 (n = 1)	0 (n = 8)	8	0	0	0	2	1	5
5.0	50 (n = 1) 200 (n = 2) 400 (n = 1) 800 (n = 2) 1600 (n = 1) 3200 (n = 1)	0 (n = 8)	8	0	0	0	1	1	6

[a]ELISA, enzyme-linked immonosorbent assay; PCA, plaque-cell forming assay.
[b]O, no response (changes in respiratory rate within 71-129% of the mean pre-challenge rate); M, moderate response (an increase in respiratory rate to 130% or more of the mean pre-challenge rate); S, severe response (decrease in respiratory rate to 70% or less of the mean pre-challenge rate).
[c]0, no erythema; 1, scattered mild erythema; 2, moderate diffuse erythema; 3, intense erythema.

Hurtenbach *et al.*, 1987; Stiller-Winkler *et al.*, 1988). Joseph *et al.* (1988), however, have questioned the reliability of this assay. They have shown that popliteal lymph node activity is associated not only with autoimmunogenic drugs such as procainamide and phenytoin, but also with irritants such as 1% acetic acid and 50% ethanol.

The development of reliable, well-validated animal models for predicting the potential of a drug or industrial chemical to cause autoimmunity is an important area for further work; however, it should be remembered that 'chemically induced autoimmunity' is a generic term for a wide range of diseases, the mechanisms of which are, in many cases, poorly understood. It is highly unlikely that a single protocol will be capable of predicting all types of autoimmunogens.

ALLERGIC CONTACT DERMATITIS

In contrast to the situation with respiratory allergy and autoimmunity, there are many predictive animal models for allergic contact dermatitis, the majority involving the guinea-pig. Eight guinea-pig tests are included in current regulatory guidelines (e.g., those of the Organisation for Economic Co-operation and Development, the European Economic Community, the US Environmental Protection Agency and the Japanese Ministry of Agriculture, Fisheries and Food); they are shown in Table 4, together with their important distinguishing features. The common basis for all the tests is an initial exposure (induction phase), in which the guinea-pigs are treated with intradermal and/or topical application of the test compound, followed by a single re-exposure (challenge phase) to the same test compound, normally after a rest period of 10-14 days. Sensitization is determined by assessing skin reactions (e.g., erythema and oedema) to the challenge exposure with a non-irritant concentration of test compound, or by comparing skin reactions following induction and challenge in individual animals.

These methods have, in general, proved to be of great value for predicting hazard of sensitization for man; however, it should be recognized that a number of significant problems are associated with the tests. For example, there is no international agreement on the conduct of the test protocols, or on the interpretation of the test results in terms of human hazard. Neither is there an agreed view, based on data from a range of chemicals, on the relative sensitivities of the tests, except that 'adjuvant tests' (see Table 4) are probably

Table 4. Predictive tests in guinea-pigs for allergic contact dermatitis in current regulatory guidelines

Test	Induction application	Challenge application
Draize test[a]	Intradermal (x10)	Intradermal
Freund's complete adjuvant test[b]	Intradermal in adjuvant (x5)	Epidermal (open)
Optimization test[b]	Intradermal (x3) Intradermal in adjuvant (x6)	Intradermal Epidermal (occluded)
Maximization test[b] (M & K)	Intradermal (x1) Intradermal in adjuvant (x1) Adjuvant (x1) Epidermal (occluded) (x1)	Epidermal (occluded)
Split adjuvant test[b]	Epidermal (occluded) (x2) Adjuvant (x1) Epidermal (occluded) (x2)	Epidermal (occluded)
Buehler test	Epidermal (occluded) (x3)	Epidermal (occluded)
Open epidermal test	Epidermal (open) (x21)	Epidermal (open)

[a]The US Environmental Protection Agency pesticide assessment guidelines include the footpad test in place of the Draize test.
[b]Adjuvant test.

more sensitive than non-adjuvant procedures. Finally, all of the tests are dependent on a subjective means of assessment (usually erythema), which can lead to problems when coloured or irritant materials are tested.

With the increasing understanding of cellular immunology in general, and of immune responses in allergic contact dermatitis in particular, more rational, objective, immunologically based predictive test methods are now beginning to emerge. Many of these new methods utilize the mouse as the experimental model, mainly because the immune system in this species is better understood than that of the guinea-pig. Application of a sensitizing chemical to mouse skin results in interaction of the chemical with epidermal Langerhans cells. These cells then actively transport the chemical, *via* the lymphatic drainage, to the lymph node that drains the site of application. Here, T lymphocytes carrying cell surface receptors which can recognize the chemical in association with the Langerhans cell undergo activation and rapid proliferation. The result is a selective expansion of chemical-specific clones of T cells which retain the memory of the encounter with the chemical. It is at this point that the mouse is sensitized. The same mechanism probably operates in the guinea-pig and in man.

If the mouse is subsequently re-exposed to the same substance, the specific memory T cells recognize the chemical at the site of application, become activated and secrete hormone-like materials called lymphokines. The lymphokines recruit to the site of exposure other lymphocytes and macrophages, and the latter become non-selectively aggressive. Local tissue destruction ensues, resulting in an inflammatory reaction, which is recognized clinically as contact dermatitis. In the guinea-pig and in man, the most common clinical sign is erythema; in the mouse it is oedema (swelling). Consequently, in the mouse, challenge is most conveniently performed on the ears, where it is possible to compare ear thickness pre- and post-challenge as a more objective assessment of the challenge reaction. Clinical signs of contact dermatitis are normally most severe 24-72 h after challenge - hence, the classification of the condition as a delayed-type (or type-IV) hypersensitivity. Details of the mechanism of allergic contact dermatitis can be found in the review of Breathnach (1986).

Three recent approaches to the prediction of contact dermatitis using the mouse are summarized in Table 5. The vitamin A acetate and the mouse ear swelling test (MEST)

Table 5. New predictive tests in the mouse for allergic contact dermatitis

Test	Pretreatment	Induction application[a]	Challenge application[a]	Assessment of reaction
Vitamin A acetate (VAA) test (Maisey & Miller, 1986)	VAA in diet	Epidermal (flank) (x6)	Epidermal (both ears)	Statistical comparison of ear thickness pre- and post-challenge
Mouse ear swelling test (Gad *et al.*, 1986)	-	Adjuvant injection Tape stripping of application site Epidermal (flank) (x1) Tape stripping of application site Epidermal (flank) (x3)	Epidermal (one ear)	≥20% increase in ear thickness above that of vehicle-treated control ear
Local lymph node assay (Kimber *et al.*, 1989)	-	Epidermal (both ears) (x3)	-	Three-fold increase in lymphocyte proliferation in draining lymph node of test animals compared with vehicle-treated control mice

[a]Applications are unoccluded in all three tests.

involve sensitization on the flank of the mouse, followed by challenge to one or both ears, and measurement of the resulting increase in ear thickness with an engineer's micrometer. In the vitamin A acetate test, sensitivity is enhanced by maintaining the mice on a diet supplemented with vitamin A acetate. In the MEST, the technique is enhanced by means of a single injection of adjuvant and by tape-stripping the site of the induction applications. On the basis of an initial validation with 72 materials, Gad et al. (1986) claimed that the MEST was at least as good a predictor of human sensitization as the guinea-pig maximization test. Cornacoff et al. (1988), however, have questioned the capacity of the MEST method for detecting weak sensitizers.

The local lymph node assay of Kimber et al. (1989) is based on a different strategy, in which, following topical exposure to the test material, the sensitizing potential of a chemical is measured as a function of the initial T-cell activation and proliferation in the draining lymph nodes. Lymphocyte proliferation is measured in situ by injection of tritiated thymidine. In common with the vitamin A acetate test and the MEST, the local lymph node assay is not subject to problems of interpretation when coloured chemicals are used. In addition, as lymphocyte proliferation does not appear to be induced by non-sensitizing irritant chemicals, this assay has added utility for testing irritant materials.

The major advantages of the new mouse tests are the following:

(1) They are based on objective endpoints.
(2) They are not influenced by the colour of the test substance.
(3) The local lymph node assay is not influenced by the irritancy of the test substance.
(4) They are of shorter duration.
(5) They require less test substance.
(6) With the exception of the MEST, they avoid the use of adjuvant.

To date, the major disadvantages are the lack of comparison with the regulatory guinea-pig tests and between laboratories. Several initiatives are under way to address these problems, but it is likely to be several years before mouse tests will replace guinea-pig procedures in regulatory guide-lines.

For the future, one of the most stimulating challenges is to define the way in which the immune response to contact sensitizers determines the potency of the allergic reaction. Guidelines for the conduct of the currently accepted guinea-pig tests do not require an assessment of the doses of a material below which it is impossible either to induce contact sensitization or to elicit a dermatitic reaction in a previously induced animal. These assessments are in any case difficult to perform, often requiring large numbers of animals and an extended testing period. Assessment of risk for allergic contact dermatitis would be improved considerably by the introduction of practical, reliable methods which were capable of determining the potency of a sensitizer on the basis of dose-response.

REFERENCES

Botham, P.A., Hext, P.M., Rattray, N.J., Walsh, S.T. & Woodcock, D.R. (1988) Sensitisation of guinea-pigs by inhalation exposure to low molecular weight chemicals. Toxicol. Lett., 41: 159-173

Botham, P.A., Rattray, N.J., Woodcock, D.R., Walsh, S.T. & Hext, P.M. (1989) The induction of respiratory allergy in guinea-pigs following intradermal injection of trimellitic anhydride: a comparison with the response to 2,4-dinitrochlorobenzene. Toxicol. Lett., 47: 25-39

Breathnach, J.M. (1986) Immunological aspects of contact dermatitis. Clin. Dermatol., 4: 5-17

Chan-Yeung, M. & Lam, S. (1986) Occupational asthma. Am. Rev. respir. Dis., 133: 686-703

Cornacoff, T.B., House, R.V. & Dean, J.H. (1988) Comparison of a radioisotopic incorporation method and the mouse ear swelling test (MEST) for contact sensitivity to weak sensitizers. Fundam. appl. Toxicol., 10: 40-44

Cronin, E. (1980) Contact Dermatitis, London, Churchill Livingstone

Doe, J.E. (1983) Animal models of sensitisation via the respiratory tract. In: Gibson, C.G., Hubbard, R. & Parke, D.V., eds, Immunotoxicology, London, Academic Press, pp. 149-160

Gad, S.C., Dunn, B.J., Dobbs, D.W., Reilly, C. & Walsh, R.D. (1986) Development and validation of an alternative dermal sensitisation test: the mouse ear swelling test (MEST). Toxicol. appl. Pharmacol., 84: 93-114

Gleichmann, H. (1981) Studies on the mechanism of drug sensitisation: T-cell-dependent popliteal lymph node reaction to diphenylhydantoin. *Clin. Immunol. Immunopathol.*, **18**: 203-211

Hurtenbach, U., Gleichmann, H., Nagata, N. & Gleichmann, E. (1987) Immunity to D-penicillamine: genetic, cellular and chemical requirements for induction of popliteal lymph node enlargement in the mouse. *J. Immunol.*, **139**: 411-416

Joseph, X., Utrecht, J.P. & Balazs, T. (1988) On the popliteal lymph node (PLN) assay for the detection of autoimmunogens in mice. *Toxicologist*, **8**, 11

Karol, M.H. & Magreni, C. (1982) Extensive skin sensitisation with mininal antibody production in guinea-pigs as a result of exposure to dicyclohexylmethane-4,4'-diisocyanate. *Toxicol. appl. Pharmacol.*, **65**: 291-301

Karol, M.H., Hauth, B.A., Riley, E.J. & Magreni, C.M. (1981) Dermal contact with toluene diisocyanate (TDI) produces respiratory tract hypersensitivity in guinea-pigs. *Toxicol. appl. Pharmacol.*, **58**: 221-230

Karol, M.H., Stadler, J. & Magreni, C. (1985) Immunotoxicological evaluation of the respiratory system: animal models for immediate- and delayed-onset pulmonary hypersensitivity. *Fundam. appl. Toxicol.*, **5**: 459-472

Kimber, I., Hilton, J. & Weisenberger, C. (1989). The murine local lymph node assay for identification of contact allergens: a preliminary evaluation of *in situ* measurement of lymphocyte proliferation. *Contact Dermatitis*, **21**: 215 -220

Maisey, J. & Miller, K. (1986) Assessment of the ability of mice fed on vitamin A supplemented diet to respond to a variety of potential contact sensitisers. *Contact Dermatitis*, **15**: 17-23

Stiller-Winkler, R., Radaszkiewicz, T. & Gleichman, E. (1988) Immunopathological signs in mice tested with mercury compounds - I. Identification by the popliteal lymph node assay of responder and non-responder strains. *Int. J. Immunopharmacol.*, **10**: 475-484

Thomas, W.R., Asherson, G.L. & Watkins, M.C. (1976) Reaginic antibody produced in mice with contact sensitivity. *J. exp. Med.*, **144**: 1386-1390

Trizio, D., Basketter, D.A., Botham, P.A., Graepel, P.H., Lambre, C., Magda, S.J., Pal, T.M., Riley, A.J., Ronneberger, H., Van Sittert, N.J. & Bontinck, W.J. (1988) Identification of immunotoxic effects of chemicals and assessment of their relevance to man. *Food. chem. Toxicol.*, **26**: 527-539

CONTACT ALLERGY TO CHROMIUM AND NICKEL

C. Avnstorp[1], T. Menné[1] & H. Maibach[2]

[1]Department of Dermatology, Gentofte Hospital, 2900 Hellerup, Denmark; and
[2]Department of Dermatology, University of California, School of Medicine,
Moffitt Hospital, San Francisco, California 94143, USA

ABSTRACT

Metal contact dermatitis is encountered daily in dermatology clinics around the world. The condition is often potentially debilitating, with a relatively pure prognosis. Chromium and nickel contact dermatides are susceptible to preventive measures. Metal contact dermatitis occurs not only in individuals who come into contact with metal products occupationally but is also prevalent in the general population. Contact allergy is never hereditary, but genetic factors may influence the tendency to develop it. Cement dermatitis can be prevented by adding ferrous sulfate to cement, thereby reducing the content of water-soluble chromate to not more than 2 ppm. Nickel dermatitis caused by exposure to nickel-plated articles, such as earrings and buttons, can be prevented by using nickel alloys that release less than 0.5 µg/cm2 per week nickel in synthetic sweat. In Denmark, recommendations are given for both the chromate content of cement and for the nickel that can be released from metals for use in direct contact with the skin.

INTRODUCTION

Chronic exposure to metals and their compounds is associated with several toxic effects, including respiratory cancer due to chromium and nickel (Nieboer & Sanford, 1985; Friberg et al., 1986). Although often overlooked by toxicologists, the skin is also a target organ for metals, resulting in irritant and allergic contact dermatitis. This disease differs from cancer in that exposure occurs mainly via external, dermal contact. Metal contact dermatitis is not limited to individuals who come into contact with metal products occupationally (especially with nickel and to a lesser extent with chromium), it is also prevalent in the general population.

Examples of situations in which exposure to chromium and nickel can cause eczematous reactions are given in Tables 1 and 2.

We illustrate that metal contact dermatitis (i) is a disease encountered daily in dermatology clinics around the world; (ii) is a potentially debilitating condition, often with a poor prognosis; and (iii), most importantly, is preventable.

CLINICAL PATTERNS

Chromium dermatitis

Most cases of chromate dermatitis start as a primary sensitization of the hands. Patients with primary hand eczema may develop shoe dermatitis from the trivalent chromium present in leather as a subsequent event, although Cr[III] is a rare cause of primary chromium sensitization, presumably due to its low water solubility and low dermal diffusibility (Haines & Nieboer, 1988). Allergic cement eczema is located primarily on the hands and fingers (Burrows & Calnan, 1965; Høvding, 1970; Avnstorp, 1983). Eczema on

Table 1. Examples of eczematogenic exposures to chromium compounds[a]

Chromium-containing material or object	Profession or place of contact	Chromium compounds responsible
Chromium ore	Industrial chromium production	Chromate
Chrome baths	Electroplating industry Graphics trade Metal industry	Chromic acid, sodium dichromate Chromates Chromates, zinc chromate
Chrome colours and dyes	Painters and decorators, graphics trades, textile rubber, glass and china industries	Chromic oxide green, chromic hydroxide green, chrome yellow (lead chromate)
Lubricating oils and greases	Metal industry	Chromic oxide, chromate
Anticorrosive agents in water systems	Diesel locomotive workshops and sheds, central heating and air-conditioning systems	Alkali dichromates
Wood preservation (Wolman salts)	Wood impregnation furniture industry, carpenters, miners	Alkali dichromates
Cement, cement products, quick-hardening agents for cement (e.g., Sika 1)	Cement production, manufacture of cement products, building trades	Chromates
Cleaning materials (eau de Javel), washing and bleaching materials	Housewives, cleaners, laundry workers	Chromates
Textiles, furs	Textile and fur industries, everyday life	Chromates
Leather and artificial leather tanned with chromium	Leather and footwear industries, everyday life	Chromium sulfate, chromium alum

[a]Derived from Haines & Nieboer (1988).

Table 2. Examples of eczematogenic exposures to nickel compounds[a]

Nickel-containing material, object or process	Profession or place of contact	Nickel compounds responsible
Nickel refineries	Labourers	Nickel-containing dust, dissolved nickel salts
Plating baths	Labourers	Dissolved nickel salts
Clips, tools, medical equipment	Hairdressers, electricians, nurses, doctors	Electroplated nickel, stainless-steel
Clothing fasteners, jewellery, watch straps, needles, pins	Public	Electroplated nickel
Coins, cooking utensils, cutlery	Public	Nickel alloys, stainless-steel
Cosmetics, detergents, tap-water	Public	Unspecified nickel contaminants
Surgical implants, prosthodontic items	Patients	Nickel alloys, stainless-steel

[a]See the following books for additional information: Cronin (1980), Fisher (1986) and Maibach and Menné (1989).

the dorsal aspects of the right hand, in particular, has been shown to be associated with sensitivity to chromium (Avnstorp, 1983). Allergic cement eczema may spread to the forearms, the feet and sometimes the face and parts of the trunk. In cases where nummular eczema is also present, systemic contact dermatitis may be suspected (Menné & Maibach, 1987).

Heat and high humidity were seen to exacerbate allergic cement eczema among workers in Kuwait, perhaps because excessive perspiration could lead to increased leaching of chromium through the skin (Kanan, 1972). In Singapore, where the climate is hot and humid all year round, the number of heat-related dermatoses was, nevertheless, lower than expected, possibly due to the use of air conditioning and good factory ventilation (Goh & Soh, 1984).

Nickel dermatitis

Primary nickel dermatitis occurs at skin sites in close contact with costume jewellery and clasps in clothing, resulting in a patchy, eventually symmetrical, pattern. The relation to metal contact sites is often so obvious that patients establish a diagnosis of nickel allergy themselves. Primary nickel dermatitis has a good medical prognosis, and individuals experience only minor discomfort; however, if the condition is neglected, and the patient continues to have intensive contact with nickel, the dermatitis may become chronic and spread to skin sites distant from the primary sensitization.

Nickel dermatitis has a tendency to spread to the hands, elbow flexures, eyelids and genital area. A population-based study established that nickel-sensitized individuals have a statistically significant risk for developing hand eczema (Menné et al., 1987b). The dissemination of nickel dermatitis may be caused by percutaneous or systemic (inhalation or oral) exposure to nickel (Menné & Maibach, 1987).

Systemic exposure to chromium and nickel

A transient state of hardening or immunological tolerance can be induced by repeated oral or parenteral exposure of contact-sensitized individuals to a hapten. This approach is, however, experimental and does not yet represent a practical therapeutic modality. Oral exposure of contact-allergic persons to haptens can induce a flare of the original dermatitis. How frequently this mechanism operates in the case of nickel and chromate dermatides is controversial. Most authors consider that the normal daily intake of nickel and chromium intake in food is an insignificant source of allergic contact dermatitis caused by these metals; however, it is scientifically difficult to establish the clinical effects of diets with low nickel and chromium contents, as double-blind studies have not been performed (Menné & Maibach, 1987).

Metal devices used in dentistry and orthopaedic surgery are usually made of stainless-steel, containing both chromium and nickel. Adverse reactions from such implants in sensitized individuals are exceptional, probably because of the low exposure concentration (Menné & Maibach, 1987).

HYPERSENSITIVITY

Immunological mechanisms

The immunological response in contact dermatitis involves specific events activated by haptens and nonspecific events triggered by irritants (Scheper et al., 1989). Allergic contact dermatitis develops in four phases: refractory, induction, elicitation and persistence (Haines & Nieboer, 1988). In the refractory period, an individual is exposed to the allergen but remains unaffected. During the induction period, the individual develops sensitized populations of lymphocytes. Elicitation, which involves secondary challenge of the antigen, results in the inflammatory skin reaction. Persistence involves continued presence of specific effector cells that can produce inflammation.

Contact allergy is never inborn, but genetic factors influence the tendency to develop this condition (Menné & Holm, 1986). Most decisive for susceptibility is the degree of cutaneous exposure. Although nickel, cobalt and chromium are ubiquitous metals, and all human beings are exposed to them in trace amounts, this in itself does not suffice to induce contact sensitization in the general population. A certain concentration threshold limit must be exceeded in order to initiate induction of sensitization. Recognition of the existence of a concentration-dependent risk for sensitization provides the basis for preventive strategies. It should be emphasized that such thresholds vary considerable from one person to another.

Chromium sensitization

Hexavalent chromium compounds are strong sensitizers (Magnusson & Kligman, 1969), whereas chromium metal itself is considered to be nonsensitizing (Cronin, 1980).

Concentration. If the content of water-soluble chromate in dry cement does not exceed 2 ppm, the risk for chromium hypersensitivity following skin contact with the cement in wet form is comparable to that seen among workers who have had no contact with wet cement (Avnstorp, 1989b). In a study in San Francisco, USA, among workers exposed to cement containing no more than 0.1 ppm water-soluble chromate, few workers became hypersensitive to chromium although more than one-third had evidence of mild to moderate cement eczema (Perone *et al.*, 1974). In the German Democratic Republic, the concentration of water-soluble chromate in cement required to induce chromium hypersensitivity was found to be between 0.4 and 24 ppm (Reifenstein *et al.*, 1986).

The risk for developing chromium hypersensitivity increases with the intensity and duration of exposure. Workers in building component factories have the most intensive exposure to wet cement; retired bricklayers have had long exposure time. Both groups had higher prevalences of chromium allergy than other groups of workers examined (Avnstorp, 1983). Høvding (1970) also found an association between duration of exposure and the development of chromium allergy.

Penetration of the hapten and antigen formation. Hexavalent chromium compounds can penetrate the skin (Mali *et al.*, 1963), so that even low concentrations of chromate in cement may induce contact sensitivity. Since trivalent chromium compounds are not soluble in a mixture of alkaline cement and water (Fregert & Gruvberger, 1972), their ability to induce hypersensitivity is limited. In addition, the high affinity of trivalent chromium salts and their tendency to form large salt complexes reduces their diffusibility through tissues (Mali *et al.*, 1963). These compounds are more likely to penetrate damaged skin (Flesh, 1965).

The reduction of Cr[VI] to Cr[III] in the epidermis and the formation of protein-Cr[III] complexes is the first possible step in sensitization (Mali *et al.*, 1963). A common antigenic determinant is probably involved in chromium contact sensitivity, rather than independent entities corresponding to each valency state. This determinant has been suggested to be formed by chromium in the trivalent form (Siegenthaler *et al.*, 1983).

The reduction of Cr[VI] to Cr[III] in the skin is brought about by sulfur-containing amino acids (Samitz & Katz, 1964). Cr[III] then binds to skin proteins (Samitz & Katz, 1969) and to components of the Langerhans cells (Shelley & Juhlin, 1976).

Nickel sensitization

Using two experimental designs, Vandenberg and Epstein (1963) and Kligman (1963) sensitized 9% and 48% of subjects, respectively, within a short period. On the basis of these limited studies, nickel was classified as a medium-to-strong contact sensitizer. Most cases of primary nickel sensitization are a consequence of prolonged (hours) nonoccupational skin contact with nickel-plated objects or nickel alloys. Short-lasting skin contact with nickel, as from coins, doorknobs and kitchen equipment, does not give rise to sensitization but might cause chronicity in individuals who are previously nickel-sensitized. At one time, suspenders and metal buttons in blue jeans caused most cases of sensitization; today, ear piercing, costume jewellery and cheap wrist watches are the main causes.

The risk for sensitization from different types of nickel coatings and alloys has been evaluated in experimental studies only recently. Menné *et al.* (1987a) examined 11 widely used nickel alloys with respect to corrosion stability and reactivity in nickel-sensitized individuals. Alloys that released more than 1 µg/cm² nickel per week in synthetic sweat induced strong patch-test reactivity in nickel-sensitive persons; alloys that released less than 0.5 µg/cm² per week, such as nickel-tin, stainless-steel and white gold, were weakly reactive. Even though the study included only patients already sensitized to nickel, it indicates the sensitizing capacity of different nickel alloys. We have observed that items that release more than 1 µg/cm² nickel per week cause the majority of cases of sensitization; nickel alloys that release less than 0.5 µg/cm² rarely produce primary nickel dermatitis.

Animal sensitization assays

As reviewed by Wahlberg (1989) over 25 methods have been used in attempts to induce contact sensitivity in experimental animals, and the sensitization rate has varied greatly. The guinea-pig maximization test (GPMT) can be regarded as the best reference method (Andersen, 1986). If this test fails, there are several alternatives; but since no comparative study has been performed it is difficult to recommend one method over another. The optimization test gives a high sensitization rate, but one drawback is that it is based on intradermal challenge. The Polak-Turk and TINA test methods give high sensitization rates but are laborious to perform; nickel toxicity has been found to be a limiting factor in the Polak-Turk method. Repeated epidermal painting gives high sensitization rates and does not seem to be toxic to animals; but this method is also laborious. Skin painting combined with injections of potassium alum gives a high sensitization rate, but this finding must be confirmed by other laboratories.

EPIDEMIOLOGY

Exposure

The epidemiology of allergic contact sensitization has been reviewed recently (Menné et al., 1987b). Since the 1930s, nickel has been the most frequent contact sensitizer in women, due to exposure to cheap nickel-plated articles such as suspenders, clasps, buttons, jewellery, earrings, zippers, glasses and wrist watches (Table 2). The putative sensitizing agent is the nickel ion, but, due to corrosion by sweat, nickel chloride is produced on the skin beneath nickel-plated articles. The risk of sensitization from a nickel-plated or nickel-containing alloy, therefore, depends upon its corrosion stability in human sweat (Menné et al., 1987b). Cobalt occurs in nature together with nickel, and in most nickel alloys there is some available cobalt; therefore, cobalt allergy is often seen in conjunction with nickel allergy. Isolated cobalt allergy is rare and occurs mainly as an occupational dermatitis in the metal and ceramic industries.

In contrast to nickel, chromate sensitivity has considerable occupational consequence (Table 1). In most countries, more than 50% of all cases of chromate dermatitis are due to contact with wet cement in the construction industry (Burrows, 1983). The first epidemics of cement eczema occurred during the construction of the Paris metro and the London underground. The existence of trace amounts of hexavalent chromium in wet cement was recognized in the 1950s as the main reason for cement dermatitis. As for nickel, cobalt and chromate, the sensitizing ability of these metals is related to their ability to generate water-soluble salts.

Prevalence and incidence

Chromium dermatitis. Chromium sensitivity affects men more often than women, reflecting the fact that sensitization occurs in jobs that are more frequently occupied by men - for example, the building industry (Burrows, 1983). In some countries, a high incidence of chromium-induced hand dermatitis has been found in women, due perhaps to the small amounts of chromate in detergents and bleaches used in houshold tasks (Feuerman, 1969; Garcia-Perez et al., 1973).

The prevalence of chromium sensitivity in men in Finland varied from 2% in the general population to 6.8% among patients in a hospital clinic to 15.5% among workers in the building industry (Peltonen & Fräki, 1983). The incidence of chromium allergy in a patch-tested population and the ratio of male to female cases remained stable in Sweden from 1969 to 1987 (Edman, 1988). In the Federal Republic of Germany (P. Frosch, personal communication) and in the German Democratic Republic (H.J. Schubert, personal communication), the incidence appeared to be stable at 2-4% during 1981-87; 20-70% of chromium-sensitive patients were thought to have allergic cement eczema, but details were not available.

Nickel dermatitis. Epidemiological studies have disclosed a prevalence of nickel allergy of 10-15% among school children, due to the piercing of ears. Some cases of dermatitis related to the wearing of metal objects next to the skin, however, might be due not to the primary irritant effects of metals but to infection. Patch testing is therefore necessary for verification of contact allergy.

Population studies in Scandinavia and the USA have established that 5-15% of the female population is nickel-sensitized (Menné *et al.*, 1989). Reports from dermatological departments and patch-test clinics in most parts of the world corroborate the general pattern that nickel and cobalt sensitivity are most prevalent in females and chromate and cobalt in males. These differences probably do not reflect differences in susceptibility to developing allergic contact dermatitis, but rather differences in hapten exposures. These studies also show that most nickel-sensitive individuals have light or intermittent contact dermatitis; only a minority develops severe dermatitis leading to sick leave and permanent impairment.

Causes of chronicity

Chromium dermatitis. In workers already hypersensitive to chromium, the concentration of water-soluble chromate in cement required to elicit allergic cement eczema is probably lower than the concentration needed to induce sensitivity (Pirilä, 1954). Elicitation of allergic cement eczema by very low concentrations may be enhanced if the skin is damaged as a result of irritation by wet cement. Concentrations of water-soluble chromate below 2 ppm may elicit a reaction, although this concentration should not induce hypersensitivity. Cement in which the chromate content has not been reduced, used as a filler in repair work, may represent a source of the hapten (Lück & Jentsch, 1988).

Chromium concentrates at the dermoepidermal junction and in the upper dermis (Lidén & Lundberg, 1979), and Cr[III] may persist in the skin for as long as four years after intracutaneous injection (Fregert,1971). Chromium compounds are ubiquitous in the human environment, and reactions may be elicited from skin contact not only with hexavalent compounds but also with trivalent ones (Zelger, 1964; Polak, 1983).

Nickel dermatitis. After primary sensitization, a person will experience a flare up of dermatitis on further exposure to the hapten, provided that the concentration threshold is surpassed (Menné *et al.*, 1987b). On repeated exposures to nickel, the severity of allergy increases and the patient runs the risk of spread of the dermatitis to secondary sites. Secondary spread of nickel and cobalt dermatitis, particularly in females, involves the hands, eyelids, elbow flexures and groin. The reason for this spread is not completely understood, but cutaneous absorption of the hapten followed by haematological dissemination is a possibility. Experimentally, secondary flares can be reproduced by giving an oral dose of nickel or cobalt salts.

Medical prognosis

The persistence of allergic contact dermatitis in cement workers is due partly to irritation of the skin by wet cement. If a worker is advised to change occupations, it is essential that the new job not involve contact with abrasive 'wet' work processes or with other irritants such as cutting oils. Whether chromium dermatitis can be avoided by changing occupation is not clearly shown in the literature. Some authors have found the medical prognosis to be poor in spite of such changes (Fregert, 1975; Dooms-Goossens *et al.*, 1980), while others have found that a job change had a favourable influence on the course of the disease (Geiser & Girard, 1965; Peter, 1968). In one study, the status of workers who had continuous contact with wet cement containing no more than 2 ppm water-soluble chromate was almost equal to that of workers who had had no contact with wet cement (Avnstorp, 1989a).

If the worker remains in the same occupation, the prognosis may also be favourable. In his cohort study of chromium-allergic bricklayers and bricklayer's assistants in Bergen, Norway, Høvding (1970) found that four of 15 cases of eczema cleared up after five years. Similarly, the cement eczema of eight of 17 bricklayers in Geneva, Switzerland, cleared up, even though the workers stayed in the same jobs (Hunziker & Musso, 1960). The chromate content of the cement used by the workers in both of these studies remained the same. No conclusive explanation has been given for this adaptive phenomenon seen in some workers; it may be that they develop immunological tolerance (Peck et al., 1945), and some may experience hyporeactivity induced by repeated irritation of the skin (Lammintausta et al., 1987). In guinea-pigs, hardened skin is characterized by a thickened stratum corneum and an epidermis which is about three times thicker than normal (McOsker & Beck, 1967).

MANAGEMENT AND PROPHYLAXIS

Diagnosis

Diagnosis of nickel and chromium allergy is established by patch testing, a technique in which patients are exposed to a small quantity of nickel or chromium under occlusion on the upper back for 48 h. A positive reaction discloses redness, oedema and, eventually, vesicles.

Chromium dermatitis

A method for reducing the amount of water-soluble chromate in cement, by adding ferrous sulfate, was suggested by Fregert et al., (1979). In 1981, Aalborg Portland A/S, the sole manufacturer of cement in Denmark, patented a method whereby the amount of chromate in the cement could be reduced using this method. As of September 1981, ferrous sulfate has been added to the cement produced by that company for use in Denmark, thus reducing the content of water-soluble chromate in cement to not more than 2 ppm at a cost of about 1% of the total value of the cement.

The addition of ferrous sulfate to the cement did not influence the medical status of workers who were already chromium-sensitive, most of whom had chronic hand eczema (Avnstorp, 1989). In contrast very few workers with irritant cement eczema developed chronic hand eczema. The prognosis of workers who develop irritant cement eczema in the future is, therefore, improved, since the risk for developing cutaneous contact sensitivity to chromium has been significantly reduced (Avnstorp, 1989b). As the risk for developing irritant cement eczema persists, these findings are important. Reduction of the chromate content of cement was also found to be significantly more effective in preventing allergic cement eczema than other methods, such as the use of gloves.

Nickel dermatitis

The primary goal in the management of nickel-sensitive patients is to instruct them how to avoid future exposure. In this respect, the dimethylglyoxime test (Fisher, 1986) has great practical impact. The spot-test kit contains 1% dimethylglyoxime in alcohol and a 10% ammonium hydroxide solution. The test is performed by adding a few drops of each solution to the object in question; the development of a cherry-red colour indicates the availability of free nickel ions. Objects that give a positive result in the dimethylglyoxime test probably produce nickel sensitization and contact dermatitis in previously sensitized individuals. Objects that give a negative result can be regarded as safe with respect to nickel allergy.

Prevention of nickel sensitization is not only rational but also realistic. Use of nickel alloys that release less than 0.5 $\mu g/cm^2$ per week in synthetic sweat will reduce the number of nickel-sensitized individuals in the population significantly.

TREATMENT

Patients with active chromium or nickel dermatitis, particularly hand eczema, are treated with topical corticoid creams for weeks or months. Short-term systemic corticoid treatment may be indicated in severe cases. Topical and systemic use of nickel chelating drugs, as well as the use of low-nickel diets, must be considered experimental approaches.

Even with effective management, however, only 20-30% of patients with hand eczema and chromium or nickel allergy are cured, according to the results of long-term follow up studies (Fregert, 1975; Christensen, 1982; Avnstorp, 1989a).

REFERENCES

Andersen, K.E. (1986) Contact allergy to chlorocresol, formaldehyde and other biocides. Guinea pig tests and clinical studies. Thesis, University of Copenhagen. *Acta dermatovenereol.*, **Suppl. 125**

Avnstorp, C. (1983) [Cement eczema among Danish workers at building sites and in industry.] (English summary), PhD Thesis, University of Copenhagen

Avnstorp, C. (1989a) Follow-up of workers from the prefabricated concrete industry after the addition of ferrous sulfate to Danish cement. *Contact Dermatitis* (in press)

Avnstorp, C. (1989b) Prevalence of cement eczema in Denmark before and since addition of ferrous sulfate to Danish cement. *Acta dermatovenereol.*, **69**: 151-155

Burrows, D. (1983) Adverse chromate reactions on the skin. In: Burrows, D., ed., *Chromium: Metabolism and Toxicity*, Boca Raton, FL, CRC Press, pp. 137-163

Burrows, D. & Calnan, C.D. (1965) Cement dermatitis. 2. Clinical aspects. *Trans. St John's Hosp. Derm. Soc.*, **51**: 27-39

Christensen, O.B. (1982) Prognosis in nickel allergy and hand eczema. *Contact Dermatitis*, **8**: 7-15

Cronin, E. (1980) *Contact Dermatitis*, Edinburgh, Churchill Livingstone, pp. 228, 338-367

Dooms-Goossens, A., Ceuterich, A., Van Maele, N. & Degreff, H. (1980) Follow-up study of patients with contact dermatitis caused by chromates, nickel and cobalt. *Dermatologica*, **160**: 249-260

Edman, B. (1988) *Computerized Patch Test Data in Contact Allergy*, Thesis, University of Lund, Sweden, pp. 28-36

Feuerman, E.J. (1969) Housewives' eczema and the role of chromates. *Acta dermatovenereol.*, **49**: 288-293

Fisher, A.A. (1986) *Contact Dermatitis*, 3rd ed., Philadelphia, Lea & Febiger, pp. 745-761

Flesch, P. (1965) The role of epidermal components in cutaneous sensitization to some chemical agents. *Proc. Congr. Hubg. Derm. Soc.*, pp. 113-115

Fregert, S. (1971) Remaining chromium in intracutaneous test sites. *Contact Dermatitis Newsl.*, **10**: 233

Fregert, S. (1975) Occupational dermatitis in a 10-year material. *Contact Dermatitis*, **1**: 96-107

Fregert, S. & Gruvberger, B. (1972) Chemical properties of cement. *Dermatosen*, **20**: 238-248

Fregert, S., Gruvberger, B. & Sandahl, E. (1979) Reduction of chromate in cement by iron sulfate. *Contact Dermatitis*, **5**: 39-42

Friberg, L., Nordberg, G.F. & Vouk, V.B., eds (1986) *Handbook on the Toxicology of Metals*, Vol. II, Amsterdam, Elsevier

Garcia-Perez, J., Martin-Pascual, A. & Sanches-Misiego, A. (1973) Chrome content in bleaches and detergents. Its relationship to hand dermatitis in women. *Acta dermatovenereol.*, **53**: 353-358

Geiser, J.D. & Girard, A. (1965) [Remarks on cases of cement eczema observed at the dermatovenereological clinic of Lausanne from 1947 to 1961.] (in French) *Dermatologica*, **131**: 93-102

Goh, C.L. & Soh, S.D. (1984) Occupational dermatoses in Singapore. *Contact Dermatitis*, **11**: 288-293

Haines, A.T. & Nieboer, E. (1988) Chromium hypersensitivity. In: Nriagu, J.O. & Nieboer, E., eds, *Chromium in the Natural and Human Environments*, New York, Wiley Interscience, pp. 497-532

Høvding, G. (1970) *Cement Eczema and Chromium Allergy, an Epidemiologic Investigation*, Thesis, University of Bergen, Norway

Hunziker, N. & Musso, E. (1960) [Cement eczema.] (in French). *Dermatologica*, **121**: 204-212

Kanan, M.W. (1972) Cement dermatitis and atmospheric parameters in Kuwait. *Br. J. Dermatol.*, **86**: 155-159

Kligman, A.M. (1966) Identification of contact allergies by human assay. III. Maximization test: a procedure for screening and rating contact sensitizers. *J. invest. Dermatol.*, **47**: 393-409

Lammintausta, K., Maibach, H.I. & Wilson, D. (1987) Human cutaneous irritation: induced hyporeactivity. *Contact Dermatitis*, **17**: 193-198

Lidén, S. & Lundberg, E. (1979) Penetration of chromium in intact human skin in vivo. *J. invest. Dermatol.*, **72**: 42-45

Lück, H. & Jentsch, G. (1988) Chromium dermatitis caused by epoxy resin. *Contact Dermatitis*, **19**: 154-155

Magnusson, B. & Kligman, A.M. (1969) The identification of contact allergens by animal assay. The guinea pig maximization test. *J. invest. Dermatol.*, **52**: 268-276

Maibach, H.I. & Menné, T. (1989) *Exogenous Dermatoses*, Boca Raton, FL, CRC Press (in press)

Mali, J.W.H., Van Kooten, W.J. & Van Neer, E.C.J. (1963) Some aspects of the behavior of chromium compounds in the skin. *J. invest. Dermatol.*, **41**: 111-112

McOsker, D.E. & Beck, L.W. (1967) Characteristics of accomodated (hardened) skin. *J. invest. Dermatol.*, **48**: 372-383

Menné, T. & Holm, N.V. (1986) Genetic susceptibility in human allergic contact sensitization. *Semin. Dermatol.*, **5**: 301-306

Menné, T. & Maibach, H.I. (1987) Systemic contact allergy reactions. *Semin. Dermatol.*, **6**: 108-118

Menné, T., Brandrup, F., Thestrup-Pedersen, K., Veien, N.K., Andersen, J.R., Yding, F. & Valeur, G. (1987a) Patch test reactivity to nickel alloys. *Contact Dermatitis*, **16**: 255-259

Menné, T., Christopherson, J. & Maibach, H.I. (1987b) Epidemiology of allergic contact sensitization. In: Schlumberger, H.D., ed., *Epidemiology of Allergic Diseases*, Basel, Karger, pp. 132-161

Menné, T., Christopherson, J. & Green, A. (1989) Epidemiology of nickel dermatitis. In: Maibach, H.I. & Menné, T., eds, *Nickel and the Skin: Immunology and Toxicology*, Boca Raton, FL, CRC Press (in press)

Nieboer, E. & Sanford, W.E. (1985) Essential, toxic and therapeutic functions of metals (including determinants of reactivity). *Rev. Biochem. Toxicol.*, **7**: 205-245

Peck, S., Gant, J.Q. & Schwartz, L. (1945) 'Hardening' in industrial allergic dermatitis. *Ind. Med.*, **14**: 214-222

Peltonen, L. & Fräki, J. (1983) Prevalence of dichromate sensitivity. *Contact Dermatitis*, **9**: 190-194

Perone, V.B., Moffitt, A.E., Possick, P.A., Key, M.M., Danzinger, S.J. & Gellin, G.A. (1974) The chromium, cobalt and nickel contents of American cement and their relationship to cement dermatitis. *Am. ind. Hyg. Assoc. J.*, **35**: 301-306

Peter, K. (1968) [Outcome of patients with occupational eczema.] (in German) *Dermatologica*, **136**: 236-256

Pirilä, V. (1954) On the role of chrome and other trace elements in cement eczema. *Acta dermatovenereol.*, **34**: 136-143

Polak, L. (1983) Immunology of chromium. In: Burrows, D., ed., *Chromium: Metabolism and Toxicity*, Boca Raton, FL, CRC Press, pp. 51-136

Reifenstein, H., Lück, H., Pätzold, M. & Harms, U. (1986) [Incidence of cement eczema in the processing of low-chromate cements.] (in German) *Z. ges. Hyg.*, **32**: 559-560

Samitz, M.H. & Katz, S. (1964) A study of the chemical reactions between chromium and skin. *J. invest. Dermatol.*, **43**: 35-42

Samitz, M.H., Katz, S., Scheiner, D.M. & Gross, P.R. (1969) Chromium-protein interactions. *Acta dermatovenereol.*, **49**: 142-146

Scheper, R.J., von Blomberg, M., Vreeburg, K.J.J. & van Hoogstraten, M.V. (1989) Recent advances in immunology of nickel sensitization. In: Maibach, H.I. & Menné, T., eds, *Nickel and the Skin: Immunology and Toxicology*, Boca Raton, FL, CRC Press (in press)

Shelley, W.B. & Juhlin, L. (1976) Langerhans cells form a reticuloendothelial trap for external contact antigens. *Nature*, **261**: 46-47

Siegenthaler, U., Laine, A. & Polak, L. (1983) Studies on contact sensitivity to chromium in the guinea pig. The role of valence in the formation of the antigenic determinant. *J. invest. Dermatol.*, **80**: 44-47

Vandenberg, J. & Epstein, W. (1963) Experimental skin contact sensitization in man. *J. invest. Dermatol.*, **41**: 413-416

Wahlberg, J.E. (1989) Nickel animal sensitization assays. In: Maibach, H.I. & Menné, T., eds, *Nickel and the Skin: Immunology and Toxicology*, Boca Raton, FL, CRC Press (in press)

Zelger, J. (1964) [Clinical and pathogenesis of chromate eczemas.] (in German) *Arch. klin. exp. Dermatol.*, **218**: 499-542

ALLERGENIC POTENTIAL OF PLATINUM COMPOUNDS

G. Rosner[1] & R. Merget[2]

[1]*Fraunhofer Institute for Toxicology and Aerosol Research, D-3000 Hanover*
[2]*Hospital of the Johann Wolfgang Goethe University, Department of Internal Medicine*
Division of Pneumology
D-6000 Frankfurt/Main, Federal Republic of Germany

ABSTRACT

Apart from the antitumour agent cis-platinum and its analogues, the toxicological relevance of platinum is confined mainly to some of its complex halide salts, which are some of the most potent sensitizers known. Symptoms of platinum-related allergy, such as rhinitis, conjunctivitis, asthma, urticaria and, occasionally, contact dermatitis, have been reported almost exclusively from occupational environments. With latency periods of a few weeks to several years, the incidence of allergic reactions was as high as 73% some 40 years ago. Despite control measures and the setting of a threshold limit value of 2 μg/m³, there is still a high risk of developing sensitivity to platinum salts. The underlying mechanism appears to be a type-I (IgE-mediated) response. Diagnosis is based mainly on the results of skin prick tests, which provide reproducible and reliable results. In-vitro tests, including the radioallergosorbent test and histamine release, are too nonspecific to be used for screening purposes. The potential health risk to the general population of exposure to platinum from emissions from car catalysts is discussed. There is at present no evidence that allergenic platinum compounds are emitted; however, further research should be done to clarify the potential health implications of increased amounts of platinum in our environment.

INTRODUCTION

Except for its use in dentistry and jewellery, most of the platinum produced is consumed in industry. This use pattern explains why health hazards from exposure to platinum compounds have been found almost exclusively in the occupational environment. Toxicological problems other than allergy, arising from medical use of the antitumour agent cis-platinum and its analogues, are out of the scope of this paper.

In 1975, platinum-containing catalysts were introduced in US cars in order to meet the stringent limits on monoxide, hydrocarbons and nitrogen oxides set by the Federal Clean Air Act. More than a decade later, the introduction of automobile catalytic converters also became an issue in western Europe. As a consequence, potential occupational exposure to platinum has undoubtedly increased, as demonstrated by the following figures: total platinum consumption in the USA between 1961 and 1972 was on average 14.3 tonnes per year (Brubaker et al., 1975). In 1987, about 26 tonnes of platinum were sold in the USA to the consuming industries, of which 71% was used in car catalysts (Loebenstein, 1988).

There was and still is concern over possible harmful effects to the general population from the attrition of platinum from car catalysts. We will discuss this subject, presenting new data on emissions. First of all, however, we will review the toxicological relevance of the potent allergenicity of some platinum compounds.

PLATINUM ALLERGY: HISTORICAL BACKGROUND

Platinum and its compounds were considered harmless for a long time, although allergic rhinitis has been known since 1804. The first scientific description of health problems arising from occupational exposure to platinum was published by Karasek and Karasek in 1911. They investigated workers in photographic studios in Chicago who handled photographic paper treated with complex platinum salts. The symptoms observed in eight workers were pronounced irritation of the nose and throat causing violent sneezing and coughing, together with difficulty in breathing. Cases of dermatitis were also noted (Harris, 1975).

More than 30 years later, Hunter *et al.* (1945) conducted the first environmental and clinical study on workers in four British platinum refineries. Out of 91 workers exposed to complex salts of platinum, 52 showed symptoms starting with repeated sneezing and a runny nose, followed by tightness of the chest, shortness of breath, cyanosis and wheezing. Scaly erythematous dermatitis of hands and forearms and sometimes of the face and neck and urticaria was observed in 13 workers. The symptoms persisted during working hours and for about 1 h after leaving the factory. The latent period from first contact with platinum and the occurrence of the first symptoms varied from some months to six years. Once sensitivity was established, symptoms tended to become worse as long as the workers remained in that environment.

In the USA, Roberts (1951) studied 21 employees of a platinum refinery for five years and confirmed the findings of Hunter *et al.* (1945). All workers showed some form of platinum-related disease, for which Roberts (1951) introduced the term 'platinosis'. According to his classification of this occupational disease, 40% of the employees did not show typical symptoms but exhibited the same inflammatory changes in the conjunctivae and the mucous membranes of the upper respiratory tract that were seen in the 60% of workers with definite symptoms (see Table 1).

These observations have since been confirmed by many investigators. The term 'platinosis' is no longer used, as it implies a chronic fibrosing lung disease such as silicosis, as was assumed by Roberts (1951) but has not been observed subsequently. Instead, 'platinum salt allergy' (Schultze-Werninghaus *et al.*, 1978), 'platinum salt sensitivity' (Linnett, 1987), 'allergy to platinum compounds containing reactive halogen ligands' (Hughes, 1980) and similar terminology is preferred.

EPIDEMIOLOGY

In early surveys, the incidence of allergic reactions due to exposure to platinum salts was as high as 73% (Table 2). Reported concentrations of platinum ranged from 0.9 to 1700 µg/m³ (Hunter *et al.*, 1945). Due to analytical deficiencies, these data cannot be used to quantify former exposure situations, but it can be assumed that workplace concentrations were definitely higher than those after adoption of the threshold limit value for

Table 1. Classification of signs and symptoms of soluble platinum salt allergy according to Roberts (1951)

Type	Severity	Signs and symptoms
Skin	Acute	Itching, redness, urticaria, usually of exposed areas
	Subacute	Early urticaria, replaced by typical contact-type dermatitis
	Chronic	Persistent contact dermatitis with secondary eczema
Respiratory	Mild	Sneezing, lachrymation, with burning of eyes
	Moderately Severe	Aggravation of mild type, extending to rest of respiratory tract producing dry cough, tightness in chest
	Severe	Frank, full-fledged bronchial asthma
Mixed		Symptoms of both the cutaneous and the respiratory type

Table 2. Incidence of soluble platinum salt allergy in surveys of platinum workers

Total no. of workers	Workers with platinum salt allergy	Incidence (%)	Reference
91	52	57	Hunter *et al.* (1945)
20	12	60	Roberts (1951)
15	11	73	Massmann & Opitz (1954)
51	35	69	Hebert (1966)
86	35	41	Dally *et al.* (1980)
65	15	23	Bolm-Audorff *et al.* (1988)
27	8	30	Merget *et al.* (1988)

soluble platinum salts of 2 $\mu g/m^3$. Today, it is also common practice to discharge or relocate sensitized workers, so that the incidence of platinum sensitivity and allergenicity should be considerably lower. However, recent reports showing work-related symptoms in 23-30% of exposed workers (Table 2) indicate that this is not the case. Analyses of airborne dust in a platinum refinery revealed levels of 0.08-0.1 $\mu g/m^3$ in a separation department. In other areas, the levels were all below 0.05 $\mu g/m^3$ (Bolm-Audorff *et al.*, 1988) or 0.08 $\mu g/m^3$ (Merget *et al.*, 1988). Thus, adoption of the threshold limit value has not been sufficient to prevent the development of sensitivity to platinum salts.

Although no unequivocal concentration-effect relationship can be deduced from the available literature, the risk of developing platinum salt sensitivity seems to be correlated with exposure intensity. In the surveys of Bolm-Audorff *et al.* (1988) and Merget *et al.* (1988), the highest incidences occurred in the groups with the highest exposures.

CLINICAL SYMPTOMATOLOGY

The latent period to first symptoms usually varies between three months and three years (Parrot *et al.*, 1969; Schultze-Werninghaus *et al.*, 1978; Ruff *et al.*, 1979), but may be less than three months (Roberts, 1951; Hughes, 1980; Merget *et al.*, 1988).

The symptoms of platinum salt allergy, as classified by Roberts (1951) (Table 1), reflect the full range of possible cutaneous and respiratory manifestations, including occupational asthma. Contact urticaria, sometimes manifesting as chronic dermatitis, is a common skin lesion and may be the first indication of sensitization (Hughes, 1980).

The symptoms usually worsen with increasing length of exposure, but most disappear when the subject is removed from exposure; however, after longer exposure periods, individuals may never become completely symptomless (Schultze-Werninghaus *et al.*, 1989).

IMMUNOLOGICAL MECHANISM AND DIAGNOSIS

The clinical manifestations of soluble platinum salt allergy reflect a true allergic response on the basis of the following criteria:

(a) the appearance of sensitivity is followed by a symptomless exposure;
(b) only a fraction of exposed subjects become sensitized;
(c) the affected persons become more and more sensitive to platinum and react to levels far below those normally encountered at work;
(d) atopic and nonatopic control persons show negative results in skin prick tests.

Platinum salt allergy appears to be a type-I (IgE-mediated) response. The possibility that IgE antibodies to platinum chloride complexes are stimulated in sensitive persons has been assumed on the basis of allergic and serological tests. It is believed that the low-molecular-weight platinum salts act as haptens, combining with serum proteins to form the complete antigen. However, the actual immunological mechanism is not yet known (Zachgo *et al.*, 1985).

Skin prick test

Skin prick tests with dilute concentrations of soluble platinum complexes appear to provide reproducible, reliable, highly sensitive biological indications of allergenicity (Cleare et al., 1976). The compounds used for routine screening of exposed workers are ammonium hexachloroplatinate, sodium hexachloroplatinate[IV] and sodium tetrachloroplatinate[II]. After sensitization by previous exposure, prick testing with concentrations of 10^{-3} to 10^{-9} g/ml of the platinum compound produces immediate wheal-and-flare reactions in highly susceptible people (Pepys et al., 1972; Pickering, 1972; Hughes, 1980; Gallagher et al., 1982; Biagini et al., 1985; Boggs, 1985; Jacobs, 1987; Linnett, 1987; Murdoch & Pepys, 1987; Schultze-Werninghaus et al., 1989). With these concentrations, nonspecific skin reactions did not occur in atopic or nonatopic controls (Pepys et al., 1972; Murdoch & Pepys, 1987; Merget et al., 1988).

Nasal test

Instillation into the nose of the same platinum solutions at the same concentrations as above is another simple method for detecting sensitivity to platinum salts. A nasal reaction was considered to be positive if itching, sneezing, nasal obstruction or discharge occurred singly or in combination within 15 min of the challenge (Pepys et al., 1972).

Inhalation test

Inhalation tests with a dust consisting of a mixture of ammonium hexachloroplatinate and lactose induced immediate asthmatic reactions and were regarded as safe tests for occupational exposure (Pepys et al., 1972). Merget et al. (1989) recently reported three cases of negative skin tests in platinum refinery workers who showed nonspecific hyperreactivity and a clearly positive immediate reaction to the inhalation provocation test. Thus, for practical purposes, an inhalation test should be carried out in the case of positive anamnesis but a negative skin test result.

Serological tests

Passive transfer of immediate reactivity to intracutaneous tests was demonstrated with the Prausnitz-Küstner test by Freedman and Krupey (1968). Schultze-Werninghaus et al. (1978) observed positive reactions in the form of passive cutaneous anaphylaxis (PCA) in monkeys tested with serum from a platinum worker. Similar tests were performed by Pepys et al. (1979) with sera from refinery workers; the results, however, were inconsistent, as positive as well as negative results were elicited in the Prausnitz-Küstner prick test and for PCA reactions in human and monkey recipients, respectively. Parish (1970) also demonstrated the presence of heat-stable short-term sensitizing IgG antibodies by PCA on monkey skin.

The sensitivity and reliability of the skin prick test has not been equalled by any in-vitro test available. IgE antibodies specific to platinum chloride complexes were found in enzyme immunoassays (Zachgo et al., 1985; Merget et al., 1988) and in radioallergosorbent tests (Cromwell et al., 1979; Pepys et al., 1979). Although a good correlation with the results of prick tests was reported (Cromwell et al., 1979), the practical application of these tests for screening purposes was questioned (Boggs, 1985; Jacobs, 1987; Merget et al., 1988) because of their nonspecifity, demonstrated in a cross-sectional survey of platinum refinery workers (Merget et al., 1988). Higher total serum IgE and platinic chloride-specific IgE levels were noted in subjects with work-related symptoms; however, not all allergic individuals showed binding in the radioallergosorbent test, and some of the controls did (Fig. 1).

Similar effects were seen in vitro by histamine release from basophils; the level was relatively high in skin test-positive workers, but even higher in the atopic control group. Histamine release with anti-IgE showed a similar pattern, indicating identical binding sites of platinic chloride and anti-IgE on the surface of cutaneous mast cells and basophils.

Since refinery workers are exposed to more than one metal salt of the platinum group, the question of cross-reactivity was investigated in PCA tests. Initial results indicated that platinum (sodium hexachloroplatinate and ammonium hexachloroplatinate) and palladium (sodium hexachloropalladate[IV]) are equally effective as eliciting agents. Five-fold concentrated sera from platinum refinery workers elicited PCA in monkeys (Biagini et al.,

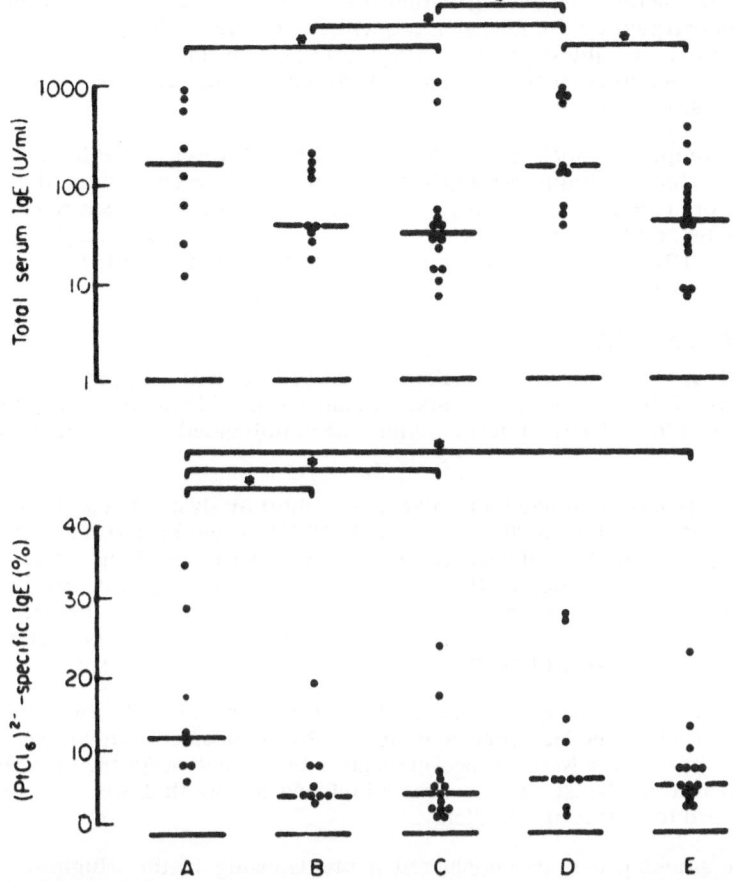

Fig. 1. Total serum IgE and platinic chloride $(PtCl_6)^{2-}$-specific IgE in refinery workers: Group A, workers with work-related symptoms, n=8; Group B, workers with symptoms not clearly work-related, n=9; Group C, asymptomatic workers, n=13; and in controls Group D, atopics, n=10; Group E, nonatopics, n=16. *, $p<0.05$. From Merget *et al.* (1988).

1982); no in-vivo reaction to palladium salts was reported. Murdoch and Pepys (1987) found only a limited cross-reactivity between platinum and palladium salts in both skin tests and the radioallergosorbent test. Reactions to platinum group metals other than platinum were seen only in platinum salt-sensitive individuals.

ALLERGENIC POTENCY OF PLATINUM COMPOUNDS

Metallic platinum appears to be nonallergenic: with the exception of a single case of an alleged contact dermatitis due to platinum metal (Sheard, 1955), no allergic reaction has been reported.

It is commonly accepted that the allergenic properties of platinum are confined to certain coordination complexes. Halogenated platinum salts are among the most potent known sensitizers, and the compounds mainly responsible for platinum sensitization are its chlorinated salts, such as the tetravalent compounds ammonium hexachloroplatinate and dipotassium tetrachloroplatinate[II], and the hexavalent dipotassium hexachloroplatinate[IV]. Sensitivity to disodium platinous chloride and to platinic chloride has also been observed. Cleare *et al.* (1976) investigated the allergenic potency of platinum complexes by means of skin prick tests in platinum refinery workers who were known to be sensitive to hexachloroplatinate. Their results suggest that platinum allergy is confined to a small group of charged compounds that contain reactive ligand systems. Most effective are chloride ligands, and the allergic response generally increases with increasing number of chloro groups as demonstrated by the following sequence of potency: $(NH_4)_2[PtCl_6] \simeq (NH_4)_2 [PtCl_4]$ > $CS_2[Pt(NO_2)Cl_3]$ > $CS_2[Pt(NO_2)Cl_2]$ > $CS_2[Pt(NO_2)_3Cl]$. $K_2[Pt(NO_2)_4]$, containing no chloro group, was inactive. Ionic platinum compounds containing bromide or iodide are also allergenic, but less effective.

Neutral complexes such as $[Pt(NH_2)_2CS_4Cl_2]$, $K_2[Pt(NO_2)_4]$, $[Pt(NH_3)_4]Cl_2$, and the antitumour agent cis-platinum, cis-$[Pt(NH_3)_2Cl_2]$, are not allergenic, since they probably do not react with proteins to form a complete antigen. Anaphylactic shock reactions observed after intravenous administration of relatively high doses of cis-platinum (Khan et al., 1975; Von Hoff et al., 1979) were probably caused by contamination with the potent hexa- or tetrachloroplatinate (Pepys, 1983).

PREDISPOSING FACTORS

Roberts (1951) considered the following characteristics to be predisposing factors: a previous history of allergy, i.e., atopic status; skin lesions like acne; blond hair, blue eyes and thin or pale skin. Since then, few data have been published that would support Roberts' views.

Dally et al. (1980) conducted a retrospective cohort analysis on a group of 86 platinum workers who started work at a UK refinery in 1973-74. They found that significantly more atopics left employment, but, apparently, irrespective of the development of platinum salt allergy. In fact, the prevalence of the disease did not differ significantly between atopic subjects (14/32; 44%) and nonatopic subjects (21/54; 39%). Thus, the increased leaving rate of atopic workers cannot be regarded as proof that atopic status is a true predisposing factor, as suggested by Linnett (1987).

Ethnic differences have also been claimed (Jacobs, 1987), on the basis of the assumption that atopy is less prevalent among black people than among whites, and, among whites, those of the Nordic type were said to be more susceptible than those from the Mediterranean littoral. No study has been published so far that would substantiate this thesis with regard to platinum salt allergy.

Whether smoking can be considered a predisposing factor (Hughes, 1980) is also controversial. Merget et al. (1988) examined 27 refinery workers and found no evidence to support this assumption; however, in a longitudinal cohort study on 91 platinum refinery workers in the UK (86 men) who started work in 1973-74 and were followed up until 1980, smoking was found to increase the risk for a positive skin test result by four to five times as compared to nonsmokers (Venables et al., 1989). Age, which varied from 15-54 years in the cohort, was certainly a confounding factor; and after taking account of age, the risk for leaving refinery work was only 1.75 times greater in smokers than in nonsmokers. The risk associated with atopy was not significant after taking smoking into consideration, confirming the idea that atopy cannot yet be confirmed as a predisposing factor for developing platinum salt allergy. However, since applicants with a history of allergy were not employed, workers found to be atopic during the study probably had only low susceptibility; hence, the risk of atopy may have been underestimated.

PREVENTION OF ALLERGY TO PLATINUM COMPOUNDS

In order to minimize the risk for developing platinum allergy, all potential employees in platinum refineries should be subjected to:
  (a) a questionnaire, with particular attention to previous asthma and allergy;
  (b) a skin prick test for examining atopic status, using house dust and mixed grass pollens;
  (c) a skin prick test using halogenated salts and platinic chloride to detect sensitization due to previous employment; and
  (d) a physical examination, including an assessment of lung function.

To detect sensitization during employment, whenever possible before symptoms appear, skin prick tests should be performed on all potentially exposed persons at three-monthly intervals. Use of protective clothing, including specially designed airstream helmets

(Boggs, 1985), has also been suggested. Since cases of platinum salt allergy still occur, despite the reduction of workplace concentrations below the established limit value of 2 µg/m³, the most effective preventive measure would be to improve control measures, such as enclosed processing and optimal ventilation, thus reducing exposure to platinum salt aerosols and dusts to the lowest feasible limit.

ALLERGENIC POTENTIAL OF PLATINUM EMISSIONS FROM CAR CATALYSTS

Until recently, exposure to platinum salts was confined to occupational settings, primarily in mining areas, platinum metal refineries and catalyst synthesis plants. However, the introduction of the automotive exhaust gas catalyst gave rise to concern that the emission of platinum could constitute a 'new' environmental pollutant. We have reviewed the available literature to assess the potential health implications of environmental exposure to platinum (Rosner & Hertel, 1986). A few data are available from experiments with one first-generation pellet-type catalyst in the USA, which indicate that the total amount of platinum emitted would be 1-2 µg/km at a speed of 50-100 km/h. Only 10% of the platinum emitted was classified as water-soluble and thus with potential biological activity.

Using dispersion models developed by the US Environmental Protection Agency (Ingalls & Garbe, 1982), we calculated the concentrations of platinum that would occur in different scenarios. As shown in Table 3, concentrations of soluble platinum near and on streets would range from 0.5 pg/m³ to 0.9 ng/m³. The figures predicted for parking and personal garages are definitely overestimates. The results of experiments in progress at the

Table 3. Estimated ambient concentrations of soluble platinum compounds in various exposure situations[a]

Exposure situation	Emission rate	Pt concentration (ng/m³)
Personal garage	0.1 µg/min[b]	
Typical (30-s run time)		0.8
Severe (5-min run time)		6.7
Parking garage	0.1 µg/min[b]	
Typical		0.4
Severe		5.6
Roadway tunnel	0.2 µg/km[c]	
Typical		0.4
Severe		0.9
Street canyon (sidewalk receptor)	0.2 µg/km[c]	
Typical, 800 vehicles per h		0.01
Typical, 1600 vehicles per h		0.03
Severe, 1200 vehicles per h		0.05
Severe, 2400 vehicles per h		0.09
On expressway	0.2 µg/km[c]	
Typical		0.07
Severe		0.16
Near expressway (short-term)	0.2 µg/km[c]	
Severe (1 m)		0.13
10 m		0.11
100 m		0.03
1000 m		0.004
Near expressway (annual)	0.2 µg/km[c]	
Severe (1 m)		0.02
10 m		0.015
100 m		0.004
1000 m		0.0005

[a]Adapted from Rosner & Hertel (1986).
[b]Assumed value; no emission data available.
[c]From Hill & Mayer (1977).

Fraunhofer Institute for Toxicology and Aerosol Research in Hanover indicate that the attrition of platinum depends on the temperature of the exhaust gas. During idling or at very low speeds, emissions would be negligible.

The predicted ambient air concentrations are lower by at least by a factor of 1000 than the threshold limit value of 2 µg/m³. However, since some halogenated platinum complexes are highly allergenic, sensitized people could develop allergic reactions even to these low concentrations.

One immunological study conducted by Cleare (1977) addressed the question of whether the emitted platinum is allergenic. They investigated the response of highly sensitive people to extracts of particulate exhaust samples with a highest total platinum content of more than 5×10^{-6} g, which would be sufficient to elicit a response. None of the five extracts, tested on only three persons using the skin prick test, elicited a positive response. No other data have been published to confirm these observations.

The Fraunhofer Institute has conducted engine test-stand experiments with the new-generation three-way catalyst of the monolith type (König et al., 1989). These experiments are part of a government programme (Federal Ministry on Research and Technology) to assess the relative risk of exposure to this new man-made environmental source. Initial results indicate that at a simulated speed of 100 km/h, total platinum attrition in the exhaust gas is about 17 ng/m³, corresponding to approximately 25 ng/km. This is lower by a factor of 100 than the data on emissions given above, lowering the theoretical ambient concentrations to the picogram to femtogram range. The emitted platinum is probably in the metallic form. Preliminary results indicated that approximately 10% of the total platinum penetrates a depth-type filter to be trapped in the condensate, but these results could not be confirmed. Experiments are under way to determine the chemical nature of the platinum emissions. It must be stressed that these data on the three-way catalyst are still preliminary, since they are derived from experiments with only one catalytic converter. Further experiments using several catalysts are to be conducted to increase the data base.

Current knowledge therefore indicates that the allergenic potential of platinum emissions from car catalysts is, if present, very low. However, to be on the safe side, further research should be done to clarify the potential health implications of increased amounts of platinum in our environment.

REFERENCES

Biagini, R.E., Clark, J.C., Gallagher, J.S., Bernstein, I.L. & Moorman, W.M. (1982) Passive transfer in the monkey of human immediate hypersensitivity to complex salts of platinum and palladium. Fed. Proc., 41: 827

Biagini, R.E., Bernstein, I.L., Gallagher, J.S., Moorman, W.J., Brooks, S. & Gann, P.H. (1985) The diversity of reaginic immune responses to platinum and palladium metallic salts. J. Allergy clin. Immunol., 76: 794-802

Boggs, P.B. (1985) Platinum allergy. Cutis, 35: 318-320

Bolm-Audorff, U., Bienfait, H.-G., Burkhard, J., Bury, A.-H., Merget, R., Pressel, G. & Schultze-Werninghaus, G. (1988) [On the frequency of respiratory allergies in a platinum processing factory]. In: Baumgartner, E., Brenner, W., Dierich, M.P. & Rutenfranz, J., eds [Report of the 28th Annual Meeting of the German Society for Occupational Medicine, 4-7 May 1988, Innsbruck, Austria], Stuttgart, Gentner Verlag, pp. 411-416 (in German)

Brubaker, P.E., Moran, J.P., Bridbord, K. & Hueter, F.G. (1975) Noble metals: a toxicological appraisal of potential new environmental contaminants. Environ. Health Perspect., 10: 39-56

Cleare, M.J. (1977) Immunological Studies on Platinum Complexes and their Possible Relevance to Autocatalysts (Society of Automotive Engineers Report No. 770061), Warrendale, PA, Society of Automotive Engineers

Cleare, M.J., Hughes, E.G., Jacoby, B. & Pepys, J. (1976) Immediate (type I) allergic responses to platinum compounds. Clin. Allergy, 6: 183-195

Cromwell, O., Pepys, J., Parish, W.E & Hughes, E.G. (1979) Specific IgE antibodies to platinum salts in sensitized workers. Clin. Allergy, 9: 109-117.

Dally, M.B., Hunter, J.V., Hughes, E.G., Stewart, M. & Newman Taylor, A.J. (1980) Hypersensitivity to platinum salts: a population study. Am. Rev. respir. Dis., 121 Suppl.: 230

Freedman, S.O. & Krupey, J. (1968) Respiratory allergy caused by platinum salts. J. Allergy, 42: 233-237

Gallagher, J.S., Baker, D., Gann, P.H., Jarabek, A.M., Brooks, S.M. & Bernstein, I.L. (1982) A cross sectional investigation of workers exposed to platinum salts. *J. Allergy clin. Immunol.*, **69**: 134

Harris, S. (1975) Nasal ulceration in workers exposed to ruthenium and platinum salts. *J. Soc. occup. Med.*, **25**: 133-134

Hebert, R. (1966) [Ailments induced by platinum compounds.] (in French) *Arch. Mal. prof. Med. Travail Sec. soc.*, **27**: 877-886

Hill, R.F. & Mayer, W.J. (1977) Radiometric determination of platinum and palladium attrition from automotive catalysts. *IEEE Trans. Nucl. Sci.*, **NS-24**: 2549-2554

Hughes, E.G. (1980) Medical surveillance of platinum refinery workers. *J. Soc. occup. Med.*, **30**: 27-30

Hunter, D., Milton, R. & Perry, K.M.A. (1945) Asthma caused by the complex salts of platinum. *Br. J. ind. Med.*, **2**: 92-98

Ingalls, M.N. & Garbe, R.J. (1982) *Ambient Pollutant Concentrations from Mobile Sources in Microscale Situations (Society of Automotive Engineers Technical Paper Series No. 820787)*, Warrendale, PA, Society of Automotive Engineers

Jacobs, L. (1987) Platinum salt sensitivity. *Nurs. Rep. S. AfricaVerpleging*, **2**: 34-37

Karasek, S.R. & Karasek, M. (1911) *The Use of Platinum Paper. Report of (Illinois) Commission on Occupational Diseases to his Excellency Governor Charles S. Deneen, January, 1911*, Chicago, Warner Printing Company, p. 97 (cited by Roberts, 1951)

Khan, A., Hill, J.M., Grater, W., Loeb, E., MacLellan, A. & Hill, N. (1975) Atopic hyper-sensitivity to cis-dichlorodiammine-platinum(II) and other platinum complexes. *Cancer Res.*, **35**: 2766-2770

König, H.P., Kock, H. & Hertel, R.F. (1989) [Analytical Determination of Platinum with Regard to the Car Catalyst Issue]. In: *Fifth CAS Colloquium Atomspektrometrische Spurenanalytik, Konstanz, FRG, 3-7 April 1989*, Überlingen, Perkin-Elmer Verlag (in German)

Linnett, P.J. (1987) Platinum salt sensitivity. A review of the health aspects of platinum refining in South Africa. *J. Mine med. Off. Assoc. S. Afr.*, **63**: 24-28

Loebenstein, J.R. (1988) Platinum-group metals. In: US Bureau of Mines, ed., *Minerals Yearbook 1987*, Vol. I, Washington DC, Department of the Interior, pp. 723-733

Massmann, W. & Opitz, H. (1954) [On platinum allergy.] *Zentralbl. Arbeitsmed. Arbeitsschutz*, **4**: 1-4 (in German)

Merget, R., Schultze-Werninghaus, G., Muthorst, T., Friedrich, W. & Meier-Sydow, J. (1988) Asthma due to the complex salts of platinum - a cross-sectional survey of workers in a platinum refinery. *Clin. Allergy*, **18**: 569-580

Merget, R., Zachgo, W., Schultze-Werninghaus, G., Bergmann, E.-M., Bolm-Audorff, U., Friedrich, W., Bury, A.H. & Meier-Sydow, J. (1989) [Quantitative skin test and inhalation provocation test in asthma associated with platinum compounds.] *Pneumologie* (in press) (in German)

Murdoch, R.D. & Pepys, J. (1987) Platinum group metal sensitivity: reactivity to platinum group metal salts in platinum halide salt-sensitive workers. *Ann. Allergy*, **59**: 464-469

Parish, W.E. (1970) Short-term anaphylactic IgG antibodies in human sera. *Lancet*, **ii**: 591-592

Parrot, J.-L., Hébert, R., Saindelle, A. & Ruff, F. (1969) Platinum and platinosis. Allergy and histamine release due to some platinum salts. *Arch. environ. Health*, **19**: 685-691

Pepys, J. (1983) Allergy of the respiratory tract to low molecular weight chemical agents. *Handb. exp. Pharmacol.*, **63**: 163-185

Pepys, J., Pickering, C.A.C., & Hughes, E.G. (1972) Asthma due to inhaled chemical agents - complex salts of platinum. *Clin. Allergy*, **2**: 391-396

Pepys, J., Parish, W.E., Cromwell, O. & Hughes, E.G. (1979) Passive transfer in man and the monkey of type I allergy due to heat labile and heat stable antibody to complex salts of platinum. *Clin. Allergy*, **9**: 99-108

Pickering, C.A.C. (1972) Inhalation tests with chemical allergens: complex salts of platinum. *Proc. R. Soc. Med.*, **65**: 272-274

Roberts, A.E. (1951) Platinosis. A five-year study of the effects of soluble platinum salts on employees in a platinum laboratory and refinery. *Arch. ind. Hyg. occup. Med.*, **4**: 549-559

Rosner, G. & Hertel, R.F. (1986) [Health risk assessment of platinum emissions from automotive exhaust gas catalysts.] *Staub-Reinhalt. Luft*, **46**: 281-285 (in German)

Ruff, F., Di Matteo, G., Dupuis, J.P., Hébert, R. & Parrot, J.-L. (1979) [Bronchopulmonary reactions and asthma due to platinum. Incidence among platinum workers in the Paris region.] *Rev. fr. Mal. respir.*, **7**: 206-208

Schultze-Werninghaus, G., Roesch, A., Wilhelms, O.-H., Gonsior, E. & Meier-Sydow, J. (1978) [Bronchial asthma due to occupational allergy of immediate type (I) to platinum salts.] *Dtsch. med. Wochenschr.*, **23**: 972-975 (in German)

Schultze-Werninghaus, G., Merget, R., Zachgo, W., Muthorst, T., Mahlesa, D., Lisson, R. & Bolm-Audorff, U. (1989) [Platinum salts as occupational allergens - a review.] *Allergologie*, **12**: 152-157 (in German)

Sheard, C. (1955) Contact dermatitis from platinum and related metals. *Arch. Dermatol. Syphilol.*, **71**: 357-360.

Venables, K.M., Dally, M.B., Nunn, A.J., Stevens, J.F., Stephens, R., Farrer, N., Hunter, J.V., Stewart, M., Hughes, E.G. & Newman Taylor, A.J. (1989) Smoking and occupational allergy in workers in a platinum refinery. *Br. med. J.*, **299**: 939-942

Von Hoff, D.D., Schilsky, R., Reichert, C.M., Reddick, R.L., Rozencweig, M., Young, R.C. & Muggia, F.M. (1979) Toxic effects of cis-dichlorodiammineplatinum(II) in man. *Cancer Treat. Rep.*, **63**: 9-10

Zachgo, W., Merget, R. & Schultze-Werninghaus, G. (1985) [Proof of specific IgE against low molecular substances (platinum salts).] *Atamw.-Lungenkr.*, **11**: 267-268 (in German)

AUTOIMMUNITY

ROLE OF CYTOKINES
IN THE INDUCTION OF AUTOIMMUNITY

M. Goldman

*Laboratoire Pluridisciplinaire de Recherche Experimentale Biomédicale
and Department of Nephrology, Hôpital Erasme
Université Libre de Bruxelles, Belgium*

ABSTRACT

Cytokines are the mediators of a wide variety of cellular interactions within and outside the immune system. In this paper, we analyse the possible roles of cytokines in the pathogenesis of experimental and human autoimmune diseases. In organ-specific autoimmunity, interferon-γ (IFN-γ) may initiate or perpetuate the activation of autoreactive T helper cells by inducing an aberrant expression of class-II molecules of the major histocompatibility complex on target cells. As in insulin-dependent diabetes mellitus, cytokines (IFN-γ, tumour necrosis factor, interleukin-l) may also be directly involved in the pathogenesis of tissue lesions. In systemic lupus erythematosus, T cell-derived cytokines appear to be responsible for the activation of autoreactive B cells. Thus, the pathobiology of cytokines could lead to the development of new therapeutic strategies in autoimmune diseases.

INTRODUCTION

In recent years, significant advances have been made in the pathobiology of autoimmune diseases. Firstly, the demonstration of the pivotal role of major histocompatibility complex (MHC) gene products in the development of immune responses has provided a molecular basis for the genetic predisposition to autoimmunity (Stasny et al., 1983). Secondly, several mechanisms by which the immune system may become reactive to self-antigens have been proposed, such as aberrant expression of class-II MHC molecules on target organs (Bottazzo et al., 1983), molecular mimicry (Dwyer et al., 1986; Gaulton & Greene, 1986) and failure of suppression circuits (Dorf & Benacerraf, 1984). Thirdly, the involvement of T helper (Th) cells in the triggering of autoreactive B cells has become apparent in several models of antibody-mediated autoimmunity (Prud'homme & Palfrey, 1988). Cytokines may be involved in these different aspects of autoimmune diseases and may also represent important mediators of the tissue damage resulting from autoimmune reactions (Dinarello & Uyer, 1987; Revel & Schattner, 1987; Prud'homme & Palfrey, 1988). The contribution of cytokines to autoimmunity is not surprising since these polypeptides govern a variety of intercellular communications within the immune system (Dinarello & Wyer, 1987). In addition, cytokines may be produced by and act on a variety of non-immune cell types (De Maeyer & De Maeyer-Guignard, 1988). Their biological effects are frequently a result of intimate cell-to-cell interactions, but, like hormones, they may also appear in the circulation and exert profound systemic effects (Dinarello & Wyer, 1987). Cytokines may interact in various ways, either synergistically or as antagonists, either at the level of their production or at the level of the target cells. They thus form a highly complex network called the cytokine network (De Maeyer & De Maeyer-Guignard, 1988). Originally, cytokines were named according to their biological activity. Since most of these substances exert pleiotropic effects, it was proposed that, once the amino acid sequence of a new cytokine was defined, it would be designated by the term 'interleukin' followed by a number. A list of the most relevant cytokines and of their major biological activities is given in Table 1.

Table 1. Properties of human lymphokines relevant to autoimmunity

Cytokine[a]	Major biological properties
IL-1 (α and β)	Activation of resting T cells; mediation of acute-phase responses and catabolic processes; induction of collagen and collagenase synthesis; activation of fibroblasts, endothelial cells and macrophages; cofactor for B-cell activation
TNF (α and β)	Cytotoxic for some cells; mediator of acute-phase responses, catabolic processes and septic shock; induction of collagen and collagenase synthesis; activation of endothelial cells and macrophages
IL-2	Growth factor for activated T cells; activation of cytotoxic T cells; induction of other lymphokines; proliferation and terminal differentiation of B cells
IL-3	Supports the growth of pluripotent bone-marrow stem cells
IL-4	Growth factor for B cells and resting T cells; enhancement of Ia antigens on B cells and preferential induction of IgE secretion; activation of cytotoxic T cells; mast-cell growth factor
IL-5	Eosinophil differentiation; induction of IgM secretion by activated B cells
IL-6	Triggers synthesis of liver acute-phase proteins; differentiation factor for B cells and T cells
IL-7	Induces the proliferation of pre-B cells
IFN-γ	Induces class-I, class-II and other surface antigens on a variety of cells; activation of endothelial cells and macrophages; exerts antiviral activity
IFN α and β	Induces class-I antigen expression; exerts antiviral properties; enhances activity of natural killer cells

[a]IL, interleukin; TNF, tumour necrosis factor; IFN, interferon.

In this review, we focus on the role of cytokines in the induction of autoimmune diseases. Since the pathogenetic mechanisms of organ-specific autoimmunity appear to be quite distinct from those involved in systemic autoimmunity, the two types of autoimmune conditions are considered separately.

ORGAN-SPECIFIC AUTOIMMUNITY

It is quite well established that tolerance to most self-antigens is maintained at the Th cell level (Cruse & Lewis, 1985). Antigen recognition by Th cells requires adequate presentation of antigenic peptides in association with class-II MHC molecules, which are selectively expressed on cells of the immune system, such as monocytes, macrophages, B cells and activated T cells (Benacerraf, 1985). Under physiological conditions, most tissues outside the immune system do not express class-I MHC molecules (also called Ia antigens), and consequently the self-antigens on their surface cannot be presented to Th cells. Bottazzo and coworkers (1983) postulated that this was an important factor in the maintenance of tolerance to self-antigens, and they suggested that aberrant expression of Ia antigens could trigger autoimmune reactions. The demonstration that interferon-γ (IFN-γ) is a potent inducer of Ia antigens on nonlymphoid cell types (Todd *et al.*, 1985; Trinchieri & Perussia, 1985) led to the consideration that this cytokine could be involved in the pathogenesis of some forms of organ-specific autoimmunity, and particularly in autoimmune endocrine diseases (Schattner, 1988).

Autoimmune thyroiditis

The human and experimental thyroiditides represent a group of diseases in which both thyroid antigen-specific autoantibodies and T cells have been identified (Volpé, 1987; Prud'homme & Palfrey, 1988). In human autoimmune thyroid diseases, immunopathological studies have demonstrated an abnormal expression of class-II MHC molecules (HLA-DR antigens) on thyrocytes (Hanafusa *et al.*, 1983; Bottazzo *et al.*, 1986). The role of this phenomenon in the induction of autoimmunity was suggested by the demonstration that thyrocytes that express class-II MHC molecules can efficiently present antigens to Th cells, in a MHC class II-restricted fashion (Londei *et al.*, 1984). Moreover, T-cell lines isolated from the thyroid gland of patients with autoimmune thyroiditis have been found to react with thyrocytes expressing class-II MHC molecules (Londei *et al.*, 1985). Along the same line, Th cells that recognize thyroglobulin in the context of class-II MHC antigens have been isolated from mice with experimental autoimmune thyroiditis and found to transfer the disease (Romball & Weigle, 1987). IFN-γ, a cytokine produced by Th cells, has been found to be the major mediator responsible for the induction of class-II MHC antigens on thyrocytes (Todd *et al.*, 1985; Feldmann, 1988). Interestingly, thyroid-stimulating hormone amplifies this effect of IFN-γ, demonstrating a possible interaction between the cytokine network and the endocrine system (Todd *et al.*, 1987). Although it has been claimed that recombinant IFN-γ can induce experimental thyroiditis (Rémy *et al.*, 1987), the temporal relationship between IFN-γ production, aberrant expression of class-II antigens and occurrence of autoimmunity is a matter of debate. Indeed, some data suggest that the expression of HLA-DR antigens on thyrocytes of patients with autoimmune thyroid diseases is a consequence of the intrathyroidal production of IFN-γ by activated lymphocytes rather than a primary event (Mowat, 1985; Volpé, 1987). Even if it is not the initiating step in the development of autoimmunity, the aberrant expression of class-II MHC molecules induced by IFN-γ can obviously play an important role in the amplification and perpetuation of anti-thyroid autoimmune responses (Volpe, 1987; Schattner, 1988). The factors responsible for local production of IFN-γ by Th remain to be defined, but it has been suggested that viruses may be involved in this process (Bottazzo *et al.*, 1983).

Insulin-dependent diabetes mellitus

There is now strong evidence to suggest that insulin-dependent diabetes mellitus (IDDM; type-I diabetes) is an autoimmune disease in which both humoral and cell-mediated immune responses are involved in the destruction of the β cells of the pancreatic islets of Langerhans. Indeed, antibodies as well as cytotoxic T cells directed against islet cells have been identified in the circulation of diabetic patients (Nerup *et al.*, 1971; Huang & MacLaren, 1981; Boitard *et al.*, 1982; Dobersen, 1985; Bottazzo *et al.*, 1986; Eisenbarth, 1986). The leukocytic infiltration of damaged islet cells (insulitis) commonly observed in IDDM (Gepts & Lecompte, 1981) is thought to be the consequence of these autoimmune phenomena. Autoantibodies, islet-specific T cells and insulitis have also been demonstrated in the spontaneous diabetes that develops in the bio-breeding rat and in the nonobese diabetic mouse (Prud'homme & Palfrey, 1988); Immunopathalogical studies have revealed that the majority of the cells infiltrating the β islets are T cells, both in human and experimental IDDM (Bottazzo *et al.*, 1985; Dean *et al.*, 1985). The crucial role of T cells in the induction of the disease has been well documented in nonobese diabetic mice since it has been possible to transfer IDDM to nondiabetic littermates by injection of purified T-cell populations (Bendelac *et al.*, 1987). In man, the successful pancreatic transplantation between identical twins by Sibley *et al.* (1985) further supports the involvement of the host immune system in the development of IDDM: after grafting, islet cells from the normal pancreas (obtained from the twin without diabetes) were rapidly destroyed, in association with massive T-cell infiltration. Along the same lines, increased levels of activated T cells have been found in the circulation of diabetic patients (Jackson *et al.*, 1982) as well as in spontaneously diabetic bio-breeding rats (Francfort *et al.*, 1985). In view of these findings, elucidation of the cause(s) of T-cell activation in IDDM and of the mechanisms by which T cells lead to the destruction of β islet cells may provide important clues for the pathogenesis as well as for the treatment of the disease.

As far as the cause of T-cell activation is concerned, a link between IDDM and viruses has been suspected for many years on the basis of epidemiological data showing an increased incidence of IDDM after some viral infections (Maugh, 1975). Subsequently, viruses were identified occasionally within the pancreases of patients dying from diabetic ketoacidosis (Yoon *et al.*, 1979; Jenson *et al.*, 1980). The demonstration that viruses can induce IDDM in mice provides an experimental basis for an interpretation of these findings (Craighead & McLane, 1968; Oldstone *et al.*, 1984; Sharpe & Fields, 1985). In this respect, the observations of autoimmune phenomena in reovirus-induced IDDM and their prevention by immunosuppressive agents are of particular interest (Onodera et al., 1982); however, the definitive evidence that viruses play a pivotal role in the pathogenesis of human IDDM is still lacking.

Cytokines produced by activated T cells could contribute in several ways to the destruction of ß islet cells. Firstly, interleukin-2 (IL-2) may activate the cytotoxic T cells involved in this process (Huang & MacLaren, 1981; Boitard et al., 1982). Secondly, IFN-γ, which stimulates monocytic cells to produce interleukin-1 (IL-1) and tumour necrosis factor (Philip & Epstein, 1986), may act synergistically with these cytokines to suppress insulin release. Indeed, Mandrup-Poulsen et al. (1985) have shown that IL-1 is markedly toxic to isolated ß islet cells, and Campbell et al. (1988a) demonstrated that IFN-γ in association with tumour necrosis factor induces profound functional and morphological effects on these cells. Thirdly, cytokines may render the ß islet cells more immunogenic and more susceptible to immunological insult by modifying the expression of MHC antigens on their surface: (1) IFN-γ alone has been found to up-regulate the expression of HLA-A, B and C antigens on human islet cells, a phenomenon which could favour the targetting of autoreactive cytotoxic T cells to the ß cells (Campbell et al., 1986); (2) in concert with tumour necrosis factor or lymphotoxin, IFN-γ can also induce the aberrant expression of HLA-DR antigens on ß cells, and this may contribute to the perpetuation of autoimmune processes involving Th cells (Pujol-Borrell et al., 1987). An abnormal expression of HLA-DR antigen on ß islet cells has indeed been found in IDDM of recent onset (Bottazzo et al., 1985; Foulis & Farquharson, 1986). As for autoimmune thyroiditis, the interpretation of these findings remains controversial, but recent experimental data suggest that IFN-γ may be involved in the pathogenesis of IDDM: systemic administration of IFN-γ was found to enhance autoimmune, streptozotocin-induced diabetes in the mouse (Campbell et al., 1988b), and transgenic mice harbouring fusion genes between the human insulin promoter and IFN-γ were shown to develop IDDM (Sarvetnick et al., 1988).

SYSTEMIC AUTOIMMUNITY

Systemic lupus erythematosus (SLE) is the prototype of systemic autoimmune diseases. The availability of experimental models of SLE has made it possible to obtain insight into the pathophysiology of SLE and related autoimmune disorders (Smith & Steinberg, 1983; Gleichmann et al., 1984; Theofilopoulos & Dixon, 1985; Goldman et al., 1988a; Prud'homme & Palfrey, 1988). Here, we concentrate on the mediators of the lymphocytic interactions involved in two types of experimental SLE-like syndromes: (i) genetically-determined SLE that develops spontaneously in particular murine strains and (ii) chronic allogeneic diseases.

Spontaneous murine SLE-like diseases

SLE-like syndromes appear spontaneously in (NZBxNZW)F1 (B/W) females, BxSB males and MRL-lpr/lpr (MRL/l) mice. The main pathological features of these syndromes include lymphoid hyperplasia (prominent in MRL/l mice), thymic atrophy and immune-complex glomerulonephritis (Andrews et al., 1978). At the immunological level, all lupus-prone mice develop hypergammaglobulinaemia and produce autoantibodies directed against nuclear components, erythrocytes, immunoglobulins, other self constituents and haptens (Andrews et al., 1978; Izui et al., 1978). They also possess more immunoglobulin-containing cells (Theofilopoulos et al., 1980) and more clonable B cells (Kincade et al., 1979) than do normal mice. Similar abnormalities have been found in human SLE (Jasin & Ziff, 1975; Blaese et al., 1980; Kumagai et al. 1982), so that polyclonal B-cell hyperactivity appears as a cardinal feature of the disease (Prud'homme and Palfrey, 1988; Table 2). Although the precise causes of the B-cell hyperactivity remain to be elucidated, several studies indicate that T cell-derived cytokines are involved in the pathogenesis of both experimental and clinical SLE.

In the NZB/W, NZB and BxSB murine strains, B cells display an increased sensitivity to T cell-derived proliferation and differentiation B-cell factors (Prud'homme et al., 1983a; Herron et al., 1988), presumably as a consequence of genetically determined B-cell defects (Prud'homme & Palfrey, 1988). Thus, highly purified B cells from adult NZB mice proliferate

Table 2. Common immunological features of murine and human systemic lupus erythematosus (SLE)

Model[a]	T cell-mediated B-cell hyperactivity	Ia hyper-expression	T-cell deficiency
NZB, NZB/NZW	+	?	+
MRL/1	+	+[b,c]	+
Chronic GVH	+	+[b]	+
HVG	+	+[b]	+
Human SLE	+	+[d]	+

[a]GVH, graft *versus* host; HVG, host *versus* graft.
[b]On B cells.
[c]On macrophages (see text for references).
[d]On T cells (Volk *et al.*, 1986).

in response to interleukin-4 (IL-4) alone, whereas additional signals are required to trigger normal B cells (Gutierrez *et al.*, 1986). Clonal analysis of splenic T cells from NZB/W mice has shown that two types of T helper cells are involved in the B-cell stimulation: the first type recognizes self-Ia and preferentially induces anti-DNA antibodies, whereas the second type triggers B cells by bystander effects (Ando *et al.*, 1987). Interestingly, anti-DNA antibodies produced in the context of abnormal T-B interactions appear to be particularly nephritogenic because of their cationic charge (Datta *et al.*, 1987). The reasons why anti-DNA antibodies are preferentially produced *in vivo* are poorly understood. On the one hand, data indicate that anti-DNA antibodies appear in the context of a generalized polyclonal activation (Klinman & Steinberg, 1987). On the other hand, circulating DNA, which has been shown to be present in normal individuals and to be increased in lupus diseases (Fournié, 1988), could play an important role in the triggering of anti-DNA producing cells (Gleichmann *et al.*, 1984). Since a particular subset of B cells, Ly-1+ B cells, has been claimed to be responsible for most of the autoantibody production in lupus-prone mice (Hayakawa *et al.*, 1984), it would be interesting to analyse the responsiveness of these particular B cells to T cell-derived cytokines.

In MRL/1 mice, Th cells spontaneously produce factors that induce the growth and differentiation of B cells (Prud'homme *et al.*, 1983b; Rosenberg *et al.*, 1986; Dobashi *et al.*, 1987). These cytokines appear to be directly involved in polyclonal B-cell hyperactivity and in the production of autoantibodies (Prud'homme & Palfrey, 1988). B151-TRF2, a factor spontaneously secreted by spleen cells from MRL/1 mice, is one of these mediators, since it induces polyclonal differentiation of unprimed B cells into IgM-secreting cells in the absence of any antigenic stimulation (Dobashi *et al.*, 1987). Although interleukin-5 (IL-5) was not detected in spleen cell supernatants containing B151-TRF2 activity (Dobashi *et al.*, 1987), Rosenberg *et al.* (1986) reported the production by T-cell lines from MRL/1 mice of a B-cell growth factor with the same physicochemical properties as IL-5. In addition, these T-cell lines were found to secrete IL-4, a cytokine which increases Ia expression on B cells and which stimulates the differentiation of activated B cells into IgG1- and IgE-producing cells (Paul & Ohara, 1987). Since interleukin 6 (IL-6) also corresponds to a B-cell maturation and differentiating factor (Kishimoto & Hirano, 1988), its role in murine SLE should be considered as well (Prud'homme & Palfrey, 1988). Indeed, the association between IL-6 production and autoimmunity has already been reported in patients with cardiac myxoma (Hirano *et al.*, 1987).

Besides these B-cell-tropic factors, T cell lines from MRL/1 mice have been shown to synthesize IL-2 (Rosenberg *et al.*, 1984a) and IFN-γ (Lu & Unanue, 1982) constitutively. These two cytokines could also participate in the process of polyclonal B-cell activation (Leibson *et al.*, 1984; Sidman *et al.*, 1984; Santoro *et al.*, 1985). Indeed, the administration of IFN-γ to lupus-prone mice has been shown to accelerate the progression of the autoimmune disease (Heremans et al., 1978; Engleman et al., 1981). Along the same line, patients treated with human recombinant IFN-γ may develop antinuclear antibodies (Seitz et al., 1988). In human SLE, there is evidence for the production of an acid-labile IFN-α (Preble et al., 1982; Schattner, 1988). Although the physiopathological role of this cytokine remains unclear, one should note that treatment in vivo of healthy volunteers or of patients with unrelated diseases with leukocyte IFN has occasionally resulted in clinico-pathological manifestations of SLE (Rich, 1981; Schattner, 1988). In addition, acid-labile IFN-α is also detected in patients infected with human immunodeficiency virus (Eyster et al., 1983; Schattner, 1988), who often present with autoimmune features (Kopelman & Zolla-Paznzer, 1988). These data provide some support for the hypothesis that viruses are etiological agents of SLE (Pincus, 1982).

The T-cell subset involved in the secretion of B cell-tropic factors in MRL/l mice has not been clearly defined. The proliferating T cells responsible for the lymphoid hyperplasia express markers similar to those of early thymocytes (Lyt-1+, Lyt2-, Thy-1.2+, L3T4-, Ly-5+; Morse et al., 1982), and Rosenberg et al. (1986) reported that T-cell lines producing IL-4 and IL-5-like factors display a similar phenotype. However, L3T4+ Th cells have also been found to contribute to the development of lymphoproliferation and of autoantibody production in MRL/l mice (Santoro et al., 1988). Whatever their phenotype, some of the T cells that secrete B cell-tropic factors appear to react with self-Ia determinants, as suggested by the data of Rosenberg et al. (1986). The increased expression of Ia antigens on macrophages (Kelley & Roths, 1982) and on B cells (Rosenberg et al., 1986) induced by IFN-γ and IL-4, respectively (Santoro et al., 1983; Rosenberg et al., 1986) could favour and amplify the activation of those T cells that recognize self-Ia determinants (Rosenberg et al., 1984b). This amplification phenomenon is obviously important for the perpetuation of the autoimmune process. Recent observations suggest that similar interactions between T cells and autologous B cells may play a role in human SLE via the release by activated T cells of helper factors for B cells (Volk et al., 1986; Huang et al., 1988).

Chronic allogeneic diseases

Graft-versus-host (GVH) disease can be induced experimentally by injecting parental lymphocytes from strain X into a semi-allogeneic (XxY) Fl hybrid. Depending on the strain combination, the GVH reaction may lead to different pathological situations (Rolink et al., 1983a,b; Gleichmann et al., 1984; Via & Shearer, 1988a). The injection of donor cells that differ from those of the Fl recipient at both class-I and class-II loci results, in most cases, in an acute, lethal, immunosuppressive syndrome characterized by skin atrophy, lesions of the gastrointestinal tract, hypoplasia of the lymphoid and haematopoietic tissues, hypogammaglobulinaemia as well as depressed T-cell function in vitro (Rolink et al., 1983a; Gleichmann et al., 1984). This syndrome is induced by alloreactive suppressor/cytotoxic T cells which recognize class-I MHC antigens on host T cells with the help of donor Th cells stimulated by host class-II MHC molecules (Rolink et al., 1983b; Gleichmann et al., 1984); however, in selected parent-Fl combinations, such as in DBA/2 mice injected with (C57Bl/6xDBA/2) spleen cells, the GVH reaction is not acute and results in a chronic autoimmune syndrome resembling human SLE (Gleichmann et al., 1982). Indeed, animals undergoing stimulatory GVH reaction develop hypergammaglobulinaemia, antibodies to nuclear antigens, erythrocytes, thymocytes and skin basement membrane as well as antibody-mediated glomerulonephritis (Lewis et al., 1968; Gleichmann et al., 1982; Bruijn et al., 1988). The lack of acute GVH in this particular model has been related to the relative inability of T cells from DBA/2 mice to mount anti-C57Bl/6 cytotoxic responses (Via & Shearer, 1988a). In contrast, donor CD4+ Th cells that recognize class-II alloantigens from the host are functional and activate host B cells to produce immunoglobulins (Rolink et al., 1983a,b). Gleichmann et al. (1982) demonstrated that these interactions between donor T cells and host B cells lead to a preferential secretion of anti-DNA antibodies, presumably because DNA provides an additional signal to alloactivated B cells. Some of the mediators involved in the interactions between T cells and B cells have been identified recently. Dobashi et al. (1987) showed that spleen cells from mice undergoing a stimulatory GVH reaction spontaneously produce IL-5 (Murakami et al., 1988) as well as B151-TRF2. The role of the latter factor in the induction of autoimmunity was demonstrated by its ability to promote the production of antibodies to bromelein-treated red blood cells after injection *in vivo*. In our laboratory, the demonstration of high IgE serum levels and of an increased expression of Ia antigens on B cells led to the consideration that IL-4 might be another mediator of B-cell activation in this model. Indeed, we found IL-4 activity in spleen cell supernatants of mice undergoing stimulatory GVH and we showed that the increased expression of Ia antigens on B cells was significantly inhibited by a monoclonal anti-IL-4 antibody (J.M. Doutrelepont and others, manuscript in preparation).

Allogeneic interactions are involved in another model of autoimmune disease that develops in X mice injected at birth with spleen cells from (XxY)F1 hybrids (Goldman *et al.*, 1983). This manipulation has been known for a long time to induce transplantation tolerance to Y alloantigens in the X host (Billingham & Brent, 1959). Tolerance can be demonstrated *in vivo* by survival of skin grafts and *in vitro* by the inability of T cells from tolerant mice to proliferate in response to or to generate cytotoxicity against Y alloantigens (Brent *et al.*, 1976). Although the mechanisms of this adoptively acquired tolerance remain a matter of controversy (Nossal, 1983), there is evidence for a clonal deletion of donor-specific cytolytic T cells as well as of donor-specific Th cells that secrete IL-2 and IFN-γ (Feng *et al.*, 1983). Since the (XxY)F1 cells injected at birth persist in the X host for a long period, tolerant mice are thus chimeric, and this chimerism was recently found to be associated with the occurrence of autoimmunity and immune complex disease (Goldman *et al.*, 1983; Luzuy *et al.*, 1986). Among the autoantibodies, there is a preferential production of anti-DNA antibodies, but anti-erythrocyte and anti-lymphocyte antibodies as well as rheumatoid factors are also detected in tolerant animals (Goldman *et al.*, 1983). These autoantibodies are produced in the context of a polyclonal B-cell hyperactivity characterized by a preferential production of IgG1 and IgE (Goldman *et al.*, 1988b) and by an increased expression of Ia antigens on B cells (D. Abramowicz and others, submitted). In two different strain combinations (Balb/c mice neonatally injected with either Balb/cxC57Bl/6 or with A/JxBalb/c cells), allotypic studies have established that the vast majority of the autoantibodies are produced by F1 donor B cells persisting in the host (Luzuy *et al.*, 1986; Abramowicz *et al.*, 1987). This F1 donor B cell activation requires CD4+ Th cells, as depletion of these Th cells *in vivo* prevents the development of the autoimmune syndrome (Merino *et al.*, 1987). Using an in-vitro approach, we recently demonstrated that host CD4+ cells that recognize donor Ia antigens are directly involved in the activation of donor B cells and that IL-4 is one of the mediators of this host-*versus*-graft reaction (Goldman *et al.*, 1989). This model offers a unique opportunity to analyse the T-cell subsets and the cytokines involved in the stimulation of autoreactive B cells. Indeed, the Th cells responsible for the donor B cell stimulation are unable to produce IL-2 or IFN-γ (see above), while they secrete IL-4 and perhaps other B cell-tropic cytokines such as IL-5. This dissociation in the secretion of lymphokines corresponds to the two non-overlapping Th subsets that have been identified recently in the mouse (Mossman & Coffman, 1987): the Th1 subset produces IL-2 and IFN-γ while the Th2 subset produces IL-4 and IL-5. Our observations therefore suggest that the donor-specific Th2 of chimeric mice selectively escapes induction of tolerance. This apparent resistance of the Th2 subset could be an important factor for the emergence of antibody-mediated autoimmune diseases. Besides its effects on the production of IgG1 and IgE antibodies (Paul & Ohara, 1987), the secretion of IL-4 by Th2 could amplify B-cell stimulation by increasing the density of Ia antigens at the B-cell surface, as suggested by experiments in MRL/1 mice (Rosenberg *et al.*, 1986). In addition, we recently found that IL-6 derived from macrophages might be involved in this model, as (i) T cell-depleted spleen cells spontananeously produce high levels of IL-6 and (ii) the hyperproduction of immuno-globulins by F1 donor B cells is enhanced by IL-6 (P. Vandenabeele and others, manuscript in preparation).

Thus, experimental allogeneic diseases represent interesting tools for investigating the role of T cell- or macrophage-derived cytokines in the triggering of autoreactive B cells and for studying the effects of cytokine synergism, e.g., between IL-4 and IL-5 (Purkerson *et al.*, 1988), or of cytokine antagonism, e.g. between IL-4 and IFN-γ (Snapper & Paul, 1987), on the development of systemic autoimmunity. These models may be particularly relevant for the understanding of autoimmune phenomena occurring in man after bone-marrow transplantation (Rouquette-Gally *et al.*, 1988) or after administration of drugs (Kolb *et al.*, 1987).

Impairment of cytokine production in autoimmune diseases

Among the immunological abnormalities found in experimental and human SLE, T-cell deficiency is a common feature (Table 2). In lupus-prone mice, several T-cell defects have been reported, and particularly an impaired production of IL-2 in response to different stimuli (Altman *et al.*, 1981; Dauphinee *et al.*, 1981; Wofsy *et al.*, 1981). In human SLE, IL-2 secretion, expression of IL-2 receptors and T-cell proliferative responses to antigens or mitogens have been found to be impaired in the active stages of the disease (Alcocer-Varela & Alarcon-Segovia, 1982; Miyasaka *et al.*, 1984; Murakawa *et al.*, 1985). These findings may appear paradoxical, since Th cells have been found to play a crucial role in the pathogenesis of murine and human SLE (Wofsy & Seaman, 1985; Huang *et al.*, 1988; Santoro *et al.*, 1988) by providing activation signals to autoreactive B cells (see above and Table 2). On the other hand, IL-2 itself may be involved in the induction of autoimmune processes, as observed in bio-breeding rats and in nude mice injected with IL-2 (Reimann & Diamantstein, 1981; Kolb *et al.*, 1986; Kroemer *et al.*, 1986).

Two non-mutually exclusive phenomena could explain these associations between systemic autoimmunity and Th deficiency. First, experiments performed in a GVH model (Moser *et al.*, 1987) and in MRL/l mice (Via & Shearer, 1988a) indicated a selective impairment of CD4[+] cells producing IL-2 during MHC-self-restricted responses. This Th defect could be related to the presence of CD4[+] suppressor T cells, and Via and Shearer (1988b) suggested that these suppressor cells arise as a consequence of the autoimmune processes. As in host-*versus*-graft disease, the dissociation between IL-2 production and B-cell help could be related to the fact that these functions are exerted by different subsets of Th cells. Indeed, Via and Shearer (1988b) postulated that suppressor cells would act selectively on Th1 cells without affecting the function of Th2 cells. Secondly, some of the T-cell defects found in *vitro* may not reflect the T-cell status in *vivo*. Indeed, T cells that display markers of activation have a decreased ability to respond to mitogens in *vitro*, as shown in human SLE (Huang *et al.*, 1988) and in patients receiving haemodialysis (Chatenoud *et al.*, 1986). Along this line, Huang *et al* (1986) demonstrated that the defective secretion of IL-2 by circulating T cells of patients with SLE is restored when the cells are rested for a few days in culture. Moreover, the same authors reported high serum levels of IL-2 in SLE patients who display a decreased production of IL-2 in *vitro* (Huang *et al.*, 1988).

THERAPEUTIC PERSPECTIVES BASED ON THE PATHOBIOLOGY OF CYTOKINES

Since cytokines produced by Th appear to play a pivotal role in the pathophysiology of both organ-specific and systemic autoimmune diseases (Table 3), they represent interesting targets for the development of new strategies of immunosuppression.

(1) One may consider eliminating the cellular source of the cytokines by the use of anti-Th (anti-CD4) antibodies, as has been done in several murine models of autoimmune diseases (Wofsy, 1988). One major obstacle to the clinical application of such treatment is the development of host immune responses to the administered Igs (Chatenoud, 1986).

(2) One may act at the level of cytokine gene expression. The beneficial effects of glucocorticoids and cyclosporin A in autoimmune diseases may in part be related to this mechanism (Taniguchi, 1988).

(3) Antibodies that neutralize cytokine activities may be efficient, as illustrated by the effects of an anti-IFN-γ antibody in murine SLE (Jacob *et al.*, 1987).

(4) Blockage of cytokine receptors is another interesting approach, since it allows selective action on the cells involved in the autoimmune processes. Thus, a monoclonal anti-IL-2 receptor antibody has proved effective in murine diabetic insulitis and lupus nephritis by blocking activated T cells (Kelley *et al.*, 1988).

(5) As the induction of an increased or aberrant expression of Ia antigens appears to be an important mechanism by which cytokines contribute to the pathophysiology of autoimmune disease, modulation of Ia expression by drugs or antibodies represents another therapeutic strategy. In this respect, prostaglandins of the E series have been shown to

Table 3. Involvement of cytokines in experimental autoimmunity

Model[a]	Cytokine[b]	Reference
Murine thyroiditis	IFN-γ	Rémy et al. (1987)
Thyroiditis of OS chickens	IL-2	Kroemer & Wick (1989)
Spontaneous IDDM in NOD mice	IL-2	Kelley et al. (1988)
IDDM in transgeneic mice	IFN-γ	Sarvetnick et al. (1988)
MRL-lpr/lpr mice	IL-5	Rosenberg et al. (1986)
MRL-lpr/lpr mice	IL-4	Rosenberg et al. (1986)
(NZBxNZW)F1 mice	IL-2	Kelley et al. (1988)
(NZBxNZW)F1 mice	IFN-γ	Jacob et al. (1987)
Chronic murine graft-*versus*-host disease	IL-5	Dobashi et al. (1987
	IL-4	Doutrelepont et al. (1989)
Host-*versus*-graft disease in mice	IL-4	Goldman et al. (1989)
Mercury-induced auto-immunity in mice	IL-4	Ochel et al. (1989)

[a]OS, obese strain; IDDM, insulin-dependent diabetes mellitus; NOD, non-obese diabetic.
[b]IFN, interferon; IL, interleukin.

inhibit Ia expression on macrophages (Snyder et al., 1982) and were used successfully to treat murine and human SLE (Kelley et al., 1981; Nagayama et al., 1988). Similarly, glucocorticoids antagonize the effects of IFN-γ on the expression of MHC antigens (Leszczinski et al., 1986). Anti-Ia antibodies have been tested successfully in experimental allergic encephalomyelitis (Sriram & Steinmen, 1982), in NZB/W mice (Adelman et al., 1983), in experimental myasthenia gravis (Waldor et al., 1983) and in type-II collagen arthritis (Wooley et al., 1985). These antibodies may act by blocking the interactions between Th cells, B cells and antigen-presenting cells and also by depleting Ia-bearing cells (Wofsy, 1988).

(6) Finally, Jacob and Mc Devitt (1988) recently observed a defect in the production of tumour necrosis factor-α in NZB/W mice, and they found that replacement therapy with recombinant material induced a significant delay in the development of the renal lesions. This paradoxical observation of the beneficial effect of a potentially pathogenic cytokine exemplifies the complexity of the relations between the cytokine network and the occurrence of autoimmunity. A better understanding of these relations is obviously required before considering the development of cytokine-specific treatment in human autoimmune diseases.

ACKNOWLEDGEMENTS

This work was supported by the Fonds National de le Recherche Scientifique Médicale (Belgium) and the David and Alice van Buuren Foundation.

REFERENCES

Abramowicz, D., Goldman, M., Bruyns, C., Lambert, P.H., Thoua, Y. & Toussaint, C. (1987) Autoimmune disease after neonatal injection of semi-allogeneic spleen cells in mice; involvement of donor B and T cells and characterization of glomerular deposits. *Clin. exp. Immunol.*, **70**: 51-67

Adelman, N.E., Watling, D.L. & McDevitt, H.O. (1983) Treatment of (NZBxNZW)F1 disease with anti-I-A monoclonal antibodies. *J. exp. Med.*, **158**: 1350-1355

Alcocer-Varela, J. & Alarcon-Segovia, D. (1982) Decreased production of and response to interleukin 2 by cultured lymphocytes from patients with systemic lupus erythematosus. *J. clin. Invest.*, **69**: 1388-1392

Altman, A., Theofilopoulos A.N., Weiner, R., Katz, D.H. & Dixon, F.J. (1981) Analysis of T cell function in autoimmune murine strains. Defects in production of and responsiveness to interleukin-2. *J. exp. Med.*, **154**: 791-808

Ando, D.G., Sercarz, E.E. & Hahn, B.H. (1987) Mechanisms of T and B cell collaboration in the in vitro production of anti-DNA antibodies in the NZB/NZW F1 murine SLE model. *J. immunol.*, **138**: 3185-3190

Andrews, B.S., Eisenberg, R.A., Theofilopoulos, A.N., Izui, S., Wilson, C.B., McConahey, P.J., Murphy, E.D., Roths, J.B. & Dixon, F.J. (1978) Spontaneous murine lupus-like syndromes. Clinical and immunopathological manifestations in several strains. *J. exp. Med.*, **148**: 1198-1215

Benacerraf, B. (1985) Significance and biological function of class II MHC molecules. *Am. J. Pathol.*, **120**: 334-343

Bendelac A., Carnaud, C., Boitard, C. & Bach, J.F. (1987) Syngeneic transfer of autoimmune diabetes from diabetic NOD mice to healthy neonates. *Am. J. Pathol.*, **166**: 823-831

Billingham, R.W. & Brent, L. (1959) Quantitative studies on tissue transplantation immunity. IV. Induction of tolerance in newborn mice and studies on the phenomenon of runt disease. *Philos. Trans. R. Soc. Lond. (Biol. Sci.)*, **242**: 439-477

Blaese, R.M., Grayson J. & Steinberg, A.D. (1980) Elevated immunoglobulin secreting cells in the blood of patients with active systemic lupus erythematosus: correlation of laboratory and clinical assessment of disease activity. *Am. J. Med.*, **69**: 345-350

Boitard, C., Chatenoud, L.M. & Debray-Sachs, M. (1982) In vitro inhibition of pancreatic B cells by T lymphocytes in diabetes. *J. Immunol.*, **129**: 2529-2531

Bottazzo, G.F., Pujol-Borell, R., Hanafusa, T. & Feldmann, M. (1983) Role of aberrant HLA-DR expression and antigen presentation in induction of endocrine autoimmunity. *Lancet*, **ii**: 1115-1119

Bottazzo, G.F., Dean, B.M., McNally, J.M., MacKay, E.H., Swift, P.G.F. & Gamble, D.R. (1985) In situ characterization of autoimmune phenomena and expression of HLA molecules in the pancreas in diabetic insulitis. *New Engl. J. Med.*, **313**: 353-360

Bottazzo, G.F., Todd, I., Mirakian, R., Belfoire, A. & Pujol-Borrell, R. (1986) Organ-specific autoimmunity: a 1986 overview. *Immunol. Rev.*, **94**: 137-169

Brent, L., Brooks, C.G., Medawar, P.B. & Simpson, E. (1976) Transplantation tolerance. *Br. med. Bull.*, **32**: 101-106

Bruijn, J.A., Van Elven, E.H., Hogendoorn, P.C.W., Corver, W.E., Hoedemaeker, P.J. & Fleuren, G.J. (1988) Murine chronic graft-versus-host disease as a model for lupus nephritis. *Am. J. Pathol.*, **130**: 639-641

Campbell, I.L., Bizilj, K., Colman, P.G., Tuch, B.E. & Harrison, L.C. (1986) Interferon-gamma induces HLA-A, B, C but not HLA-DR on human pancreatic B cells. *J. clin. Endocrinol. Metab.*, **62**: 1101-1109

Campbell, I.L., Iscaro, A. & Harrison, L.C. (1988a) Interferon-gamma and tumor necrosis factor-alpha: cytotoxicity to murine islets of Langerhans. *J. Immunol.*, **141**: 2325-2329

Cambell, I.L., Oxbrow, L., Koulmanda, M. & Harrison, L.C. (1988b) Interferon-gamma induces islet cell MHC antigens and enhances autoimmune, streptozotocin-induced diabetes in the mouse. *J. Immunol.*, **140**: 1111-1115

Chatenoud, L. (1986) The immune response against therapeutic monoclonal antibodies. *Immunol. Today*, **7**: 367-368

Chatenoud, L., Dugas, B., Beaurain, G., Touam, M., Drueke, T., Vasquez, A., Galanaud, P., Bach, J.F. & Delfraissy, J.F. (1986) Presence of preactivated T cells in hemodialyzed patients: their possible role in altered immunity. *Proc. natl Acad. Sci. USA*, **83**: 7457-7461

Craighead, J.E. & McLane, M.F. (1968) Diabetes mellitus: induction in mice by encephalomyocarditis virus. *Science*, **162**: 913-914

Cruse, J.M. & Lewis, R.E. (1985). Contemporary concepts of autoimmunity. *Concepts Immunopathol.*, **1**: 1-31

Datta, S.K., Patel, H. & Berry, D. (1987) Induction of a cationic shift in IgG anti-DNA antibodies. Role of T helper cells with classical and novel phenotypes in three murine models of lupus nephritis. *J. exp. Med.*, **165**: 1252-1268

Dauphinee, M.J., Kipper, S.B., Wofsy, D. & Talal, N. (1981) Interleukin 2 deficiency is a common feature of autoimmune mice. *J. Immunol.*, **127**: 2483-2487

Dean, B.M., Walker, R., Boen, A.J., Baird, J.D. & Cooke, A. (1985) Prediabetes in the spontaneously diabetic BB/E rat: lymphocyte subpopulations in the pancreatic infiltrate and expression of rat MHC class II molecules in endocrine cells. *Diabetologia*, **28**: 464-466

De Maeyer E. & De Maeyer-Guignard, J. (1988) *Interferons and Other Regulatory Cytokines*, New York, Wiley

Dinarello, C.A. & Wyer, J.W. (1987) Current concepts: lymphokines. *New Engl. J. Med.*, **317**: 940-845

Dobashi, K., Ono, S., Murakami, S., Takahama, Y., Katoh, Y. & Hamaoka, T. (1987) Polyclonal B cell activation by a B cell differentiation factor, B151-TRF2. III. B151-TRF2 as a B cell differentiation factor closely associated with autoimmune disease. *J. Immunol.*, **138**: 780-787

Doberson, M. (1985) Humural autoimmune aspects of insulin-dependent (type I) diabetes mellitus. *Concepts Immunopathol.*, **2**: 47-64

Dorf, M.E. & Benacerraf, B. (1984) Suppressor cells and immunoregulation. *Ann. Rev. Immunol.*, 2:127-157

Dwyer, D.S., Vakil, M. & Kearney, J.F. (1986) Idiotypic network connectivity and a possible cause of myasthenia gravis. *J. exp. Med.*, **164**: 1310-1319

Eisenbarth, G.S. (1986) Type I diabetes mellitus: a chronic autoimmune disease. *New Engl. J. Med.*, **314**: 1360-1368

Engleman, E.G., Sonnenfeld, G., Dauphinee, M., Greenspan J.S., Talal, N., McDevitt, H.O. & Merigan, T.C. (1981) Treatment of NZW Fl mice with mycobacterium bovis strain BCG or type II interferon preparations accelerates autoimmune disease. *Arthritis Rheum.*, **24**: 1396-1402

Eyster, M.E., Goedert, J.J., Poon, M.C. & Preble, O.T. (1983) Acid-labile alpha interferon: a possible preclinical marker for the acquired immunodeficiency syndrome in hemophilia. *New Engl. J. Med.*, **309**: 583-586

Feldmann, M. (1988) Regulation of HLA class II expression and its role in autoimmune diseases. In: Evered, D. & Whelan, W., eds, *Autoimmunity and Autoimmune Disease* (*Ciba Foundation Symposium 129*), Chichester, Wiley, pp. 88-97

Feng, H.M., Glasebrook, A.L., Engers, H.D. & Louis, J.A. (1983) Clonal analysis of T cell unresponsiveness to alloantigens induced by neonatal injection of Fl spleen cells into parental mice. *J. Immunol.*, **131**: 2165-2169

Foulis, A.K. & Farquharson, M.A. (1986) Aberrant expression of HLA-DR antigens by insulin-containing beta-cells in recent-onset type I diabetes mellitus. *Diabetes*, **35**: 1215-1224

Fournié, G.J. (1988) Circulating DNA and lupus nephritis. *Kidney Int.*, **33**: 487-497

Francfort, J.W., Barker, C.F., Kimura, H., Silvers, W.K., Frohman, M. & Naji, A. (1985) Increased incidence of Ia antigen-bearing T lymphocytes in the spontaneously diabetic BB rat. *J. Immunol.*, **134**: 1577-1582

Gaulton, G.N. & Greene, M.I. (1986) Idiotypic mimicry of biological receptors. *Ann. Rev. Immunol.*, **4**: 253-280

Gepts, W. & Lecompte, P.M. (1981) The pancreatic islets in diabetes. *Am. J. Med.*, **70**: 105-115

Gleichmann, E., Van Elven, E.H. & Van der Veen, J.P.W. (1982) A systemic lupus erythematosus (SLE)-like disease in mice induced by abnormal T-B cell cooperation. Preferential formation of autoantibodies characteristic of SLE. *Eur. J. Immunol.*, **12**: 152-159

Gleichmann, E., Pals, S.T., Rolink, A.G., Radaskiewicz, T. & Gleichmann, H. (1984) Graft-versus-host reactions: clues to the etiology of a spectrum of immunological diseases. *Immunol. Today*, **5**: 324-332

Goldman, M., Feng, H.M., Engers, H., Hochmann, A., Louis, J. & Lambert, P.H. (1983) Autoimmunity and immune complex disease after neonatal induction of transplantation tolerance in mice. *J. Immunol.*, **131**: 251-258

Goldman, M., Abramowicz, D., Lambert, P., Van der Vorst, P., Bruyns, C. & Toussaint, C. (1988a) Hyperactivity of donor B cells after neonatal induction of lymphoid chimerism in mice. *Clin. exp. Immunol.*, **72**: 79-83

Goldman, M., Baran, D. & Druet, P. (1988) Polyclonal activation and experimental nephropathies. *Kidney Int.*, **34**: 141-150

Goldman, M., Van der Vorst, P., Lambert, P., Doutrelepont, J.M., Bruyns, C. & Abramowicz, D. (1989) Persistence of allohelper T cells secreting interleukin-4 after neonatal induction of transplantation tolerance. *Transplant. Proc.*, **21**: 238-239

Gutierrez, C., Howard, M., Gaspar, M.L. & Raveche, E.S. (1986) Differential proliferative responses of B cells from Balb/c and autoimmune NZB mice to B-cell growth factor(s). *Clin. Immunol. Immunopathol.*, **39**: 319-328

Hanafusa, T., Pujol-Borrel, R., Chovato, L., Russell, R.C.G., Doniach, D. & Bottazzo, G.F. (1983) Aberrant expression of HLA-DR antigen on thyrocytes in Graves' disease: relevance for autoimmunity. *Lancet*, **ii**: 1111-1115

Hayakawa, K., Hardy, R.R., Honda, M., Herzenberg, L.A., Steinberg, A.D. & Herzenberg, L.A. (1984) Ly-1 B cells: functionally distinct lymphocytes that secrete IgM autoantibodies. *Proc. natl Acad. Sci. USA*, **81**: 2494-2498

Heremans, S., Billiau, A., Colombatti, A., Hilgers, J. & De Somer, P. (1978) Interferon treatment of NZB mice: accelerated progression of autoimmune disease. *Infect. Immun.*, **21**: 925-930

Herron, L.R., Coffman, R.L. & Kotzin, B.L. (1988) Enhanced response of autoantibody-secreting B cells from young NZB/NZW mice to T cell-derived differentiation signals. *Clin. Immunol. Immunopathol.*, **46**: 314-327

Hirano, T., Taga, T., Yasukawa, K., Nakajima, K., Nakano, N., Takatsuki, F., Shimizu, M., Murashima, A., Tsunasawa, S., Sakiyama, F. & Kishimoto, T. (1987) Human B cell differentiation factor defined by an anti-peptide antibody and its possible role in autoantibody production. *Proc. natl Acad. Sci. USA*, **84**: 228-231

Huang, S.W. & MacLaren, N.K. (1981) Insulin-dependent diabetes. A disease of autoaggression. *Science*, **21**: 41-46

Huang, Y.P., Miescher, P.A. & Zubler, R.H. (1986) The interleukin 2 secretion defect in vitro in systemic lupus erythematosus is reversible in rested cultured cells. *J. Immunol.*, **137**: 3515-3520

Huang, Y.P., Perrin, L.H., Miescher, P.A. & Zubler, R.H (1988) Correlation of T and B cell activities in vitro and serum IL-2 levels in systemic lupus eryhtematosus. *J. Immunol.*, **141**: 827-833

Izui, S., McConahey, P.J. & Dixon, F.J. (1978) Increased spontaneous polyclonal activation of B lymphocytes in mice with spontaneous autoimmune disease. *J. Immunol.*, **121**: 2213-2219

Jackson, R.A., Morris, M.A., Haynes, B.F. & Eisenbarth, G.S. (1982) Increased circulating Ia-antigen-bearing T cells in type I diabetes mellitus. *New Engl. J. Med.*, **306**: 785-788

Jacob, C.D. & McDevitt, H.O. (1988) Tumour necrosis factor-alpha in murine autoimmune lupus nephritis. *Nature*, **331**: 356-358

Jacob, C.D., van der Meicle, P.H. & McDevitt, H.O. (1987) In vivo treatment of (NZBxNZW) F1 lupus-like nephritis with monoclonal antibody to gamma-interferon *J. exp. Med.*, **166**: 798-803

Jasin, H.E. & Ziff, M. (1975) Immunoglobulin synthesis by peripheral blood cells in systemic lupus erythematosus. *Arthritis Rheum.*, **18**: 219-228

Jenson, A.B., Rosenberg, H.S. & Notkins, A.L. (1980) Virus-induced diabetes mellitus. XVII. Pancreatic islet cell damage in children with fatal viral infections. *Lancet*, **ii**: 354-358

Kelley, V.E. & Roths, J.B. (1982) Increase in macrophage Ia expression in autoimmune mice: role of the lpr gene. *J. Immunol.*, **129**: 923-925

Kelley, V.E., Winkelstein, A., Izui, S. & Dixon, F.J. (1981) Prostaglandin El inhibits T-cell proliferation and renal disease in MRL/l mice. *Clin. Immunol. Immunopathol.*, **21**: 190-195

Kelley, V.E., Gaulton, G.N., Hattori, M., Ikegami, H., Eisenbarth, G. & Strom, T.B. (1988) Anti-interleukin 2 receptor antibody suppresses murine diabetic insulitis and lupus nephritis. *J. Immunol.*, **140**: 59-61

Kincade, P.W., Lee, G., Fernandes, G., Moore, M.A.S., Williams, N. & Good, R.A. (1979) Abnormalities in clonable B lymphocytes and myeloid progenitors in autoimmune NZB mice. *Proc. natl Acad. Sci. USA*, **76**: 3464-3468

Kishimoto, T. & Hirano, T. (1988) Molecular regulation of B lymphocyte response. *Ann. Rev. Immunol.*, **6**: 485-512

Klinman, D.S. & Steinberg, A.D. (1987) Systemic autoimmune disease arises from polyclonal B cell activation. *J. exp. Med.*, **165**: 1755-1760

Kolb, H., Zielasek, J., Treichel, U., Freytag, G., Wrann, M., & Kiesel, U. (1986) Recombinant interleukin-2 enhances spontaneous insulin-dependent diabetes in BB rats. *Eur. J. Immunol.*, **16**: 209-212

Kolb, U., Toyka, K.V. & Gleichmann, E. (1987) Histocompatibility antigens and chemical reactivity in autoimmunity. *Immunol. Today*, **8**: 3-6

Kopelman, R.G. & Zolla-Paznzer, S. (1988) Association of human immunodeficiency virus infection and autoimmune phenomena. *Am. J. Med.*, **84**: 82-88

Kroemer, G. & Wick, G. (1989) The role of interleukin-2 in autoimmunity. *Immunol. Today*, **10**: 246-251

Kroemer, G., Schauenstein, K. & Wick, G. (1986) Is autoimmunity a side-effect of interleukin 2 production? *Immunol. Today*, **7**: 199-200

Kumagai, S., Sredni, B., House, S., Steinberg, A.D. & Green, I. (1982) Defective regulation of B lymphocyte colony formation in patients with systemic lupus erythematosus. *J. Immunol.*, **128**: 258-262

Leibson, H.J., Gefter, M., Zlotnik, A., Marrack, P. & Kappler, J.W. (1984) Role of gamma-interferon in antibody-producing responses. *Nature*, **309**: 799-802

Leszczinski, D., Ferry, B., Schellekens, H., Meide, P.H. & Hayry, P. (1986) Antagonistic effects of gamma-interferon and steroids on tissue antigenicity. *J. exp. Med.*, **164**: 1470-1477

Lewis, R.M., Armstrong, M.Y.K., André-Schwartz, J., Muftouglu, A., Beldotti, L. & Schwartz, R.S. (1968) Chronic allogeneic disease. I. Development of glomerulonephritis. *J. exp. Med.*, **128**: 653-679

Londei, M., Lamb, J.R., Bottazzo, G.F. & Feldmann, M. (1984) Epithelial cells expressing aberrant MHC class II determinants can present antigen to cloned human T cells. *Nature*, **312**: 639-641

Londei, M., Bottazzo, G.F. & Feldmann, M. (1985) Human T cell clones from autoimmune thyroid gland: specific recognition of autologous thyroid cells. *Science*, **228**: 85-89

Lu, C.Y. & Unanue, E.R. (1982) Spontaneous T cell lymphokine production and enhanced macrophage Ia expression and tumoricidal activity in MRL-lpr/lpr mice. *Clin. Immunol. Immunopathol.*, **25**: 213-22

Luzuy, S., Merino, J., Engers, H., Izui, S. & Lambert, P.H. (1986) Autoimmunity after induction of neonatal tolerance to alloantigens: role of B cell chimerism and F1 donor B cell activation. *J. Immunol.*, **136**: 4420-4426

Mandrup-Poulsen, T., Bendtzen, K., Nielsen, J.H., Bendixen, G. & Nerup, J. (1985) Cytokines cause functional and structural damage to isolated islets of Langerhans. *Allergy*, **40**: 424-429

Maugh,T.H. (1975) Diabetes: epidemiology suggests a viral connection. *Science*, **188**: 347-351

Merino, J., Schurmans, S., Luzuy, S., Izui, S., Vassalli, P. & Lambert, P.H. (1987) Autoimmune syndrome after induction of neonatal tolerance to alloantigens. Effects of in vivo treatment with anti-T cell subset monoclonal antibodies. *J. Immunol.*, **139**: 1426-1431

Miyasaka, N., Nakamura, T., Russel, I.J. & Talal, N. (1984) Interleukin-2 deficiencies in rheumatoid arthritis and systemic lupus erythematosus. *Clin. Immunol. Immunopathol.*, **31**: 109-117

Morse, H.C., Davidson, W.F., Yetter, R.A., Murphy, E., Roths, J.B. & Coffman, R.L. (1982) Abnormalities induced by the mutant gene lpr: expansion of a unique lymphocyte subset. *J. Immunol.*, **129**: 2612-2615

Moser, M., Mizouchi, T., Sharrow, S.O., Singer, A.S. & Shearer, G.M. (1987) Graft-vs-host reaction limited to a class II MHC difference results in a selective deficiency in L3T4 but not in Lyt-2 helper T cell function. *J. Immunol.*, **138**: 1355-1364

Mossman, T.R. & Coffman, R.L. (1987) Two types of mouse helper T cell clones: implications for immune regulation. *Immunol. Today*, **8**: 223-227

Mowat, A.M. (1985) Interferon and class II MHC expression in autoimmunity. *Lancet*, **ii**: 283

Murakami, S., Ono, S., Harada, N., Hara, Y., Katoh, Y., Dobashi, K., Takatsu, K. & Hamaoka, T. (1988) T Cell-derived factor Bl5l-TRFl/IL-5 activates blastoid cells among unprimed B cells to induce a polyclonal differentiation into immunoglobulin M-secreting cells. *Immunology*, **65**: 221-228

Murakawa, Y., Takada, S., Ueda, Y., Suzuki, N., Hoshino, T. & Sakane, T. (1985) Characterization of T lymphocyte subpopulations responsible for deficient interleukin 2 activity in patients with systemic lupus erythematosus. *J. Immunol.*, **134**: 187-195

Nagayama, Y., Namura, Y., Tamura, T. & Muso, R. (1988) Beneficial effect of prostaglandin El in three cases of lupus nephritis with nephrotic syndrome. *Ann. Allergy*, **61**: 289-295

Nerup, J., Andersen, O.O., Bendixen, G., Egeverg, J. & Poulsen, J.E. (1971) Antipancreatic cellular hypersensitivity in diabetes mellitus. *Diabetes*, **20**: 424-427

Nossal, G.J.V. (1983) Cellular mechanisms of immunologic tolerance. *Ann. Rev. Immunol.*, **1**: 33-62

Ochel, M., Pfeiffer, C., Vohr, H.-W. & Gleichmann, E. (1989) The increased IgE formation inducible by mercuric chloride is inhibited by anti-IL-4. In: *7th International Congress of Immunology, July 30 - August 5, 1989, Berlin (West), Abstracts,* Stuttgart, Gustav Fischer, Abstract 75-27

Oldstone, M.B.A., Southern, P., Rodriguez, M. & Lampert, P. (1984) Virus persists in B cells of islets of Langerhans and is associated with chemical manifestations of diabetes. *Science*, **224**: 1440-1442

Onodera, T., Ray, U.R., Melez, K.A., Suzuki, H., Toniolo, A. & Notkins, A.L. (1982) Virus-induced diabetes mellitus: autoimmunity and polyendocrine disease prevented by immunosuppression. *Nature*, **297**: 66-68

Paul, W.E. & Ohara, J. (1987) B Cell-stimulatory factor-l or interleukin-4. *Ann. Rev. Immunol.*, **5**: 429-459

Philip, R. & Epstein, L.B. (1986) Tumour necrosis factor as immunomodulator and mediator of monocyte cytotoxicity induced by itself, gamma-interferon and interleukin-l. *Nature*, **323**: 86-89

Pincus, T. (1982) Studies regarding a possible function for viruses in the pathogenesis of systemic lupus erythematosus. *Arthritis Rheum.*, **25**: 847-856

Preble, O.T., Black, R.J., Friedman, R.M., Klippel, J.H. & Vilcek, J. (1982) Systemic lupus erythematosus: presence in human serum of an unusual acid-labile leukocyte interferon. *Science*, **216**: 429-431

Prud'homme, G.J. & Palfrey, N.A. (1988) Biology of disease: role of T helper lymphocytes in autoimmune diseases. *Lab. Invest.*, **59**: 158-172

Prud'homme, G.J., Balderas, R.S., Dixon, F.J. & Theofilopoulos, A.N. (1983a) B Cell dependence on and response to accessory signals in murine lupus strains. *J. exp. Med.*, **157**: 1815-1827

Prud'homme, G.J., Park, C.L., Fieser, T.M., Kofler, R., Dixon, F.J. & Theofilopoulos, A.N. (1983b) Identification of a B cell differentiation factor(s) spontaneously produced by proliferating T cells in murine lupus strains of the lpr/lpr genotype. *J. exp. Med.*, **157**: 730-742

Pujol-Borrell, R., Todd, I., Doshi, M., Bottazzo, G.F., Sutton, R., Gray, D., Adolf, G.R. & Feldman, M. (1987) HLA class II induction in human islet cells by interferon-gamma plus tumour necrosis factor or lymphotoxin. *Nature*, **326**: 304-306

Purkerson, J.M., Newberg, M., Wise, G., Lynch, K.R. & Isakson, P.C. (1988) Interleukin 5 and interleukin 2 cooperate with interleukin 4 to induce IgGl secretion from anti-Ig-treated B cells. *J. exp. Med.*, **168**: 1175-1180

Reimann, J. & Diamantstein, T. (1981) Interleukin-2 allows in vivo induction of anti-erythrocyte autoantibody production in nude mice in association with the injection of rat erythrocytes. *Clin. exp. Immunol.*, **43**: 641-644

Rémy, J.J., Salamero, J., Michel-Bechet, M. & Charriere, J. (1987) Experimental auto-immune thyroiditis induced by recombinant interferon-gamma. *Immunol. Today*, **8**: 73

Revel, M. & Schattner, A. (1987) Interferons: cytokines in autoimmunity. In: Evered, D. & Whelan, W., eds, *Autoimmunity and Autoimmune Disease (Ciba Foundation Symposium 129),* Chichester, Wiley, pp. 223-229

Rich, S.A. (1981) Human lupus inclusions and interferon. *Science*, **213**: 772-775

Rolink, A.G., Pals, S.T. & Gleichmann, E. (1983a) Allosuppressor and allohelper T cells in acute and chronic graft-versus-host disease. II. Fl recipients carrying mutations at H-2K and/or I-A. *J. exp. Med.*, **157**: 755-771

Rolink, A.G., Pals, S.T. & Gleichmann, E. (1983b) Allosuppressor and allohelper T cells in acute and chronic graft-versus-host disease. III. Different Lyt subsets of donor T cells induce different pathological syndromes. *J. exp. Med.*, **158**: 546-558

Romball, C.G. & Weigle, W.O. (1987) Transfer of experimental autoimmune thyroiditis with T cell clones. *J. Immunol.*, **138**: 1092-1097

Rosenberg, Y.J., Steinberg, A.D. & Santoro, T.J. (1984a) T Cells from autoimmune IL2 defective MRL-lpr/lpr mice continue to grow in vitro and produce IL2 constitutively. *J. Immunol.*, **133**: 2545-2548

Rosenberg, Y.J., Steinberg, A.D. & Santoro, T.J. (1984b) The basis of autoimmunity in MRL-lpr/lpr mice: a role for self Ia-reactive T cells. *Immunol. Today*, **5**: 64-67

Rosenberg, Y.J., Goldsmith, P.K., Ohara, J., Steinberg, A.D. & Ohriner, W. (1986) Ia antigen expression and autoimmunity in MRL-lpr/lpr mice. *Ann. N.Y. Acad. Sci.*, **475**: 251-265

Rouquette-Gally, A.M., Boyeldieu, D., Prost, A.C. & Gluckman, E. (1988) Autoimmunity after allogeneic bone marrow transplantation. A study of 53 long-term-surviving patients. *Transplantation*, **46**: 238-240

Santoro, T.J., Benjamin, W.R., Oppenheim, J.J. & Steinberg, A.D. (1983) The cellular basis for immune interferon production in autoimmune MRL-lpr/lpr mice. *J. Immunol.*, **131**: 265-268

Santoro, T.J., Lotzin, T.R., Malek, T.R. & Lehmann, K.R. (1985) Interleukin 2 as a proliferative signal for autoimmune B cells. *Fed. Proc.*, **44**: 603

Santoro, T.J., Portnova, J.P. & Kotzin, B.L. (1988) The contribution of L3T4+ cells to lymphoproliferation and autoantibody production in MRL-lpr/lpr mice. *J. exp. Med.*, **167**: 1713-1719

Sarvetnick, N., Liggit, D., Pitts, S.L., Hansen, S.E. & Stewart, T.A. (1988) Insulin-dependent diabetes mellitus induced in transgenic mice by ectopic expression of class II MHC and interferon-gamma. *Cell*, **52**: 773-782

Schattner, A. (1988) Review: interferons and autoimmunity. *Am. J. med. Sci.*, **295**: 532-544

Seitz, M., Franke, M. & Kirchner, H. (1988) Induction of antinuclear antibodies in patients receiving treatment with human recombinant interferon gamma. *Ann. rheum. Dis.*, **47**: 642-644

Sharpe, A.H. & Fields, N. (1985) Pathogenesis of viral infections. Basic concepts derived from the reovirus model. *New Engl. J. Med.*, **312**: 486-497

Sibley, R.K., Sutherland, D.E.R., Goetz, F. & Michael, A.K. (1985) Recurrent diabetes mellitus in the pancreas iso- and allograft. *Lab. Invest.*, **63**: 132-138

Sidman, C.L., Marshall, J.D., Shulz, L.D., Gray, P.W. & Johnson, H.M. (1984) Gamma-interferon is one of several B cell-maturing lymphokines. *Nature*, **309**: 801-803

Smith, H.R. & Steinberg, A.D. (1983) Autoimmunity. A perspective. *Ann. Rev. Immunol.*, **1**: 175-210

Snapper, C. & Paul, W.E (1987) Interferon-gamma and B cell stimulatory factor-1 reciprocally regulate Ig isotype production. *Science*, **236**: 944-947

Snyder, D.S., Beller, D.I. & Unanue, E.R. (1982) Prostaglandins modulate macrophage Ia expression. *Nature*, **299**: 163-165

Sriram, S. & Steinman, L. (1982) Anti-I-A antibody suppresses active encephalomyelitis. *J. exp. Med.*, **158**: 1362-1367

Stasny, P., Ball, E.J., Dry, P.J. & Nunez, G. (1983) The human immune response region (HLA-D) and disease susceptibility. *Immunol. Rev.*, **70**: 11-153

Taniguchi, T. (1988) Regulation of cytokine gene expression. *Ann. Rev. Immunol.*, **6**: 439-464

Theofilopoulos, A.N. & Dixon F.J. (1985) Murine models of systemic lupus erythematosus. *Adv. Immunol.*, **37**: 269-390

Theofilopoulos, A.N., Shawler D.L., Eisenberg, R.A. & Dixon F.J. (1980) Splenic immunoglobulin secreting cells and their regulation in autoimmune mice. *J. exp. Med.*, **158**: 446-466

Todd, I., Pujol-Borrell, R., Hammond, L.J., Bottazzo, G.F. & Feldmann, M. (1985) Interferon-gamma induces HLA-DR expression by thyroid epithelium. *Clin. exp. Immunol.*, **61**: 265-273

Todd, I., Pujol-Borrell, R., Hammond, L.J., McNally, J.M., Feldmann, M. & Bottazzo, G.F. (1987) Enhancement of thyrocyte class II expression by thyroid stimulating hormone. *Clin. exp. Immunol.*, **69**: 524-531

Trinchieri, G. & Perussia, B. (1985) Immune interferon: a pleiotropic lymphokine with multiple effects. *Immunol. Today*, **6**: 131-136

Via, C.S. & Shearer, G.M. (1988a) T Cell interactions in autoimmunity: insights from a murine model of graft-versus-host disease. *Immunol. Today*, **9**: 207-213

Via, C.S. & Shearer, G.M. (1988b) Functional heterogeneity of L3T4+ cells in MRL-lpr/lpr mice. L3T4+ cells suppress major histocompatibility complex-self-restricted L3T4+ T helper cell function in association with autoimmunity. *J. exp. Med.*, **168**: 2165-2181

Volk, H.D., Kopp, J., Korner, J., Jahn, S., Grunow, R., Barthelmes, H. & Fiebig, H. (1986) Correlation between the phenotype and the functional capacity of activated T cells in patients with active systemic lupus erythematosus. *Scand. J. Immunol.*, **24**: 109-114

Volpé, R. (1987) Immunoregulation in autoimmune thyroid disease. *New Engl. J. Med.*, **316**: 44-46

Waldor, M.K., Sriram, S., McDevitt, H.O. & Steinman, L. (1983) In vivo therapy with monoclonal anti-I-A antibody suppresses responses to acetylcholine receptor. *Proc. natl Acad. Sci. USA*, **80**: 2713-2717

Wofsy, D. (1988) Treatment of autoimmune diseases with monoclonal antibodies. *Prog. Allergy*, **45**: 106-120

Wofsy, D. & Seaman, E. (1985) Successful treatment of autoimmunity in NZB/W Fl mice with monoclonal antibody to L3T4. *J. exp. Med.*, **161**: 378-391

Wofsy, D., Murphy, E.D., Roths, J.B., Dauphinee, M.J., Kipper, S.B. & Talal, N. (1981) Deficient interleukin 2 activity in MRL/Mp and C57Bl/6J mice bearing the lpr gene. *J. exp. Med.*, **154**: 1671-1679

Wooley, P.H., Luthra, H.S., Lafuse, W.P., Huse, A., Stuart, J.M. & David, C.S. (1985) Type-II collagen-induced arthritis in mice. III. Suppression of arthritis by using monoclonal and polyclonal anti-Ia antisera. *J. Immunol.*, **134**: 2366-2371

Yoon, J.W., Austin, M., Onodera, T. & Notkins, A.L. (1979) Virus-induced diabetes mellitus: isolation of a virus from the pancreas of a child with diabetic ketoacidosis. *New Engl. J. Med.*, **300**: 1176-1179

IMMUNOLOGICALLY MEDIATED
MANIFESTATIONS OF METALS

L. Pelletier, H. Tournade & P. Druet

INSERM U 28, Hopital Brôussais
75674 Paris Cedex 14, France

ABSTRACT

Exposure to metals is frequently responsible for immunological reactions. *In vitro*, almost all metals can modify the responses of T or B cells. Experimental models of metal-induced autoimmunity have been developed in rats, mice and guinea-pigs, and metal-induced autoreactive T cells have been found in most of them. These cells recognize either class-II (Ia) molecules encoded by the major histocompatibility complex and modified by the metal, native Ia molecules, or both. T-Cell clones have been obtained from patients with nickel contact dermatitis, and most of these also recognize nickel-modified Ia molecules. Some strains of rats and mice, such as Brown Norway rats and A.SW mice, are particularly prone to metal-induced autoimmunity and exhibit similar autoimmune manifestations after administration of mercury or gold.

INTRODUCTION

Several metals have immunologically mediated manifestations that are either organ specific or systemic; some metals may also be responsible for immunosuppression. In this review, we first report some known effects of metals on cells and particularly those that may be related to the occurrence of autoimmunity. Metal-induced autoimmunity is then considered. Manifestations in humans are described and then those in experimental models. A large section is devoted to the mechanisms that have been proposed. In the third part of the review, immunosuppression phenomena related to exposure to metals are discussed.

EFFECTS OF METALS ON CELL CONSTITUENTS

Physiologically, metals can bind covalently to several groups and play a role in numerous enzymatic reactions that are essential to the cell, such as Mg^{2+}-dependent ATPase, DNA polymerase with Zn^{2+} as a cofactor, and zinc finger proteins. The last molecules interact with DNA and play a role in the regulation of transcription (Helbecque & Henichart, 1988). Metals can modify cellular metabolism in several ways:

(1) Cationic metals may replace physiological cations and block corresponding enzymatic reactions (Passow, 1970); they may mimic the behaviour of protons, and anionic metals may replace ions (such as PO_4^{2-}) in chemical reactions.

(2) Metals may themselves catalyse enzymatic reactions (Passow, 1970).

(3) Cationic metals bind to sulfhydryl, phosphoryl, carboxyl and nitryl groups with different affinities: mercury and gold bind sulfhydryl groups with affinity constants of 10^{15-20} and 10^5, respectively (Simpson, 1961; Shaw, 1980). Mercury also has substantial affinity for chloride, hydroxyl, carboxyl and phosphoryl groups, with a constant of the order of 10^{15} or more (Passow, 1970; Clarkson 1972). Binding of a metal to a chemical group may have several consequences; the binding of metals to molecules with a free thiol group can modify

their physiological role in transport, secretory processes, interaction with hormones and cell activation. Thus, cell-surface thiol reactive sites play a role in the control of cell proliferation (Noelle & Lawrence, 1981). A thiol group has also been shown to play a crucial role in the function of some proton pumps (Motais & Sola, 1973); for example, heavy metals can inhibit glucose transport, and many enzymes (referred to by Reardon & Lucas, 1987) and mercurial compounds modulate water exchange and rates of proton flux (explaining their diuretic effect). It has been shown that mercurials can bind to the SH groups of a proton-pump and block it. Cationic metals can interfere with oxidases, reductases, peroxidases and glutathione. Lead binds more easily to phosphoryl than to sulfhydryl groups, which explains the fact that lead and mercury activate cells in different ways (Lawrence et al., 1987).

(4) Metals can act on lipid peroxidation of membrane phospholipids, modifying the red-ox activity of the cells and generating free sulfhydryl groups (Lawrence, 1985; Lawrence et al., 1987). In the same way, they can modulate prostaglandin synthesis and thus influence the immune response (Lawrence et al., 1987).

We will now try to correlate the ability of a metal to induce autoimmunity and its effect on protein kinase C and adenylate cyclase transduction systems (Figs 1 and 2). Metals can affect these activation pathways in different ways (Lawrence, 1985; Warner & Lawrence, 1986a,b; Lawrence et al., 1987; Warner & Lawrence, 1988). Lead, zinc and lithium act on the Ca^{2+}-dependent pathway, while mercurials preferentially act on the pH-dependent pathway (Fig. 1). Lead can stimulate brain protein kinase C even at picomolar concentrations while nanomolar concentrations of Ca^{2+} are required to activate this enzyme (Markovac & Goldstein, 1988). Chelation of cations (essentially Ca^{2+}) by ethylenediaminetetraacetic acid (EDTA) or ortho-phenantroline inhibits mitogen-induced T cell proliferation. This inhibition

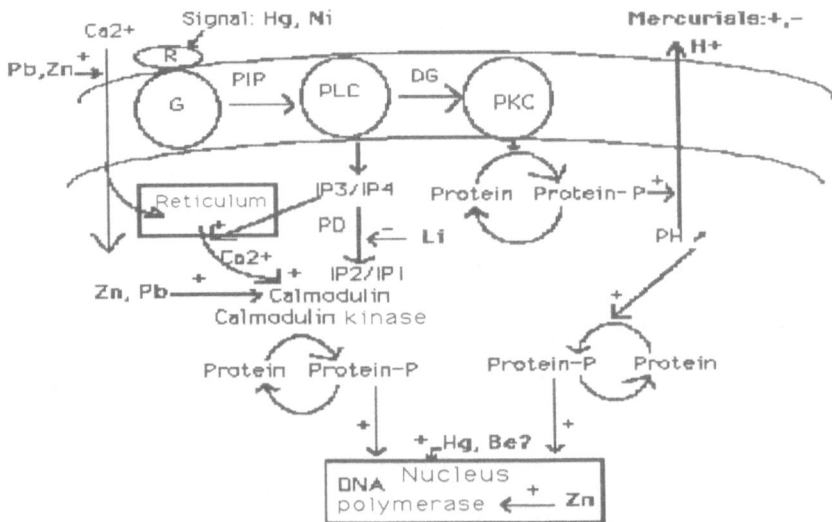

Fig. 1. Phosphatidyl inositol phosphate-mediated cell activation

Adapted from Isakov *et al.* (1986) and Enjalbert (1988). R, antigen receptor; PIP, phosphatidylinositol 4, 5-biphosphate; DG, diacylglycerol; G, GTP-binding protein; PLC, phospholipase C; PKC, phosphokinase C; IP$_3$, inositol 1,4,5-triphosphate; IP$_2$, inositol diphosphate; IP$_1$, inositol monophosphate; IP$_4$, inositol tetraphosphate; protein-P, phosphorylated protein. The binding between the ligand and the T-cell receptor activates PLC, which hydrolyses PIP into IP$_3$ and DG, the second cellular messengers. These trigger Ca- and pH-dependent phosphorylation of proteins, which can induce DNA replication.

is completely reversed by Ca²⁺ but also by Zn²⁺ and Pb²⁺ (Warner & Lawrence, 1986a), suggesting that Zn²⁺ and Pb²⁺ can mimic Ca²⁺ or can themselves deliver an activation signal to cells. Modulation of membrane phospholipids could also be involved in lead-induced lymphocyte activation (Lawrence et al., 1987) through production of a protooncogen or through protein kinase C (not shown in Fig. 1). Mercury and nickel could directly interact with T-cell receptor and activate T cells in the same way as antigens (Kapsenberg et al., 1988; Rossert et al., 1988). Mercurials can interfere with the transport of protons through the plasma membrane; they can block some proton pumps and enhance the permeability of membranes to protons (Pitterich & Lawaczeck, 1985). If mercurials enhance the permeation of T-cell membranes, they could interfere with the activation of pH-dependent kinases and modulate the production of phosphorylated proteins and DNA synthesis (Fig. 1). Lead and zinc may also increase the concentration of calmodulin, which is the substrate for calmodulin kinase (Warner & Lawrence, 1986a), an enzyme involved in the Ca-dependent phosphorylation of proteins and thus leading to an increase in DNA synthesis (Fig. 1). Calmodulin also increases phosphodiesterase activity, which allows inositol 1,4,5-triphosphate to be degraded to inositol diphosphate; the activation induced by lead and zinc could thus be antagonized by this process. Lithium inhibits the phosphodiesterase and prevents the transformation of inositol 1,4,5-triphosphate to inositol diphosphate and therefore increases the cytosol concentration of the former (Enjalbert, 1988). This molecule increases Ca release from the reticulum, which activates Ca-dependent protein kinases, phosphorylation of proteins and DNA synthesis (Isakov et al., 1986).

Little is known about interactions between metals and nuclear compounds; however, nuclear receptors have been described for mercury (Nordlind, 1984) and beryllium (Skilleter & Price, 1984). Zinc is a normal cofactor of DNA polymerase; exogenous zinc can increase the activity of this enzyme and promotes DNA synthesis (Warner & Lawrence, 1986a). Metals also play a role in the activation pathway through the adenylate cyclase-mediated phosphorylation of proteins (Fig. 2). Lithium can interfere with ion transport, since it can mimic Na⁺ in the Na-K membrane transport system (Isakov et al., 1986; Fig. 2). Lead, zinc and cadmium can inhibit membrane ouabain-sensitive ATPase, which may favour the

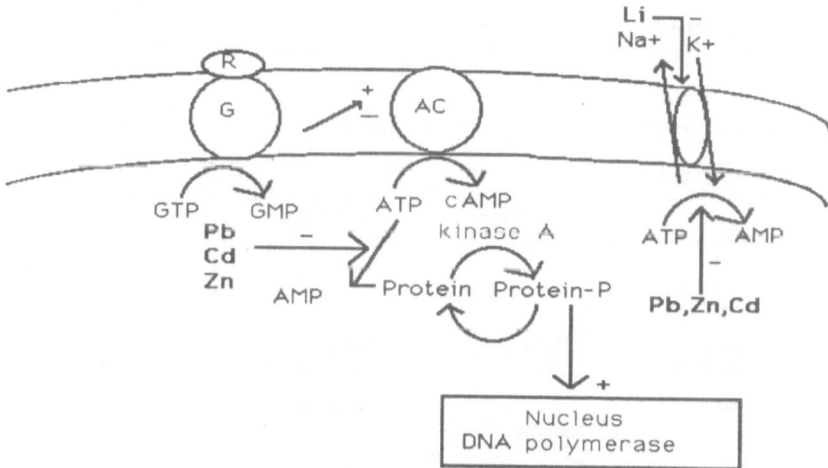

Fig. 2. Adenylate cyclase-mediated cell activation

Adapted from Enjalbert (1988). R, antigen receptor; G, GTP-binding protein; AC, adenylate cyclase; protein-P, phosphorylated protein. The binding of the ligand to its receptor activates adenylate cyclase, which generates cAMP. This in turn triggers kinase A-mediated protein phosphorylation.

transformation of ATP to cAMP and enhances kinase A-induced protein phosphorylation (Fig. 2). These phosphorylated proteins are involved in enzymatic activity, in ion transport and in the induction of DNA synthesis. It is of note, however, that inhibition of ATPase leads to cell death by blocking the ouabain-sensitive Na-K pump and the energetic metabolism of the cell.

We cannot review all the possible effects of metals on the metabolic pathways of cells, which depend upon the oxidative status of the metal, its concentration and the target cell. Therefore, it is nearly impossible to predict the net effect of a metal on a cell.

IMMUNOLOGICALLY MEDIATED MANIFESTATIONS OF METALS IN HUMANS

The skin and the kidney are the preferential targets of metals (Tables 1 and 2). Skin hypersensitivity has been described following exposure to nickel and chromium and also after beryllium, gold salts and mercurials (reviewed by Treagan, 1975). Interestingly, although nickel and chromium have been reported to be responsible for numerous cases of contact dermatitis, other organs seem to be spared: we found only one case report of nickel-induced glomerulopathy (Strauss & Eggleston, 1985). Pulmonary berylliosis is considered to be a manifestation of granulomatous hypersensitivity to beryllium (Reeves, 1983). Gold salts, mercurials and lithium salts have been associated with immunologically mediated manifestations, affecting mainly the kidney (Fillastre et al., 1988), which are described briefly.

Table 1. Metal-induced hypersensitivity and autoimmunity in man and animals

Metal	Effect in man	Effect in animals
Nickel	Contact dermatitis, glomerulonephropathy (?)	
Chromium	Contact dermatitis	Contact sensitivity (guinea-pig)
Beryllium	Contact dermatitis, pneumonitis (granulomas)	Contact sensitivity (guinea-pig)
Gold	Glomerulopathy, rashes, cytopenia, pneumonitis, hepatitis	Systemic autoimmunity (rat, mouse), glomerulopathy (rat, guinea-pig)
Mercurials	Contact dermatitis, glomerulopathy	Systemic autoimmunity (rat, mouse), glomerulopathy (rat, rabbit, mouse), contact sensitivity (guinea-pig)
Cadmium		Glomerulopathy (rat)
Lithium	Glomerulopathy, cardiomyopathy	

Table 2. Nephropathies associated with exposure to metals

Species	Nephropathy[a]				
	MGP	Anti-TBM[b]	Anti-GBM	MGC	ICGN
Human	Gold, mercurials, lithium		Mercurials	Gold, litthium	Nickel
Rat	Gold, mercurials	Gold, mercurials	Gold, mercurials		Cadmium
Rabbit	Mercurials		Mercurials		
Guinea-pig		Gold			Gold
Mouse					Gold, mercurials

[a]MGP, membranous glomerulopathy; anti-GBM (TBM), anti-glomerular (tubular) basement membrane-mediated glomerulonephritis; MGC, nephrotic syndrome with minimal glomerular changes; ICGN, immune complex type glomerulonephritis.
[b]Usually associated with MGP, anti-GBM or ICGN.

Proteinuria is observed in 6-17% of rheumatoid arthritis patients treated with gold salts. Most of them (89.5%) develop a membranous glomerulopathy, while the nephrotic syndrome with minimal glomerular changes is observed in 9.6% (reviewed by Fillastre *et al.*, 1988). The former manifestation is considered to be immune complex-mediated, while the latter is considered to be a T cell-mediated disease (Shaloub, 1974). Gold inclusions have been observed in both conditions, mainly in the lysosomes of epithelial cells of the proximal convoluted tubule and in glomerular cells (Shaw, 1980), but gold has not been co-localized with immune deposits in patients with membranous glomerulopathy (Watanabe *et al.*, 1976).

Proteinuria usually disappears following withdrawal of toxic exposure. Gold-induced proteinuria appears preferentially in patients with the DR3 antigen and among poor sulfoxidators (Wooley *et al.*, 1980). Gold salts can also induce fever, hypereosinophilia and rashes (Empire Rheumatism Council, Research Subcommottee, 1961). Cytopenia (anaemia, thrombopenia), pneumonitis and hepatitis have also been observed in patients treated with gold salts (Alcalay *et al.*, 1979; Coblyn *et al.*, 1981). These manifestations have been considered to be immunologically mediated, although thus has not been proven. Interestingly, an increase in total serum IgE level was reported in 10 of 11 patients with dermatological side-effects (Davis *et al.*, 1973).

Mercurials were used in the past as therapeutic agents, and several cases of mercury-induced membranous glomerulopathy have been published (reviewed by Fillastre *et al.*, 1988). Ointments containing mercury have also been reported to be responsible for immunologically mediated glomerulonephritis (Kibukamusoke *et al.*, 1974; Lindqvist *et al.*, 1974). Environmental and occupational exposure to mercury appear to induce similar manifestations (Fillastre *et al.*, 1988). A few cases of the nephrotic syndrome with minimal glomerular changes have also been reported (reviewed by Fillastre *et al.*, 1988). This metal is also known to induce contact hypersensitivity (Treagan, 1975).

Finally, lithium salts have been reported to be associated with the occurrence of the nephrotic syndrome with minimal glomerular changes and with one case of membranous glomerulopathy (reviewed by Fillastre *et al.*, 1988) and a few of myocardiopathy.

EXPERIMENTAL MODELS OF METAL-INDUCED AUTOIMMUNITY

Mercurials and gold salts are the most widely used metals in developing experimental models (Tables 2 and 3).

Table 3. Mercury- and gold-induced autoimmunity in rats and mice

Observation	Rat		Mouse	
	Mercury	Gold	Mercury	Gold
Autoimmunity				
Lymphoproliferation	+	+	+	+
Hyperimmunoglobulin (IgE)	+	+	+	+
Anti-nuclear antibodies	+	+	+	+
Anti-glomerular basement membrane antibodies	+	+	+	?
Autoimmune glomerulonephritis	+	+	+	+
Autoregulation	+	+	+	+
Genetic control[a]	BN: S LEW: R	BN: S LEW: R	A.SW: S DBA2: R	A.SW: S DBA2: R
Mechanism				
Anti-Ia T cells	+	+	Modified Ia (?)	Modified Ia (?)

[a]S, susceptible; R, resistant.

Mercury-induced autoimmunity in Brown-Norway rats

Nontoxic amounts (50-100 µg/100 g body weight thrice weekly) of mercuric chloride induce lymphoproliferation in Brown-Norway (BN) rats due to an increase in the number of CD4$^+$ helper T lymphocytes and B lymphocytes (Pelletier et al., 1988a). A hyperimmuno-globulinaemia affecting mainly IgE is observed (Prouvost-Danon et al., 1981). The preferential production of IgE suggests that interleukin-4 is involved. Autoantibodies are produced against glomerular basement membrane components (Bellon et al., 1982), IgG (P. Druet, unpublished data) and DNA, together with antibodies towards exogenous antigens (trinitrophenol, sheep red blood cells) (Hirsch et al., 1982). Anti-glomerular basement membrane antibodies are responsible for the appearance of an autoimmune glomerulonephritis (Sapin et al., 1977; Druet et al., 1978). These autoantibodies, which are deposited from day 10 in a linear pattern along the glomerular capillary wall (Fig. 3a), are probably responsible for the proteinuria and the nephrotic syndrome observed in this model. There is no renal failure. A membranous glomerulopathy is observed later (Fig. 3a), the pathogenesis of which has not yet been elucidated. BN rats also exhibit mucositis and Sjogren's syndrome (Aten et al., 1988). Mercuric chloride induces polyclonal activation of B cells in which T cells are required, as shown by the fact that T cell-depleted BN rats did not develop autoimmune abnormalities (Pelletier et al., 1987). The involvement of T cells was further demonstrated by transfer of autoimmunity from mercury-injected BN rats to naive syngeneic recipients with T cells. However, the recipients must be treated with an anti-CD8 antibody for full-blown expression of the disease (Pelletier et al., 1988b). Mercury-induced autoimmunity can be prevented and even cured by treatment with low doses (5-7 mg/kg per day) of ciclosporin A (Baran et al., 1986), again indicating a role for T cells. It is of note that the disease can be induced with doses of mercuric chloride as low as 5 µg/100 g body weight; the higher the dose used, the more severe was the disease (Druet et al., 1978 and unpublished). Several other mercurials, including organomercurials (Bernaudin et al., 1981) and mercury-containing pharmaceutical agents (Druet et al., 1981), were also effective.

This autoimmune disease is characterized by two other essential features. First, susceptibility is genetically controlled. Indeed, the four strains of rats tested, which bore RT1^1 haplotype (LEW, F344, BS, AS), did not develop autoimmune abnormality, in contrast to BN rats which bear the RT1^n haplotype. A study of segregants in BN and LEW (RT1^1) rats indicated that susceptibility is inherited as an autosomal dominant trait and depends upon three to four genes, one of which is within the major histocompatibility complex (MHC) (Druet et al, 1977). Study of the susceptibility of congenic LEW rats with the MHC of BN rats (LEW.1N) and of congenic BN rats with the MHC of LEW rats (BN.1L) clearly showed that both MHC and non-MHC genes are required. Indeed, LEW.1N and BN.1L rats were resistant when (LEW.1N x BN.1L) F1 hybrids were susceptible (Table 4). Second, this autoimmune disease is regulated spontaneously. Autoantibodies disappear even when mercuric chloride injections are continued, and suppressor T cells and/or auto-anti-idiotypic antibodies seem to be involved (Bowman et al., 1984; Chalopin et al., 1984). Moreover, rats that recover are resistant to challenge for two to three months (Pusey et al., 1983).

Mercury-induced autoimmunity in other strains of rats and other species

The susceptibility of several strains of rats has been tested (Table 4). Some developed an immune complex-type autoimmune glomerulonephritis but without linear IgG deposits, suggesting that anti-glomerular basement membrane antibodies were present only in BN rats (Table 4). A disease quite similar to that observed in BN rats occurred in rabbits injected with mercuric chloride (Roman-Franco et al, 1978). The susceptibility of several strains of mice has been investigated more recently (Eneström & Hultman, 1984; Hultman & Eneström, 1987; Pietsch et al.,1989): A.SW (H-2^s) mice developed lymphoproliferation, increased total serum IgG and IgE levels, IgG anti-nucleolar autoantibodies and an autoimmune glomerulonephritis, while C57Bl/6 (H-2^b) were less susceptible and DBA/2 (H-2^d) were resistant (Table 3). Other strains of mice bearing the H-2^s haplotype (B10-S and SJL) were also susceptible. Strain XIII guinea-pigs developed allergic contact sensitivity to mercuric chloride, while strain II guinea-pigs did not (Polak et al., 1968).

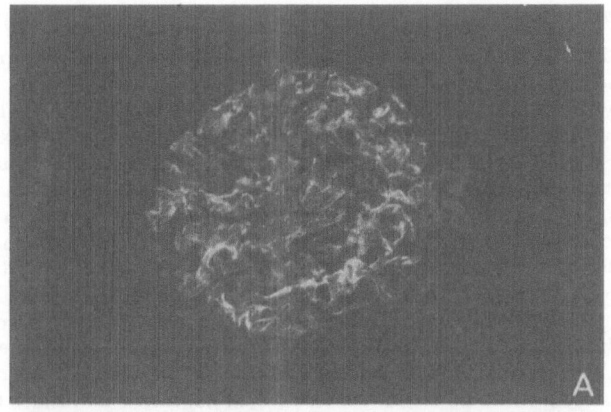

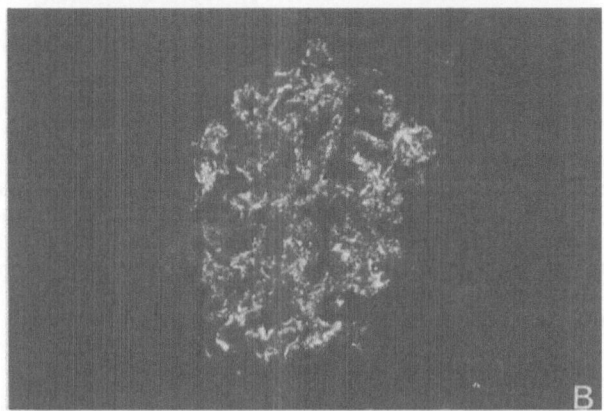

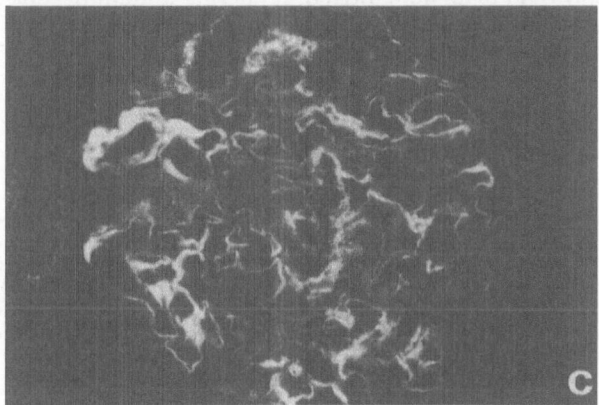

Fig. 3. Autoimmune glomerulonephritis induced in Brown-Norway rats by mercuric chloride, characterized on day 14 by linear deposits of anti-glomerular basement membrane antibodies along the glomerular capillary wall (a). On day 35, granular, immune complex-type deposits are also detected in the glomerulus (b). Aurothio-propanolsulfonate induces linear deposits of anti-glomerular basement membrane antibodies along the glomerular capillary wall and granular deposits in the vessel walls in the same strain (c).

Gold-induced autoimmunity

Wistar rats injected with aurothiomalate develop a membranous glomerulopathy (Nagi et al., 1971), the pathogenesis of which has not been studied further. We found recently that BN rats injected with sodium aurothiopropanolsulfonate (2 mg/100 g body weight thrice weekly) developed an autoimmune disease similar to that observed in BN rats injected with mercuric chloride (Table 3). BN rats exhibit a transient lymphoproliferation, a hyper-immunoglobulinaemia affecting mainly IgE, antinuclear antibodies and an autoimmune glomerulonephritis, with the successive appearance of glomerular linear and granular IgG deposits (Tournade et al., 1990). LEW rats are resistant. Gold sodium thiomalate has a similar effect in BN rats (Balazs et al., 1986). Susceptible mice with the H-2^a haplotype (A.SW) also develop increased total serum IgG, IgE and IgM levels and antinuclear antibodies when injected with gold sodium thiomalate (Table 3) (Pietsch et al., 1989). There are therefore striking similarities between the autoimmune phenomena obtained with mercury and gold in BN rats and in susceptible mice (Table 3). An autoimmune nephritis was induced in Hartley guinea-pigs that received gold sodium thiomalate (Ueda et al., 1986). Anti-tubular basement membrane antibodies were found linearly deposited along the tubular basement membrane in association, with an immune complex type glomerulonephritis. Anti-brush border antibodies are considered to be involved in the pathogenesis of the glomerular disease.

Experimental models with other metals

Low doses (3-3000 ppm for ten weeks) of cadmium have been reported to induce antinuclear antibodies in ICR mice (Ohsawa et al., 1988); Balb/c mice were resistant. Cadmium has also been considered to be responsible for an immune complex-type glomerulonephritis (Joshi et al., 1981) in rats, and autoantibodies to laminin and type-IV collagen were found in Sprague-Dawley rats injected with cadmium. Chromium and beryllium are responsible for an allergic contact sensitivity in strain II guinea-pigs, while strain XIII is resistant (Polak et al., 1968).

MECHANISMS OF METAL-INDUCED AUTOIMMUNITY

At least three mechanisms could explain metal-induced autoimmunity:
(1) A metal may bind to an autoantigen, rendering it immunogenic.
(2) A metal may be toxic for certain structures, which are then released into the circulation and become immunogenic.
(3) A metal may dysregulate the immune system, leading to a polyclonal B-cell activation.

Table 4. Mercury-induced glomerulonephritis in various strains of rat

Strain	RT-1 haplotype	Glomerular disease[a]
BN	n	Anti-GBM GN, MGP
LEW.1N	n	No anti-GBM GN
ACl.1N	n	No anti-GBM GN
LEW, F 344	l	No GN
AS, BS	l	No GN
BN. 1L	l	No GN
LEW.1NxBN.1L	n/l	Anti-GBM GN, MGP
LOU, WAG	u	No GN
Wistar Furth	u	MGP
PVG/c, AUG	c	Immune complex GN
DA, AVN	a	Immune complex GN
BDV	d	Immune complex GN
BUF	b	Immune complex GN
OKA	k	Immune complex GN
AS 2	f	Immune complex GN

[a]Anti-GBM GN, anti-glomerular basement membrane-mediated glomerulonephritis; GN, glomerulonephritis; MGP, membranous glomerulopathy.

Modified autoantigen

This mechanism could explain the immune-type complex glomerulonephritis induced by mercuric chloride in PVG/c rats (Weening *et al.*, 1980). Circulating anti-nuclear autoantibodies specific for the non-histone fraction are present in these rats, and mercury has also been found in this nuclear fraction. Weening *et al.* (1980) considered that nuclear antigens modified by mercury could become immunogenic. The glomerulopathy observed could result from deposition of immune complexes consisting of nuclear antigens and anti-nuclear antibodies, since anti-nuclear antibodies have been detected in immune-type deposits.

Immune response triggered by the release of an autoantigen

This mechanism has been proposed to explain gold-induced nephropathy in guinea-pigs (Ueda *et al.*, 1986). In this species, gold salt thiomalate provokes an autoimmune tubulointerstitial nephritis. Anti-tubular basement membrane antibodies that are produced and deposited along the membrane could be of pathogenic significance. Moreover, in some guinea-pigs, an immune complex-type nephropathy is observed that could be due to the deposition of immune complexes consisting of renal tubular epithelial antigens and of autoantibodies against these antigens. According to Ueda *et al.*, tubular basement membrane and epithelial tubular antigens could be released from renal tubules that are directly damaged by gold. Antigens thus released would lead to the production of autoantibodies.

Dysregulation of the immune system

This mechanism may be hypothesized when there is evidence that B cells are polyclonally activated, that is, when lymphoproliferation and hyperimmunoglobulinaemia are observed, together with various autoantibodies. Several mechanisms may be at play.

Direct effect on B cells. It has been shown, for example, that lithium salts increase the polyclonal activation of B cells triggered by lipopolysaccharide in mice (Ishizaka & Moller, 1982). Moreover, lithium allows B cells from nonresponder strains of mice to proliferate in the presence of lipopolysaccharide. In this situation, lithium induces RNA synthesis, while lipopolysaccharide alone does not. Zinc has also been reported to activate B cells polyclonally (Cunningham-Rundles *et al.*, 1980).

Induction of T cells able to generate a polyclonal activation of B cells. The best candidates for such an effect would be T cells that recognize class-II determinants encoded by class-II genes within the MHC. Class-II determinants are also called 'Ia determinants', and this is the denomination that will be used in this paper. Since Ia molecules are expressed at the cell surface of all B cells, these cells could be triggered by Ia-specific T cells. It is noteworthy that numerous metals can induce autoreactive anti-Ia T cells which can recognize either Ia modified by the metal or native Ia molecules (Table 5). In most cases, however, it is very difficult to discriminate between anti-'self' Ia and anti-'modified' Ia T cells.

(i) Anti-'modified' Ia autoreactive T cells: In this situation, Ia molecules modified by the metal would be recognized as alloantigens. This hypothesis was raised following the elegant, extensive work of Gleichmann and Gleichmann (1987) using the chronic graft-*versus*-host reaction model in mice. When T cells from a parent X are injected into an F1 (X x Y) hybrid, they are not rejected but they recognize as foreign the alloantigens inherited from the Y parent. A chronic graft-*versus*-host reaction is observed when parents X and Y are only class-II incompatible. Donor CD4+ T cells (from donor X), specific for the Y Ia alloantigen inherited from parent Y in the F1 hybrid, are stimulated. In turn, these anti-allo Ia T cells activate polyclonally hybrid B cells, which express class-II antigens inherited from parent Y. A lupus-like autoimmune disease appears in these animals (Fig. 4).

Gleichmann *et al.* (1984) suggested that a virus or toxin could bind Ia molecules and modify them so that they are recognized as allogeneic by autologous T cells. These T cells could then activate the 'modified' Ia-positive B cells polyclonally (Fig. 5). Several metals have been reported to induce anti-'modified' Ia T cells. Kapsenberg *et al.* (1988) cloned T cells from patients with nickel-induced contact dermatitis obtained either from peripheral blood lymphocytes or from skin lesions. These authors demonstrated that the majority of the cells were stimulated by autologous Ia-positive cells and nickel. Moreover, there was no proliferation when cells were cultured in the presence of a monoclonal anti-Ia antibody. These results are in agreement with those of Warner and Lawrence (1986a) and of Sinigaglia *et al.* (1985). The latter showed in addition that the anti-Ia-positive nickel T-cell clones could activate autologous B cells polyclonally. This B-cell activation was also blocked by an anti-Ia monoclonal antibody. All of the clones were CD4$^+$ helper T cells. Warner and Lawrence (1986b) showed *in vitro* that zinc and lead trigger the proliferation of normal mice CD4$^+$ and CD8$^+$ T cells; Ia-positive cells were required for this phenomenon to occur. The proliferation was completely abolished in the presence of an anti-Ia or anti-CD4 monoclonal antibody, suggesting that activation of CD4$^+$ T cells is required for the proliferation to occur. In these two situations, however, anti-Ia T cells have not been shown to mediate B-cell polyclonal activation. Although this has been suggested, it has not been demonstrated whether anti-Ia T cells recognize only 'modified' Ia molecules or, in addition, native Ia antigens.

(ii) Induction of anti-Ia native T cells: Recent studies by Kappler *et al.* (1987) offer convincing evidence that clonal deletion of self-MHC reactive lymphocytes takes place within the thymus. 'However, T cells exist in the peripheral lymphoid compartment that can be activated by autologous Ia antigens alone and autoreactive anti-Ia T cells develop in lymph nodes and spleens during the immune response to foreign antigens. This suggests 'that clonal deletion in the thymus is incomplete and that peripheral mechanisms of self-tolerance also exist' (Kennedy *et al.*, 1988). Moreover, peripheral anti-Ia T cells have been cloned from normal animals, whether immunized (Faherty *et al.*, 1985; Tilkin *et al.*, 1987) or not (Nagarkatti *et al.*, 1985a); however, their frequency is very low and they are controlled by suppressor/cytotoxic T cells (Sano *et al.*, 1987; Fig. 6). Such clones may induce polyclonal activation of B cells (Corley, 1985; Saito & Rajewsky, 1985), modify the antibody isotype (Clayberger *et al.*, 1985; Leung *et al.*, 1986), or inhibit the immune response (Clayberger *et al.*, 1984). *In vivo*, injection of anti-Ia T-cell clones into mice induced a lichen planus-type skin disease known to be of autoimmune origin (Saito *et al.*, 1986).

A metal could generate anti-native Ia T cells in at least three different ways. First, it could act by modifying a T lymphocyte specific for an exogenous antigen in such a way that it became specific for the Ia determinant alone. The initial antigen recognized is no longer required for the T-cell clone to proliferate. For example, a tetanus toxoid CD4$^+$ T-cell clone has been rendered specific for autologous Ia when cultured in the presence of 5-azacytidine (Richardson, 1986), which inhibits methylation of DNA. The ensuing gene de-repression is probably responsible for expression of silent genes and for the appearance of autoreactivity.

Table 5. Metal-induced anti-Ia T cells

Metal	Mechanism	Experimental system
Nickel	Anti-modified Ia T cells (and/or anti-self Ia)	Human T-cell clones
Cadmium	Anti-modified Ia T cells (or anti-self Ia ?)	Spleen cells cultured in the presence of metal
Lead	Anti-modified Ia T cells (or anti-self Ia ?)	Spleen cells cultured in the presence of metal
Zinc	Anti-modified Ia T cells (or anti-self Ia ?)	Spleen cells cultured in the presence of metal
Mercury	Anti-self Ia	Limiting dilution analysis of T cells from diseased rats
Gold	Anti-self Ia	Limiting dilution analysis of T cells from diseased rats
Beryllium	Anti-(Ia+ pulmonary antigen)	Absent

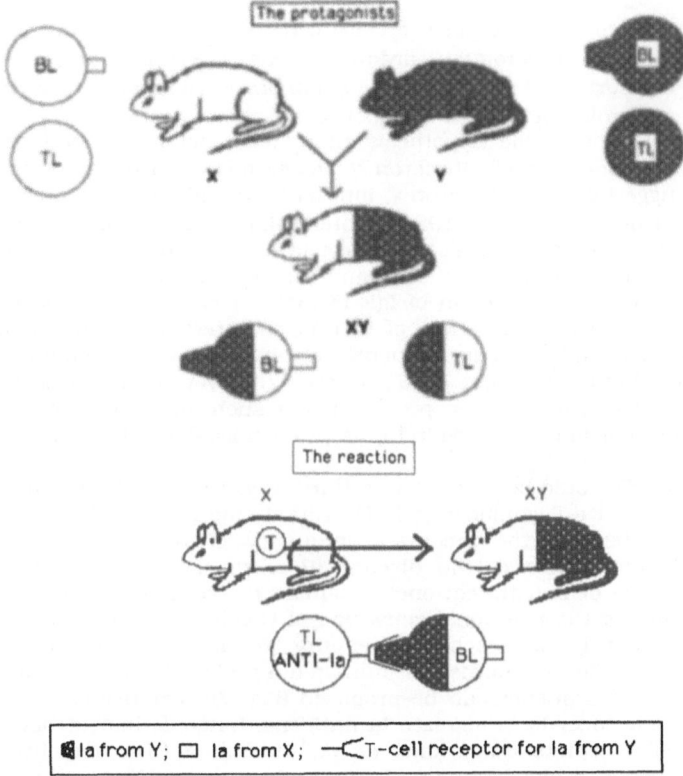

Fig. 4. Chronic graft-*versus*-host reaction. T Cells from parent X are injected into an F1 hybrid obtained by crossing X and Y. The two parents, X and Y, differ only in class-II determinants (encoded by the major histocompatibility complex). T Cells from parent X that recognize the allo-Ia of parent Y in the F1 hybrid will stimulate polyclonal B cells in the hybrid. BL, B lymphocytes; TL, T lymphocytes

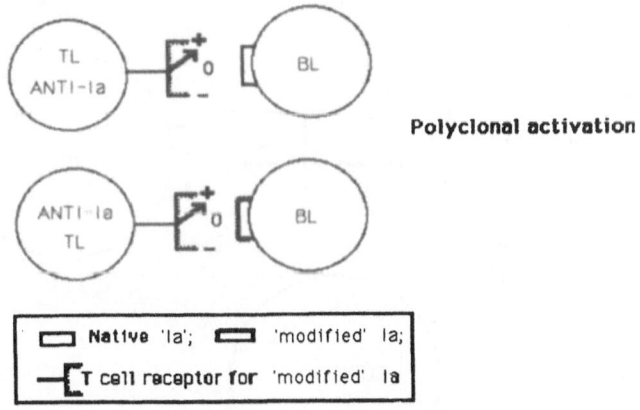

Fig. 5. Anti-'modified' Ia T cells. A metal can modify a class-II determinant so that it is recognized as an allo-Ia molecule by autologous T cells (lower panel); T cells that have a receptor for the modified Ia can also recognize native Ia (upper panel). BL, B lymphocytes; TL, T lymphocytes

131

Procainamide and hydralazine, known to induce autoimmunity, may act similarly (Cornacchia *et al.*, 1988).

Second, a metal could induce Ia expression. It has been shown in mice *in vitro* that mercury and zinc induce interferon γ (Reardon & Lucas, 1987); lead and nickel increase Ia expression at the cell surface of normal mouse lymphocytes (Warner & Lawrence, 1988) and also induce a T-cell proliferation that is blocked by an anti-interferon γ antibody. These expriments strongly support the hypothesis that some metals can induce increased Ia expression through production of interferon γ. Heavy metals also induce metallothionein, and it has been suggested that interferon γ, interleukin-1 and metallothionein are regulated in coordination (Warner & Lawrence, 1986a). Interleukin-4, the cytokine responsible for the preferential production of IgE, can also increase Ia expression at the B-cell surface. It is noteworthy that autoreactive anti-Ia T cells and mercury-induced autoreactive T cells are responsible for preferential production of IgE (Kimata *et al.*, 1983; Leung *et al.*, 1986). It would be interesting to test the effect of metals on interleukin-4 production, since an increase in total serum IgE level is frequently observed in metal-induced autoimmunity (Davis *et al.*, 1973; Prouvost-Danon *et al.*, 1981). Whatever the cytokine involved in the increase in Ia expression, it has been proposed that such an increase could enhance the production of autologous anti-Ia T cells in lupus-prone mice (Weston *et al.*, 1987).

Anti-self Ia T cells could be induced in a third way. Mercury, for example, induces the appearance of autoreactive T lymphocytes in BN rats. Using limiting dilution analysis, it has been possible to determine the precursor frequency of these lymphocytes and their phenotype at different stages of the disease (Rossert *et al.*, 1988). Two autoreactive lymphocytes have been demonstrated: one recognizes native Ia on syngeneic B cells and is probably responsible for the polyclonal activation of B cells that takes place in this model; the other is triggered by T cells exposed to mercury. The latter interaction is blocked by an anti-CD4 antibody, while the former is inhibited specifically by an anti-Ia monclonal antibody. The following sequence can be proposed (Fig. 7): mercury could first act on the CD4 molecule, which normally recognizes Ia antigens. Since 'Ia-like' structures have been described on T-cell receptors (Nagarkatti *et al.*, 1985b), a CD4 'modified' T cell could stimulate T cells bearing Ia-like determinants and induce anti-self Ia T cells.

T-Cell clones have been obtained from patients with nickel-induced contact dermatitis, and some of these recognize nickel associated with class-II molecules while others (a minor proportion) are stimulated by nickel alone. The interpretation that nickel interacts with a

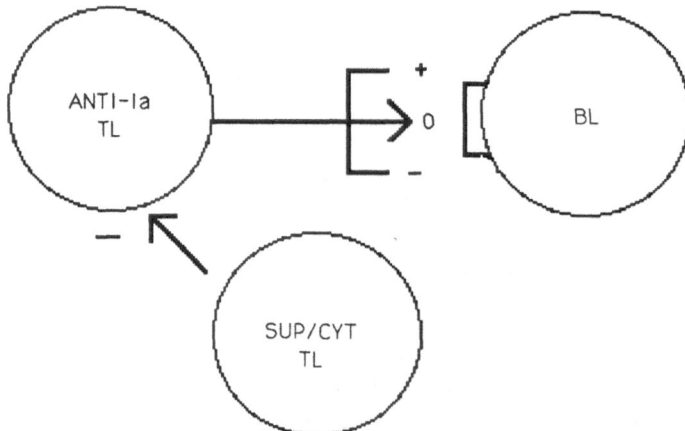

Fig. 6. Anti-native Ia T cells (TL) from normal animals. Rarely, T cells that recognize native Ia molecules are present in normal animals. These are probably controlled by suppressor/ cytotoxic (sup/cyt) T cells. BL, B lymphocytes

variable structure on these T cells is favoured by Kapsenberg *et al.* (1988). High-affinity binding of nickel to protein is selective; nickel ions bind human albumin but not dog albumin; however, dog and human albumin differ only slightly at the nickel binding site (tyrosine in human albumin replaces histidine in dog albumin). An attractive explanation for direct stimulation of a limited repertoire of T cells (putatively anti-Ia T cells) is direct cross-linkage of the antigen receptor molecules of these T cells by nickel. This hypothesis is schematized in Figure 8.

(*iii*) *Defect at the T suppressor level:* Such a defect has been suggested to be associated with exposure to nickel, lead and zinc. Mercuric chloride could also affect suppressor T cells, which would also favour the emergence of anti-self Ia T cells (Fig. 8).

IMMUNOSUPPRESSION INDUCED BY METALS

All of the metals mentioned above that can induce autoimmune phenomena can also induce immunosuppression *in vitro.* As a consequence, one would expect to observe an increased susceptibility to infections and cancers in persons exposed to them, but this has not been demonstrated. Several metals (chromium, lead, zinc, copper, cadmium, cobalt and nickel) have been reported to induce increased susceptibility to infections or cancers in mice and rats (Descotes, 1988), and exposure of rats and rabbits to beryllium leads to the occurrence of neoplasia attributed to a T-cell defect (Reeves, 1983). Interestingly, rats and rabbits do not exhibit hypersensitivity reactions to beryllium, while guinea-pigs, which do not seem to be prone to the appearance of neoplasia, develop hypersensitivity reactions.

It is not clear whether the various effects of metals on T and B cells *in vitro* (reviewed by Descotes, 1988) are relevant to what happens *in vivo.* Metals can interfere with the mitogen-induced proliferative response of T and B cells; they can decrease the response to alloantigens; and T-dependent and -independent B-cell differentiation may be affected. The

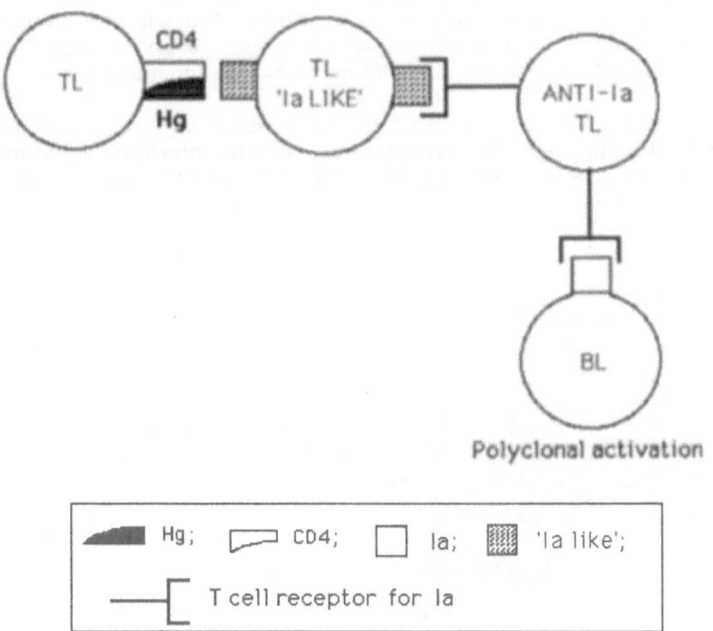

Fig. 7. Hypothetical mechanism of action of mercuric chloride-induced autoimmunity in Brown-Norway rats. The toxin would modify the CD4 determinant in T cells which normally recognizes class-II antigens or 'class II-like' antigens. T Cells that recognize both the 'Ia-like' structure and native Ia are stimulated. TL, T lymphocytes; BL, B lymphocytes

133

effects depend upon several factors, including the concentration of metal, duration of culture, oxidation status, and strain or species tested. Most of the reports have been only descriptive, and the mechanisms involved have not been explored.

Normal LEW rats are highly susceptible to the induction of various autoimmune disorders, such as experimental allergic encephalomyelitis and Heymann's nephritis, but pretreatment with mercuric chloride protects LEW rats from the occurrence of these diseases (Pelletier *et al.*, 1987). In that strain, mercury induces the appearance of non-antigen-specific CD8⁺ suppressor T cells, and it is these cells that are responsible for the protective effect observed because administration of an anti-CD8 monoclonal antibody removes the protection. Interestingly, the protective effect of mercuric chloride may also depend upon humoral factors: (LEW x BN) F1 hybrids injected with mercuric chloride are protected against the occurrence of autoimmune uveitis, and experiments in progress suggest that this protection may be related to the high total serum IgE level induced by mercury (B. Bellon and others, in preparation). Other experiments using this model have shown that mastocyte degranulation, putatively triggered by specific IgE, increases vascular permeability, thus allowing activated T cells to reach their target.

CONCLUSIONS AND RECOMMENDATIONS FOR FUTURE RESEARCH

Immunologically mediated diseases are the most frequent immunotoxic effects observed following exposure to various metals. It has been shown in humans and in experimental models that recognition of class-II encoded molecules (Ia determinants) is frequently at play. Depending upon the species considered and the metal used, the Ia molecules recognized may be either Ia 'modified' by the metal or 'native' Ia molecules. These mechanisms are not mutually exclusive. In addition, it is also possible that anti-Ia T cells recognize both the 'modified' and 'native' molecules. In order to confirm the role of anti-class-II T cells, T-cell lines and clones must be obtained in experimental models.

Animal models will allow better understanding of these mechanisms, mainly because susceptible strains of rats (BN) and mice (A.SW) have been found. These susceptible strains develop similar manifestations when given metals that are known to induce autoimmunity in patients susceptible to mercury and gold. Experimental models will be extremely useful in developing predictive assays, in determining which genes govern susceptibility and in evaluating the respective roles of the metal itself and of various chemical groups.

The fact that the total serum IgE level increases markedly in several experimental models as well as in humans suggests that cytokines such as interferon γ and interleukin-4 may play a role. It would also be interesting to test the effect of treatment with monoclonal

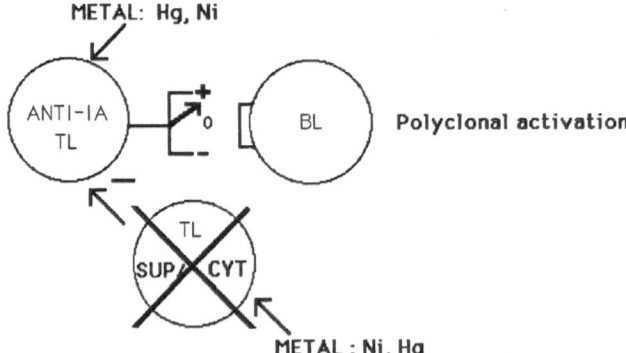

Fig. 8. Metal-induced anti-native Ia T cells. A metal could act directly on anti-Ia T cells (upper part) and expand these clones. It could also inhibit suppressor/cytotoxic (sup/cyt) T cells (lower part). TL, T lymphocytes; BL, B lymphocytes

antibodies against Ia, interleukin-2 receptor and interferon γ and with cytokines such as interferon γ.

Experiments should also be initiated to dissect further the action of metals on modification of membrane molecules (such as CD4 and Ia) and of gene expression and regulation (e.g., DNA methylation). Molecular biological techniques (such as transfection of CD4-negative cells with the gene that encodes for CD4) might be very helpful in solving these problems.

Mercurials induce an immunosuppressive effect in LEW rats, but the mechanism of this effect remain to be elucidated.

Finally, since most autoimmune disorders, such as membranous glomerulopathy, in humans are still of unknown origin, it would be interesting to test the role of unsuspected exposure to metals in prospective, European multicentre studies.

REFERENCES

Alcalay, M., Touchard, G., Patte, F., Babin, P., Reboux, J F., Thomas, P., Patte, D. & Bontoux, D. (1979) [Nephropathy, pneumopathy and hepatopathy of gold salts occurring simultaneously with ultrastructural study of pulmonary and renal lesions.] (in French) *Rev. Rhum.*, **46**: 491-498

Aten, J., Bosman, C.B., Rozing, J., Stijnen, T., Hoedemaeker, P.J. & Weening, J.J. (1988) Mercuric chloride-induced autoimmunity in the Brown Norway rat. Cellular kinetics and major histocompatibility complex antigen expression. *Am. J. Pathol.*, **133**: 127-138

Balazs, T., Robinson, C. & Abraham, A. (1986) Drug-induced autoimmunity in rats. In: *Abstracts, Sixth International Congress of Immunology, Toronto, Canada*, Ottawa, National Research Council Canada

Baran, D., Vendeville, B., Vial, M.C., Bascou, C., Teychenne, P. & Druet, P. (1986) Effect of cyclosporine A on mercury-induced autoimmune glomerulonephritis in the Brown-Norway rat. *Clin. Nephrol.*, **25 (Suppl.)**:175-180

Bellon, B., Capron, M., Druet, E., Verroust, P., Vial, M.C., Sapin, C., Girard, J.F., Foidart, J.M., Mahieu, P. & Druet, P. (1982) Mercuric chloride induced autoimmune disease in Brown-Norway rats: sequential search for anti-basement membrane antibodies. *Eur. J. clin. Invest.*, **12**: 127-133

Bernaudin, J.F., Druet, E., Druet, P. & Masse, R. (1981) Inhalation or ingestion of organic or inorganic mercurials produces auto-immune disease in rats. *Clin. Immunol. Immunopathol.*, **20**: 129-135

Bowman, C., Mason, D.W., Pusey, C.D. & Lockwood, C.M. (1984) Autoregulation of antibody synthesis in mercuric chloride nephritis in the Brown-Norway rat. I. A role for T suppressor cells. *Eur. J. Immunol.*, **14**: 464-470

Chalopin, J.M. & Lockwood, C.M. (1984) Autoregulation of antibody synthesis in mercuric chloride nephritis in the Brown-Norway rat. II. Presence of antigen augmentable plaque forming cells in the spleen is associated with humoral factors behaving as auto-antiidiotypic antibodies. *Eur. J. Immunol.*, **14**: 470-475

Clarkson, T.W. (1972) The pharmacology of mercury compounds. *Ann. Rev. Pharmacol.*, **12**: 375-406

Clayberger, C., DeKruyff, R.H. & Cantor, H. (1984) Immunoregulatory activities of autoreactive T cells: an I-a-specific T cell clone mediates both help and suppression of antibody responses. *J. Immunol.*, **132**: 2237-2243

Clayberger, C., DeKruyff, R.H. & Cantor, H. (1985) T Cell regulation of antibody responses: an I-a-specific autoreactive T cell collaborates with antigen-specific helper T cells to promote IgG responses. *J. Immunol.*, **134**: 691-694

Coblyn, J.S., Weinblatt, M., Holdsworth, D. & Glass, D. (1981) Gold-induced thrombocytopenia. A clinical and immunogenetic study of twenty-three patients. *Ann. intern. Med.*, **95**: 178-181

Corley, R.B. (1985) Somatic diversification of B cells: a role for autoreactive T lymphocytes. *Immunol. Today*, **6**: 178-180

Cornacchia, E., Golbus, J., Maybaum, J., Strahler, J., Hanash, S. & Richardson, B. (1988) Hydralazine and procainamide inhibit T cell DNA methylation and induce autoreactivity. *J. Immunol.*, **140**: 2197-2200

Cunningham-Rundles, S., Cunningham-Rundles, C., Dupont, B. & Good, R.A. (1980) Zinc-induced activation of human B lymphocytes. *Clin. Immunol. Immunopathol.*, **16**: 115-121

Davis, P., Ezeoke, A., Munro, J., Hobbs, J.R. & Hughes, G.R.V. (1973) Immunological studies on the mechanism of gold hypersensitivity reactions. *Br. med. J.*, **iii**: 676-678

Descotes, J. (1988) *Immunotoxicology of Drugs and Chemicals*, Amsterdam, Elsevier

Druet, E., Sapin, C., Gunther, E., Feingold, N. & Druet, P. (1977) Mercuric chloride-induced anti-glomerular basement membrane antibodies in the rat. Genetic control. *Eur. J. Immunol.*, **7**: 348-351

Druet, P., Druet, E., Potdevin, F. & Sapin, C. (1978) Immune type glomerulonephritis induced by HgCl$_2$ in the Brown Norway rat. *Ann. Immunol. (Inst. Pasteur),* **129C**: 777-792

Druet, P., Teychenne, P., Mandet, C., Bascou, C. & Druet, E. (1981) Immune-type glomerulonephritis induced in the Brown-Norway rat with mercury-containing pharmaceutical products. *Nephron,* **28**: 145-148

Empire Rheumatism Council. Research Subcommittee (1961) Gold therapy in rheumatoid arthritis. Final report of a multicentre controlled trial. *Ann. rheum. Dis.,* **20**: 315-334

Eneström, S. & Hultman, P. (1984) Immune-mediated glomerulonephritis induced by mercuric chloride in mice. *Experientia,* **40**: 1234-1240

Enjalbert, A. (1988) [Membrane receptors and mechanisms of transduction.] (in French) *Med. Sci.,* **Special no.**: 40-48

Faherty, D.A., Johnson, D.R. & Zauderer, M. (1985) Origin and specificity of autoreactive cells in antigen-induced populations. *J. exp. Med.,* **161**: 1293-1301

Fillastre, J.P., Druet P. & Mery, J.P. (1988) Proteinuric nephropathies associated with drugs and substances of abuse. In: Cameron, J.S. & Glassock, R.J., eds, *The Nephrotic Syndrome,* New York, Wiley, pp. 697-744

Gleichmann, H. & Gleichmann, E. (1987) Pathways to immunological diseases induced by various etiologic agents. In: Berlin, A., Dean, J., Draper, M.H., Smith, E.M.B. & Spreafico, F., eds, *Immunotoxicology. Proceedings of the International Seminar on the Immunological System as a Target for Toxic Damage,* Dordrecht, Martinus Nijhoff

Gleichmann, E., Pals, S.T., Rolink, A.G., Radaszkiewicz, T. & Gleichmann, H. (1984) Graft-versus-host reactions: clues to the etiopathology of a spectrum of immunological diseases. *Immunol. Today,* **5**: 324-332

Helbecque, N. & Henichart, J.P. (1988) ['Zinc fingers', DNA recognition elements.] (in French) *Med. Sci.,* **10**: 624-628

Hirsch, F., Couderc, J., Sapin, C., Fournie, G. & Druet, P. (1982) Polyclonal effect of HgCl$_2$ in the rat, its possible role in an experimental auto-immune disease. *Eur. J. Immunol.,* **12**: 620-625

Hultman, P. & Eneström, S. (1987) The induction of immune complex deposits in mice by peroral and parenteral administration of mercuric chloride: strain dependent susceptibility. *Clin. exp. Immunol.,* **67**: 283-292

Isakov, N., Scholz, W. & Altman, A. (1986) Signal transduction and intracellular events in T-lymphocyte activation. *Immunol. Today,* **7**: 271-277

Ishizaka, S. & Möller, G. (1982) Lithium chloride induces partial responsiveness to LPS in nonresponder B cells. *Nature,* **299**: 363-365

Joshi, B.C., Dwivedi, C., Powell, A. & Holscher, M. (1981) Immune complex nephritis in rats induced by long-term oral exposure to cadmium. *J. comp. Pathol.,* **91**: 11-15

Kappler, J.W., Roehm, N. & Marrack, P. (1987) T Cell tolerance by clonal elimination in the thymus. *Cell,* **49**: 273-280

Kapsenberg, M.L., Van der Pouw-Kraan, T., Stiekema, F.E., Schootememeijer, A. & Bos, J.D. (1988) Direct and indirect nickel-specific stimulation of T lymphocytes from patients with allergic contact dermatitis to nickel. *Eur. J. Immunol.,* **18**: 977-982

Kennedy, D.W., Weksler, M.E. & Russo, C. (1988) Peripheral but not thymic T cells participate in an autoreactive T cell network. *Cell. Immunol.,* **117**: 177-187

Kibukamusoke, J.W., Davies, D.R. & Hutt, M.S.R. (1974) Membranous nephropathy due to skin-lightening cream. *Br. med. J.,* **ii**: 646-647

Kimata, H., Shinomiya, K. & Mikawa, H. (1983) Selective enhancement of human IgE production in vitro by synergy of pokeweed mitogen and mercuric chloride. *Clin. exp. Immunol.,* **53**: 183-191

Lawrence, D.A. (1985) Immunotoxicity of heavy metals. In: Dean, J.H., Luster, M.I., Munson, A.E. & Amos, H., eds, *Immunotoxicity and Immunopharmacology,* New York, Raven Press, pp. 341-360

Lawrence, D., Mudzinski, S., Rudofsky, U. & Warner, G. (1987) Mechanisms of metal-induced immunotoxicity. In: Berlin, A., Dean, J., Draper, M.H., Smith, E.M.B. & Spreafico, F., eds, *Immunotoxicology. Proceedings of the International Seminar on the Immunological System as a Target for Toxic Damage,* Dordrecht, Martinus Nijhoff

Leung, D.Y.M., Young, M.C. & Geha, R.S. (1986) Induction of IgG and IgE synthesis in normal B cells by autoreactive T cell clones. *J. Immunol.,* **136**: 2851-2855

Lindqvist, K.J., Makene, W.J., Shaba, J.K. & Nantulya, V. (1974) Immunofluorescence and electron microscopic studies of kidney biopsies from patients with nephrotic syndrome, possibly induced by skin-lightening creams containing mercury. *East Afr. med. J.,* **51**: 168-169

Markovac, J. & Goldstein, G.W. (1988) Picomolar concentrations of lead stimulate brain protein kinase C. *Nature,* **334**: 71-73

Motais, R. & Sola, F. (1973) Characteristics of a sulphydryl group essential for sodium exchange diffusion in beef erythrocytes. *J. Physiol.,* **233**: 423-438

Nagarkatti, P.S., Snow, E.C. & Kaplan, A.M. (1985a) Characterization and function of autoreactive T-lymphocyte clones isolated from normal, unprimed mice. *Cell. Immunol.,* **94**: 32-48

Nagarkatti, P.S., Nagarkatti, M. & Kaplan, A.M. (1985b) Normal Lyt-1+2- T cells have the unique capacity to respond to syngeneic autoreactive T cells. Demonstration of a T cell network. *J. exp. Med.,* **162**: 375-380

Nagi, A.H., Alexander, F. & Barabas, A.Z. (1971) Gold nephropathy in rats. Light and electron microscopic studies. *Exp. mol. Pathol.*, **15**: 354-362

Noelle, R.J. & Lawrence D.A. (1981) Modulation of T-cell functions. II. Chemical basis for the involvement of cell surface thiol-reactive sites in control of T-cell proliferation. *Cell. Immunol.*, **60**: 453-469

Nordlind, K. (1984) Binding and uptake of mercuric chloride in human lymphoid cells. *Int. Arch. Allergy appl. Immunol.*, **77**: 405-408

Ohsawa, M., Takahashi, K. & Otsuka, F. (1988) Induction of anti-nuclear antibodies in mice orally exposed to cadmium at low concentrations. *Clin. exp. Immunol.*, **73**: 98-102

Passow, H. (1970) The red blood cell: penetration, distribution, and toxic actions of heavy metals. In: Maniloff, J., Coleman, J.R. & Miller, M., eds, *Effects of Metals on Cells, Subcellular Elements and Macromolecules*, Springfield, IL, Charles C. Thomas, pp. 291-340

Pelletier, L., Hirsch, F., Rossert, J., Druet, E. & Druet, P. (1987) Experimental mercury-induced glomerulonephritis. *Springer Semin. Immunopathol.*, **9**: 359-369

Pelletier, L., Pasquier, R., Guettier, C., Vial, M.C., Mandet, C., Nochy, D., Bazin, H. & Druet, P. (1988a) HgCl$_2$ induces T and B cells to proliferate and differentiate in BN rats. *Clin. exp. Immunol.*, **71**: 336-342

Pelletier, L., Pasquier, R., Rossert, J., Vial, M.C., Mandet, C. & Druet, P. (1988b) Autoreactive T cells in mercury-induced autoimmune disease. Ability to induce the autoimmune disease. *J. Immunol.*, **140**: 750-754

Pietsch, P., Vohr, H.W., Degitz, K. & Gleichmann, E. (1989) Immunopathological signs inducible by mercury compounds. II. HgCl$_2$ and gold sodium thiomalate enhance serum IgE and IgG concentrations in susceptible mouse strains. *Int. Arch. Allergy appl. Immunol.*, **90**: 47-53

Pitterich, H. & Lawaczeck, R. (1985) On the water and proton permeabilities across membranes from erythrocyte ghosts. *Biochim. biophys. Acta*, **821**: 233-242

Polak, L., Barnes, J.M. & Turk, J.L. (1968) The genetic control of contact sensitization to inorganic metal compounds in guinea-pigs. *Immunology*, **14**: 707-711

Prouvost-Danon, A., Abadie, A., Sapin, C., Bazin, H. & Druet, P. (1981) Induction of IgE synthesis and potentiation of anti-ovalbumin IgE response by HgCl$_2$ in the rat. *J. Immunol.*, **126**: 699-702

Pusey, C.D., Bowman, C., Peters, D.K. & Lockwood, C.M. (1983) Effects of cyclophosphamide on autoantibody synthesis in the Brown Norway rat. *Clin. exp. Immunol.*, **54**: 697-704

Reardon, C.L. & Lucas, D.O. (1987) Heavy-metal mitogenesis: Zn++ and Hg++ induce cellular cytotoxicity and interferon production in murine T lymphocytes. *Immunobiology*, **175**: 455-469

Reeves, A.L. (1983) Immunotoxicology of beryllium. In: Gibson, G.G., Hubbard, R. & Parke, D.V., eds, *Immunotoxicology*, London, Academic Press, pp. 261-282

Richardson, B. (1986) Effect of an inhibitor of DNA methylation on T cells. II. 5-Azacytidine induces self reactivity in antigen-specific T4+ cells. *Human Immunol.*, **17**: 456-470

Roman-Franco, A., Turiello, A., Albini, M., Ossi, E., Milgrom, F. & Andres, G.A. (1978) Anti-basement membrane antibodies and antigen-antibody complexes in rabbits injected with mercuric chloride. *Clin. Immunol. Immunopathol.*, **9**: 464-481

Rossert, J., Pelletier, L., Pasquier, R. & Druet, P. (1988) Autoreactive T cells in mercury-induced autoimmunity. Demonstration by limiting dilution analysis. *Eur. J. Immunol.*, **18**: 1761-1766

Saito, T. & Rajewsky, K. (1985) A self-Ia reactive T cell clone directly stimulates every hundredth B cells and helps antigen-specific B cell responses. *Eur. J. Immunol.*, **15**: 927-934

Saito, K., Tamura, K., Narimatsu, H., Tadakuma, T. & Nagashima, M. (1986) Cloned auto-Ia-reactive T cells elicit lichen planus-like lesion in the skin of syngeneic mice. *J. Immunol.*, **137**: 2485-2495

Sano, K., Fujisawa, I., Abe, R., Asano, Y. & Tada, T. (1987) MHC-restricted minimal regulatory circuit initiated by a class II-autoreactive T cell clone. *J. exp. Med.*, **165**: 1284-1295

Sapin, C., Druet, E. & Druet P. (1977) Induction of anti-glomerular basement membrane antibodies in the Brown-Norway rat by mercuric chloride. *Clin. exp. Immunol.*, **28**: 173-179

Shaloub, R.J. (1974) Pathogenesis of lipoid nephrosis: a disorder of T-cell function. *Lancet*, **ii**: 556-559

Shaw, C.F. (1980) The biochemistry and subcellular distribution of gold in kidney tissue: implications for chrysotherapy and nephrotoxicity. *Agents Actions*, **Suppl. 8**: 509-528

Simpson, R.B. (1961) Association constants of methylmercury with sulfhydryl and other bases. *J. Am. chem. Soc.*, **83**: 4711-4717

Sinigaglia, F., Scheidegger, D., Garotta, G., Scheper, R., Pletscher, M. & Lanzavecchia, A. (1985) Isolation and characterization of Ni-specific T cell clones from patients with Ni-contact dermatitis. *J. Immunol.*, **135**: 3929-3932

Skilleter, D.N. & Price, R.J. (1984) Lymphocyte beryllium binding: relationship to development of delayed beryllium hypersensitivity. *Int. Arch. Allergy appl. Immunol.*, **73**: 181-183

Strauss, F.G. & Eggleston, D.W. (1985) IgA nephropathy associated with dental nickel alloy sensitization. *Am. J. Nephrol.*, **5**: 395-397

Tilkin, A.F., Michon, J., Juy, D., Kayibanda, M., Henin, Y., Sterkers, G., Betuel, H. & Levy, J.P. (1987) Autoreactive T clones of MHC class II specificities are produced during responses against foreign antigens in man. *J. Immunol.*, **138**: 674-679

Tournade, H., Pelletier, L., Pasquier, R., Vial, M.C., Mandet, C. & Druet, P. (1990) D-Penicillamine-induced autoimmunity in Brown-Norway rats: similarities with HgCl$_2$-induced autoimmunity. *J. Immunol.* (in press)

Treagan, L. (1975) Metals and the immune response. A review. *Res. Commun. Chem. Pathol. Pharmacol.*, **12**: 189-219

Ueda, S., Wakashin, M., Wakashin, Y., Yoshida, H., Iesato, K., Mori, T., Mori, Y., Akikusa, B. & Okuda, K. (1986) Experimental gold nephropathy in guinea pigs: detection of autoantibodies to renal tubular antigens. *Kidney Int.*, **29**: 539-548

Warner, G.L. & Lawrence, D.A. (1986a) Stimulation of murine lymphocyte responses by cations. *Cell. Immunol.*, **101**: 425-439

Warner, G.L. & Lawrence, D.A. (1986b) Cell surface and cell cycle analysis of metal-induced murine T cell proliferation. *Eur. J. Immunol.*, **16**: 1337-1342

Warner, G.L. & Lawrence, D.A. (1988) The effect of metals on IL-2 related lymphocyte proliferation. *Int. J. Immunopharmacol.*, **10**: 629-637

Watanabe, I., Whittier, F.C., Moore, J. & Cuppage, F.E. (1976) Gold nephropathy: ultrastructural fluorescence and microanalytic studies of two patients. *Arch. Pathol. lab. Med.*, **100**: 632-635

Weening, J.J., Grond, J., Van der Top, D. & Hoedemaeker, P.J. (1980) Identification of the nuclear antigen involved in mercury-induced glomerulopathy in the rat. *Invest. cell. Pathol.*, **3**: 129-134

Weston, K.M., Yeh, E.T.H. & Sy, M.-S. (1987) Autoreactivity accelerates the development of autoimmunity and lymphoproliferation in MRL/MP-lpr/lpr mice. *J. Immunol.*, **139**: 734-742

Wooley, P.H., Griffin, J., Panayi, G.S., Batchelor, J.R., Welsh, K.I. & Gibson, T.J. (1980) HLA-DR antigens and toxic reaction to sodium aurothiomalate and D-penicillamine in patients with rheumatoid arthritis. *New Engl. J. Med.*, **303**: 300-302

TESTS FOR PREDICTING SENSITIZATION TO CHEMICALS
AND THEIR METABOLITES,
WITH SPECIAL REFERENCE TO HEAVY METALS

E. Gleichmann[1], P. Kind[2], H.-C. Schuppe[2] & H. Merk[3]

[1]Division of Immunology, Medical Institute of Environmental Hygiene, and [2]Dermatological Clinic, Heinrich Heine University Düsseldorf D-4000 Düsseldorf 1; and [3]Dermatological Clinic, University of Cologne D-5000 Köln 41, Federal Republic of Germany

ABSTRACT

Predictive tests for assessing the sensitizing potential of chemicals are reviewed. The methods used most frequently are those in which the capacity of chemicals to cause allergic contact dermatitis is assessed in guinea-pigs. The limitations of these tests may be overcome by use of the popliteal lymph node assay (PLNA) in rodents. The direct PLNA indicates primary and secondary T-cell responses to immunogenic compounds but can also detect nonspecific immunostimulatory and immunosuppressive effects of chemicals. The adoptive transfer PLNA lends itself to detection of sensitizing metabolites in conjugation with routine toxicology. Other tests, including those in man, are also discussed.

INTRODUCTION

Adverse immune reactions are among the most frequent untoward side-effects of drugs and other chemicals. They consist of allergic and autoimmune reactions which impair the patient's health and, occasionally, are fatal. In addition, adverse immune reactions to drugs can result in considerable costs for industry when the drug has to be withdrawn from the market. Thus, during the past five years, a number of major drugs, such as practolol (Amos, 1983), nomifensine (Anon., 1986) and zimeldine (Kristofferson & Nilsson, 1989), had to be withdrawn because they induced reactions that resembled autoimmune diseases.

One of the reasons for the frequency of untoward immunological effects of drugs and other chemicals must be sought in the fact that insufficient attention is paid to these effects during the preclinical toxicological testing of new chemical compounds. At present, only the weights of spleens and lymph nodes of test animals are determined, and, at best, this is complemented by histopathological examination of these organs. Such histological examinations are inapt, however, to detect sensitized T lymphocytes in these organs, as illustrated by studies on murine sensitization to streptozotocin (see below). Apart from routine testing for contact sensitization of cosmetics, functional immunological tests capable of detecting the sensitizing potentials of drugs (let alone other chemicals) are not usually performed during the premarketing test phase.

Ideally, a functional immunological test would be available that allowed the sensitizing potential of new chemicals to be detected during the early phase of preclinical and premarketing testing. Such a test must be simple, cost-effective and objective, and it must be possible to perform in the context of routine toxicological examination. As we shall outline below, the popliteal lymph node assay (PLNA), in particular the adoptive transfer PLNA, in rodents looks promising in this respect. According to present knowledge, it is very likely that most of the allergic and autoimmune reactions to chemicals are initiated by T-cell

Immunotoxicity of Metals and Immunotoxicology, Edited by
A. D. Dayan *et al.,* Plenum Press, New York, 1990

reactions towards the chemical or its metabolite. As we shall review here, the PLNA is capable of detecting T-cell reactions against low-molecular-weight chemicals.

Types I-IV of immunological effector mechanisms involved in allergic and autoimmune reactions, and the central role of T cells in the induction of these reactions

Since 1963, four basic types of effector mechanism have been distinguished. It should be noted that both the physiological and pathological immune reactions that the body mounts to antigen involve the types-I-IV effector mechanisms. Originally, however, Gell and Coombs (1963) used their classification for pathological immune reactions only, e.g., for allergies and autoimmune diseases. Therefore, these effector mechanisms are also referred to as types-I-IV hypersensitivity reactions:

Type I: Anaphylactic or immediate hypersensitivity reactions are mediated by IgE antibodies and cause allergic asthma, urticaria and allergic shock. In a sensitized individual, the reaction starts within minutes after secondary exposure to the sensitizing antigen.

Type II: Cytotoxic reactions involve the combination of IgG or IgM antibodies with antigenic determinants on a cell membrane. Cytolysis is caused by complement fixation or antibody-dependent cell-mediated cytotoxicity. An example is (drug-induced) autoimmune haemolytic anaemia.

Type III: Reactions mediated by soluble immune complexes. Most often, the participating antibodies belong to the IgG isotype. An example is (drug-induced) systemic lupus erythematosus.

Type IV: Cell-mediated or delayed-type hypersensitivity in which the majority of inflammatory cells consist of macrophages; antibodies are not involved. A classical example is contact dermatitis. In a sensitized individual, the reaction starts after hours and usually peaks at 24-48 h after secondary exposure to the sensitizing antigen.

While this classification is still useful, it must be emphasized that it stems from a time when T and B lymphocytes had not yet been distinguished. Today, we know that antibodies are produced by B cells and that antibody responses to the vast majority of antigens require T-cell help; this is certainly so if the antibodies are to be of the IgA, IgE and IgG isotype (with the possible exception of IgG_3). Upon contact with their specific antigen, $CD4^+$ T cells produce a variety of interleukins, which then determine whether or not a delayed-type hypersensitivity reaction ensues and, if antibodies are produced, to which Ig isotype a given antibody will belong (Fig. 1). In other words, it is the T cells that determine whether a type I, II, III or IV reaction will be made against a given antigen. In addition, interleukins have multiple effects on other cell types. Therefore, $CD4^+$ T cells play a pivotal role in that they qualitatively and quantitatively regulate almost all immune responses.

Upon first contact with an antigen, clonal proliferation of specific T and B lymphocytes ensues, which gives rise to the development of both effector and memory T and B cells. Upon second exposure to the same antigen, therefore, a secondary immune response ensues which is stronger and faster than the primary response. The immune system then attempts to destroy and eliminate the antigen by the mechanisms outlined briefly above. Which of these effector mechanisms is chosen depends on a variety of different factors, such as the type of antigen, the route of exposure to that antigen, and, last but not least, the genetic predisposition of the individual to react to that antigen.

PREDICTIVE TESTS IN ANIMALS

The direct popliteal lymph node assay (PLNA): description of the method and results obtained

In view of the central role of T cells, preclinical testing of the sensitizing effects of chemicals will be most economic when it encompasses T-cell responses to the test compounds. The PLNA in rodents is capable of doing so. Since the test procedure and the results obtained thus far have recently been reviewed (Gleichmann & Gleichmann, 1989; Gleichmann *et al.*, 1989a,b; Vohr *et al.*, 1989), we will repeat only the major findings here.

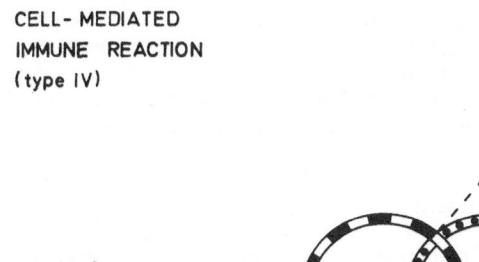

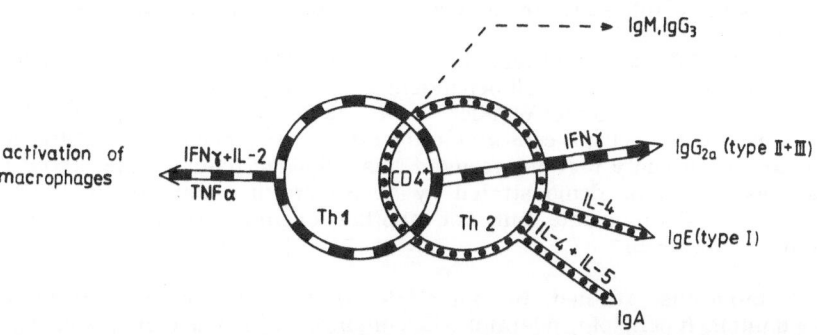

CELL- MEDIATED
IMMUNE REACTION
(type IV)

ANTIBODY MEDIATED
IMMUNE REACTIONS
(type I, II, and III)

Fig. 1. Schematic representation of the central role of CD4⁺ T helper (Th) or T regulator cells in almost all types of immune reactions, including the activation of CD8⁺ T killer cells (not shown). Upon recognition of antigen (not shown), CD4⁺ T cells secrete different interleukins, such as interferon-γ (IFN-γ) and interleukin-4 (IL-4). The pattern of secreted interleukins decides which type of immune reaction ensues. Often, the immune response against a given antigen comprises more than one type of reaction. In the mouse, two types of CD4⁺ T cells can be distinguished, Th1 and Th2 cells (Mosmann & Coffman, 1987). Th1 cells secrete IFN-γ (in addition to other interleukins); this leads to activation of macrophages, resulting in a type-IV reaction and/or production of IgG$_{2a}$ antibodies which may participate in type-II and -III reactions. Th2 cells secrete IL-4 and IL-5 (in addition to other interleukins) and thus help B cells to produce IgE and IgA. Production of IgM and IgG$_3$ can be T cell-independent.

(1) In the direct PLNA (Fig. 2), the test compound is administered subcutaneously without adjuvant into one hind footpad of a rat or mouse. The contralateral footpad is not injected or is injected with solvent only, and thus serves as an internal control. On day X

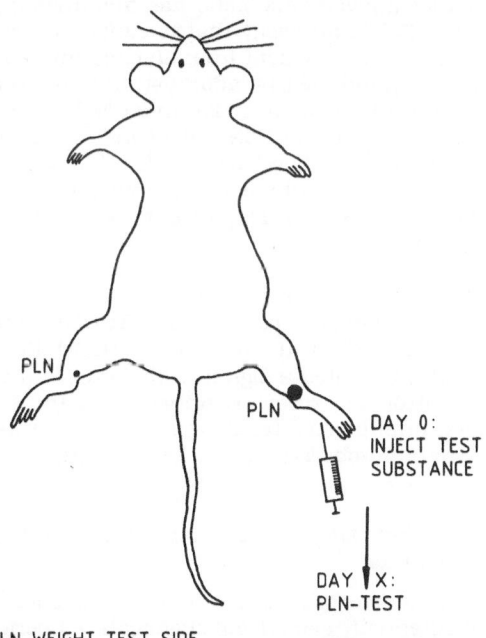

Fig. 2. Scheme of the direct popliteal lymph node (PLN) assay in rodents. The test compound is injected subcutaneously without adjuvant into one hind footpad of a test animal. The contralateral side is left untreated, or inoculated with the solvent of the test compound, and thus serves as an internal control. Days thereafter, an ensuing immune reaction can be assessed by removing the PLNs and determining either their weight index, or, more sensitively, the number of cells or ³H-thymidine incorporation. PLN may also be analysed by flow cytometry.

141

(usually day 7), both popliteal lymph nodes (PLNs) are removed and weighed. Other measurements can be included, such as cell count, ^{3}H-thymidine incorporation into the PLN, and immune flow cytometry. From the respective results, a PLN index is calculated by dividing the results obtained from the experimental side by those obtained from the control side. PLN responses of rats generally are two to three times higher than those of mice.

(2) While the PLNA is capable of indicating specific T-cell responses to small chemicals, at the same time it measures T cell-dependent B-cell responses (Gleichmann et al., 1983; Hurtenbach et al., 1987; Stiller-Winkler et al., 1988). This is due to the lymph node architecture, in which T cells, B cells and antigen-presenting cells lodge together in intimate contact. When the primary PLN enlargement has subsided (usually after about four to six weeks), specificity can be demonstrated by an enhanced secondary PLN response to a suboptimal dose of the same, but not another chemical (Hurtenbach et al., 1987; Klinkhammer et al., 1988).

(3) Compounds studied in some detail in the direct murine PLNA are diphenylhydantoin (phenytoin, dilantin) (Gleichmann, 1981; Gleichmann et al., 1983), D-penicillamine (Hurtenbach et al., 1987), streptozotocin (Klinkhammer et al., 1988), mercuric chloride and methylmercury (Stiller-Winkler et al., 1988), and gold compounds (Schuhmann et al., 1989). In these and other studies (Kammüller & Seinen, 1988; Kammüller et al., 1989), a total of more than 60 different chemicals, most of them drugs, have been tested. The combined results indicate that the PLNA is capable of indicating structure-function relationships: in general, compounds known to be sensitizers in man gave positive PLN reactions, whereas compounds without sensitizing potential in man did not induce PLNA enlargement. However, two false-negative and two false-positive results have been obtained as well (Kammüller et al., 1989).

(4) In all cases in which it was studied, PLN enlargement was caused mainly by proliferation of lymphocytes within the PLN rather than by trapping of lymphocytes from the circulation. Moreover, with the exception of quartz (SiO$_2$), which is not an antigen (Stark et al., 1988), PLN responses to chemicals were T cell-dependent, whenever this was tested (Gleichmann & Gleichmann, 1989).

(5) Immunotoxicologists are asked not only about the potential sensitizing effects of xenobiotics, but also frequently about whether a given xenobiotic has immunosuppressive potential. It is noteworthy, therefore, that the PLNA, an assay that is simple to perform, is also capable of indicating immunosuppression. This is evident from an experiment in which the direct PLN response to streptozotocin was suppressed by administration of cyclosporin A. On day 0, BALB/c mice received a single subcutaneous injection into one hind footpad of 0.5 mg streptozotocin, the test antigen. This resulted in a PLN weight index of about 4 on day 7. Other groups of mice received an additional daily dose of 25, 50 or 75 mg/kg cyclosporin A, administered on days 0-7 either intraperitoneally or orally. This treatment resulted in a dose-dependent suppression of the PLN response to streptozotocin (C. Klinkhammer and others, unpublished results).

Recently, the usefulness of the PLNA also became apparent in studies on the immunosuppressive effect of 2,3,7,8-tetrachlorodibenzo-*para*-dioxin (TCDD). Adult rats which, on day -7, had received a single intraperitoneal injection of TCDD (in the low picogram dose range per kilogram body weight) mounted a significantly lower PLN response (cell count index) to a test antigen than control rats receiving antigen and the solvent of TCDD only (M. Kubicka-Muranyi and others, unpublished results). If confirmed, this finding will be of significance for determining accurate no-observed-effect levels for this dangerous environmental pollutant.

The adoptive transfer PLNA: demonstrating specific sensitization upon specific exposure to heavy metals and other compounds

T-Cell sensitization following repeated injections of streptozotocin and mercuric chloride. Subcutaneous injection into a hind foot of potentially sensitizing chemicals, as performed in the direct PLNA, is an artificial manoeuvre. The recently developed adoptive transfer PLNA

(Klinkhammer *et al.*, 1988; Fig. 3) is more relevant because it makes it possible to look for T-cell sensitization arising (in the donor animal) during the course of routine toxicological testing, i.e., by using the same conditions, such as route of application and duration of treatment, as those planned for human use of that chemical. This test system also allows detection of sensitizing metabolites (see below). In this context, it should be noted that the spleens and lymph nodes of sensitized mice may appear completely normal by histopathological criteria although by means of the adoptive transfer PLNA they were shown to harbour sensitized T cells. Thus, the adoptive transfer PLNA, which is a functional test, is clearly superior to histopathology in demonstrating specifically sensitized T cells.

The adoptive transfer PLNA has so far been successfully used to demonstrate T-cell sensitization following repeated systemic exposure to streptozotocin, a diabetogenic compound (Klinkhammer *et al.*, 1988), mercuric chloride (Vohr *et al.*, 1989) and gold disodium thiomalate (Schuhmann *et al.*, 1989). The results obtained with gold (Au) are discussed in more detail below.

T-Cell sensitization not to Au[I] but to Au[III] following chronic treatment with an Au[I] drug: indirect evidence for biooxidation of gold. Compounds containing gold in the Au[I] state, such as gold disodium thiomalate, are widely used for the treatment of rheumatoid arthritis. These slow-acting drugs cause an unusually high frequency of adverse immune reactions, most of which involve stimulation of the immune system. After several months of treatment, adverse immune reactions necessitate discontinuation of gold therapy in up to 40% of patients (Davis, 1979; Lockie & Smith, 1985).

On the basis of a classification developed during studies of murine graft-*versus*-host disease (Gleichmann *et al.*, 1984), the adverse immune reactions to Au[I] drugs may be divided into stimulatory and hypoplastic immunopathological alterations. Stimulatory alterations induced by Au[I] drugs include dermatitis, stomatitis, eosinophilia, and, at lower

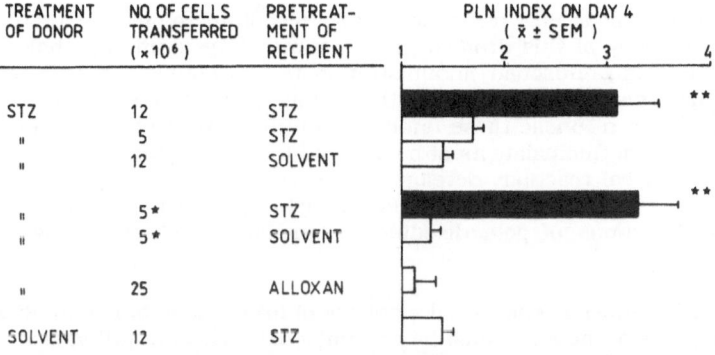

Fig. 3. **Experimental design and results of an adoptive transfer popliteal lymph node (PLN) assay performed with streptozotocin (STZ). Mean values (± SEM) of the PLN weight index are shown. Spleen cells of BALB/c donor mice, which had received five intraperitoneal injections of either STZ (40 mg/kg body weight) or the solvent of STZ, on five consecutive days, were inoculated subcutaneously into one hind footpad of syngeneic mice. The recipients had received a subcutaneous injection of either alloxan, a sub-immunogenic dose (0.1 mg) of STZ, or solvent into the same footpad 24 h before the cell transfer. Groups of seven mice each were used as recipients. *, enriched for T cells; **, $p < 0.005$ versus controls. Reproduced from Klinkhammer et al. (1988) with kind permission of the authors and the American Diabetes Association Inc. Occasionally, high background values are obtained in the control group, i.e., by transferring spleen cells from untreated donors to untreated recipients. This can be prevented by (i) irradiating the donor cells with 2000 rad in vitro and (ii) calculating the PLN indices on the basis of cell counts (M. Kubicka-Muranyi and others, unpublished results).**

frequency, immune complex glomerulonephritis, alveolitis, lymphadenopathy, hypergamma-globulinaemia, increased serum IgE levels, and formation of antinuclear autoantibodies; hypoplastic alterations include hypogammaglobulinaemia and aplastic anaemia (Davis, 1979; Scherak et al., 1984; Cohnen, 1985; Lockie & Smith, 1985; Rothschild & Marshall, 1986; Stollenwerk et al., 1986). Usually, it takes at least several weeks after the onset of Au[I] treatment before adverse reactions develop, and in some patients it may take more than a year. HLA B8 and DR3 as well as the non-HLA-linked status of slow sulfoxidizers increase the risk for adverse immune reactions (Scherak et al., 1984; Ayesh et al., 1987). The pathogenic mechanisms that trigger these reactions are unknown.

At least some of the immunological side-effects seen in man also develop in susceptible mouse strains treated with weekly intramuscular injections of gold sodium thiomalate, and, as in man, genes linked to the major histocompatibility complex as well as non-major histocompatibility complex genes are involved (Robinson et al., 1986; Pietsch et al., 1989). Both the graft-versus-host-like immunopathological picture of adverse immune reactions to chronic treatment with gold disodium thiomalate and their genetic association with the major histocompatibility complex suggest that T cells play a central role in their pathogenesis (Gleichmann et al., 1984), however, there are very few data to support or reject this hypothesis. The number of patients reported to show a positive lymphocyte transformation test in response to Au[I] drugs is surprisingly small considering the large number of cases of adverse reactions to these drugs (Denman & Denman, 1969; Schöpf et al., 1970; Louyot et al., 1974). The lymphocyte transformation test, however, is a notoriously difficult method for detecting sensitization to drugs (Rotmensch et al., 1981; Victorino & Maria, 1985).

Schuhmann et al. (1989) performed a study in which they systemically compared the T cell-sensitizing potential of various gold compounds in susceptible mouse strains. By using the direct PLNA they showed that Au[III] compounds are potent sensitizers of T cells, whereas Au[I] compounds are not. PLN reactions to Au[III] were dose-dependent, T cell-dependent, and specific; however, when Au[III] was reduced to Au[I] by addition of disodium thiomalate or methionine prior to testing in the PLNA, its immunogenicity was significantly decreased. Thus, the oxidation state of gold, i.e., Au[III] or Au[I], plays a major role in its T-cell immunogenicity.

The absent or poor PLN response to gold disodium thiomalate therefore contrasted with the high potency of this drug to induce stimulatory immunopathological alterations following repeated intramuscular administration to susceptible mouse strains, i.e., under conditions of treatment comparable with those that elicit adverse immune reactions to this drug in humans. To reconcile these findings, Schuhmann et al. (1989) proposed that the Au[I] of gold disodium thiomalate must be oxidized to Au[III] before T cells are sensitized and adverse immunological reactions develop. This speculation was supported by their results obtained with the adoptive transfer PLNA, which indicated that, indeed, repeated intramuscular injections of gold disodium thiomalate sensitized mouse spleen cells to Au[III].

Thus, the anamnestic spleen cell response of mice undergoing chronic Au[I] treatment indicates that some of the Au[I] must be gradually oxidized to Au[III] in vivo. The most likely anatomical site for this biooxidation to occur is the phagolysosomes of macrophages. As discussed in detail elsewhere (Schuhmann et al., 1989), this assumption is supported by the following lines of indirect evidence. In vitro, oxidation of gold requires O_2, low pH, thiols and time. Under these conditions, even colloidal gold, which is much less reactive than Au[I], can be oxidized to Au[III]. In vivo, the gold moiety of Au[I] drugs is preferentially taken up by the phagolysosomes of macrophages, including those of the spleen, so that, with time, their lysosomes turn into 'aurosomes'. Lysosomes have an acid pH and contain reactive oxygen species and also some of the thiols, such as metallothionein, to which gold is bound in vivo. Thus, lysosomes are candidates for generation of Au[III]. Macrophages, in addition to phagocytizing, storing and presumably oxidizing Au[I], can 'present' antigen to T cells. If, indeed, macrophages in the spleen, lymph nodes and elsewhere in the body present Au[III] to T cells, the stage would be set for development of graft-versus- host-like disease.

Interestingly, similar observations were made in rheumatoid arthritis patients who had developed adverse immune reactions after treatment with Au[I] drugs. Upon epicutaneous testing (patch test), these patients failed to react to Au[I] but developed a type-IV hypersensitivity reaction to Au[III], indicating that their T cells had been sensitized to Au[III] (G. Bäurle, personal communication, 1989).

The concept that immunogenic metabolites are generated by reactive oxygen species in phagocytes is a novel one and may be of general importance for immunotoxicology. In view of the ubiquitous presence of macrophages in the body, in particular in the lung, which is exposed to a great variety of xenobiotics, this concept needs further investigation (see Rubin & Curnutte, 1989).

Might alteration in vivo *of the oxidation state of platinum enhance sensitization?* The potent sensitizing properties of certain complex salts of platinum are well documented in workers involved in refining this metal (Roberts, 1951; Biagini *et al.*, 1985; Murdoch *et al.*, 1986; Merget *et al.*, 1988). More than 50% of exposed persons may develop symptoms of type-I hypersensitivity, such as conjunctivitis, rhinitis, bronchial asthma and, occasionally, urticaria (Roberts, 1951). Contact dermatitis has been observed less frequently. The diagnosis can be confirmed only by skin tests or bronchoprovocation (Merget *et al.*, 1988), which may lead to anaphylaxis (Freedman & Krupey, 1968). In individuals sensitized to platinum, the main eliciting agents are tetra- and hexachloroplatinate complexes, i.e., Pt[II] and Pt[IV] (Cleare *et al.*, 1976), while Pt[0] (metallic platinum) is believed to be nonallergenic (Bradford, 1987). Many attempts have been made to establish reliable in-vitro tests, such as detection of putative platinum-specific serum IgE by means of radioallergosorbent tests (Biagini *et al.*, 1985); however, specificity was lacking (Merget *et al.*, 1988), presumably because of the protein-binding property of platinum compounds (Bradford, 1987).

The precise mechanism of sensitization to platinum complexes is unclear. The allergenicity of different complexes was compared only by performing skin tests in persons already sensitized to hexachloroplatinate (Cleare *et al.*, 1976). Systematic studies aimed at predicting the sensitizing potential of various platinum compounds have not yet been performed. In addition, possible nonspecific stimulatory effects, such as the adjuvant activity for IgE production described in rats (Murdoch *et al.*, 1986), require further investigation.

Given these uncertainties, possible health hazards arising from the increasing use of platinum-containing automobile catalysts cannot be excluded. A detailed analysis of the platinum compounds released into the environment is not yet available (Bartsch & Schlatter, 1988). While most of the platinum thus released is assumed to consist of metallic Pt[0] and Pt[IV]O_2, about 10% of the estimated platinum emissions are soluble in water (Rosner & Hertel, 1986). The possible role of release of minute doses of platinum complex salts is unresolved. Moreover, the long-term chemical fate of extracorporeal as well as incorporated Pt[0] and Pt[IV]O_2 is unknown. In view of the evidence for biooxidation of Au[I] to Au[III] and subsequent sensitization (see above), alteration of the platinum oxidation state and complex formation *in vivo* might have similar importance. Before large-scale pollution by platinum reaches the 'point of no return', more research is necessary to exclude possible immunopathological hazards - the more so as epidemiological studies have already revealed higher total serum IgE levels in people living in areas with high air pollution, in particular the inner cities, than in those living in less polluted areas (Hallauer *et al.*, 1989). Moreover, in Japan the incidence of type-I hypersensitivity to cedar pollen allergens appears to be rising due to increasing air pollution, and motor car exhausts seem to contribute to this effect (Miyamoto *et al.*, 1989).

Evaluation of the PLNA and comparison with other predictive methods

Comparing guinea-pig tests for contact sensitization with the murine PLNA. Currently, the most frequently used methods for assessing the immunogenicity of new chemicals, if immunogenicity is tested at all, are those which assess the potential of a compound to induce contact dermatitis in the guinea-pig. Reactivity is measured as local erythema induced following topical challenge of sensitized animals. An example is the test described by Magnusson and Kligman (1969). Although well standardized, the guinea-pig tests have a number of limitations (Andersen & Maibach, 1985):

(1) While the skin is a relevant target organ in immunotoxicology and allergy, topical administration to the skin is not the only and not the most frequent route of exposure to chemicals in man.

(2) In order to be a contact sensitizer, a chemical must bind to Langerhans cells in the skin and thus be presented to circulating T cells for a secondary response. It is likely, however, that a number of soluble xenobiotics do not fulfil this requirement because they readily penetrate the skin, so that sensitization is manifest only in the lymphoid organs but not the skin.

(3) Testing for contact dermatitis involves subjective scoring of the lesion. Moreover, the visual assessment of erythema may be obscured when irritant or dye chemicals are examined.

(4) Testing for contact dermatitis does not automatically provide access to the sensitized lymphocytes; these are needed for advanced immunological and toxicological studies.

(5) The rat and the mouse are the two species that are most frequently used in toxicology and immunology, but they are relatively insensitive with respect to contact hypersensitivity when compared with the guinea-pig. Nonetheless, in the case of zimeldine, the direct PLNA in mice proved to be superior to the Magnusson Kligman test in detecting its immunogenicity (Kristofferson & Nilsson, 1989).

The PLNA in laboratory rodents may overcome some of the limitations related to assessment of contact dermatitis in the guinea-pig. The essential features of the PLNA can be summarized as follows:

(1) There is no anatomical variation in either the localization or the number of PLN in one hind leg; thus, preparation of the PLN is a simple and reliable procedure.

(2) In the same animal, the contralateral PLN provides an internal control.

(3) To elicit a primary reaction in the direct PLNA, the test compound is administered as a single injection without adjuvant; for induction of a secondary reaction, this manoeuvre must be repeated once.

(4) Measurement of PLN weight is an objective parameter. The same is true for other parameters that can be used in conjunction with the PLN weight assay, such as determination of the cell number in the PLN, ^{3}H-thymidine uptake and analysis of PLN cells by flow immunocytometry. As we propose use of the PLNA in conjunction with routine toxicological studies, it is worthwhile mentioning that in the rat the values of PLN indices are usually higher than those in the mouse.

(5) It should be emphasized that by no means all the compounds tested in the direct PLNA were able to induce a primary PLN reaction (Gleichmann, 1981; Kammüller & Seinen, 1988). Therefore, the PLNA is suitable for comparing the immunogenicity and/or immunostimulatory effect of closely related chemical compounds and thus for establishing structure-activity relationships (Gleichmann et al., 1983; Kammüller & Seinen, 1988; Kammüller et al, 1989). Moreover, in the case of zimeldine, the direct PLNA in mice indicated that the immunogenic site of the molecule can be separated from the site that carries the pharmacological activity (Kristofferson & Nilsson, 1989).

(6) In untreated mice, the PLN weight index ranges from about 0.8 to about 1.2; indices above 1.5 suggest and those above 2.0 indicate an immunological reaction to the test compound. During the primary PLN response to small chemicals or conventional antigens, the maximal response in the mouse very rarely exceeds a PLN weight index of 10.

However, determination of cell number in and ^{3}H-thymidine uptake by the PLN are more sensitive methods, so that the corresponding PLN indices calculated from such determinations are higher than the PLN weight index. The primary PLN response to most immunogenic chemicals tested peaked within the first ten days after injection and returned to normal by week 3 to 4; exceptions to this rule were seen with high dosages of heavy metals, such as mercuric chloride (Stiller-Winkler *et al.*, 1988), and, in particular, with quartz (SiO$_2$).

(7) Quartz also proved to be exceptional in that the direct PLN response to this agent did not require the presence of T lymphocytes (Stark *et al.*, 1988). By contrast, in all other instances in which this was tested, the PLN response to xenobiotics was T cell-dependent (Gleichmann, 1981; Gleichmann *et al.*, 1983; Hurtenbach *et al.*, 1987; Kammüller & Seinen, 1988; Klinkhammer *et al.*, 1988; Kammüller *et al.*, 1989).

(8) With the exception of quartz, which consists of nondegradable crystals, PLN responses to small chemicals proved to be antigen-specific, whenever this was tested.

(9) As discussed above, the adoptive transfer PLNA is a very promising method for detecting immunologically relevant metabolites, and it can be used in conjunction with routine toxicological testing. A prerequisite for this is, however, that the routine testing be done in inbred animals so that there is no interference by T-cell alloreactivity.

Limitations of the PLNA. These can be summarized as follows:

(1) Only material capable of passing through a small hypodermic needle can be tested in the PLNA; water-insoluble material cannot be tested or can be tested only with difficulty. When such material can be solubilized in solvents, such as dimethylsulfoxide, controls to assess the immunogenic and/or immunostimulatory effect of the solvent must be performed (Kammüller & Seinen, 1988; Kammüller *et al.*, 1989).

(2) There may be 'false' negative reactions. Most of a variety of different drugs known to have adverse immunological side-effects in man induced a primary PLN enlargement. Exceptions included the notorious autoimmunizing agent procainamide. The reasons for obtaining 'false' negative results are not known. There is a general impression that the immunogenic and/or immunostimulatory effects of chemical compounds, as detected by the PLNA, increase with their lipophilicity (Kammüller & Seinen, 1988). Moreover, as demonstrated with D-penicillamine, the pH of the solvent can influence the immunogenicity of a drug screened by the PLNA (Hurtenbach *et al.*, 1987). It is also possible, however, that hydralazine and procainamide must be metabolized before becoming immunogenic (Rubin & Curnutte, 1989) and that the direct PLNA does not provide an opportunity for metabolism. In contrast, the adoptive transfer PLNA might provide such an opportunity, as discussed above.

(3) Detecting the immunogenic and/or immunostimulatory property of a given chemical in the PLNA does not necessarily predict, of course, that this material will induce clinically relevant immunological side-effects in humans exposed to that chemical. A positive PLN reaction merely indicates that the compound tested may carry a risk with respect to such side-effects. (In the case of immunotoxicological testing of new drugs, therefore, the PLNA should be used during the early preclinical test phase.) Considering the complexity of immunological and pharmacological processes involved in chemical-induced immuno-pathological disorders, no conclusion can be drawn on the basis of one set of data alone, and additional immunological tests must be performed in such cases. In our experience, measuring specific T-cell responses to simple chemicals *in vivo* , such as with the PLNA, will give one a much greater chance of succeeding than will specific (re)stimulation of T cells *in vitro* using the same chemicals, e.g., mercuric dichloride, diphenylhydantoin, D-penicillamine and streptozotocin. A major problem with T-cell proliferation tests performed *in vitro* seems to be the proper presentation of the chemical, or its relevant metabolite, to the T cells.

Concluding remarks concerning the PLNA. The direct PLNA is a rapid, cost-effective and objective, but also adaptable method for assessing the immunogenicity of xenobiotics. It can detect specific T-cell responses to test compounds and, in this respect, is superior to both histopathological examination of lymphoid tissues and assessment of specific T-cell responses *in vitro*. In addition, the direct PLNA can detect immunosuppressive effects of chemical compounds as well as nonspecific, T cell-independent responses to immunological response modifiers, such as quartz, which is immunostimulatory without being an antigen. In the form of the adoptive transfer PLNA, the method lends itself to provide answers to the critical question of whether T cells of animals undergoing a repeated exposure regimen in routine toxicology are sensitized to the parent compound or to a metabolite. Therefore, efforts should be undertaken to determine if, indeed, the PLNA is of general use for routine testing in immunotoxicology. Such efforts should include (i) further standardization of the PLNA, (ii) comparison with other predictive assays, (iii) further evaluation of the adoptive transfer protocol using known metabolites of test compounds, and (iv) validation of the PLNA.

Other predictive tests in mice. Recently, Kimber and Weisenberger (1989) described the auricular lymph node assay (ALNA) in mice and recommended it as a predictive test for the identification of contact sensitizing chemicals. The method is based upon the fact that, following epicutaneous application, sensitizing chemicals initiate a primary immune response in the draining auricular lymph node(s) (ALN), which is characterized by lymphocyte proliferation. In their study, CBA/Ca strain mice were exposed daily for three consecutive days to various concentrations of the test chemical, or to vehicle alone, on the dorsum of the ear. Local lymph node activation was measured subsequently as a function of increased ALN weight, the frequency of large pyroninophilic cells, and lymphocyte proliferation in the presence or absence of an exogenous source of interleukin-2. The results of a validation study were reported in which 22 well-characterized sensitizing chemicals of varying potency were examined. With the exception of three chemicals, for which water was used as the application vehicle, positive responses (defined as a substantial increase in lymphocyte proliferative activity) were recorded with all the test materials. Under the conditions employed, nonsensitizing chemicals, including nonsensititzing irritant chemicals, failed to influence the immunological status of the draining ALN. From these results, Kimber and Weisenberger (1989) concluded that the ALNA provides the basis for a rapid, cost-effective alternative to the currently available predictive test methods in guinea-pigs. Moreover, like the PLNA, the ALNA may be of particular value for the evaluation of coloured or irritant chemicals which are difficult to evaluate using guinea-pig predictive tests (Andersen & Maibach, 1985).

No comparison has been made between the ALNA and the PLNA; however, as discussed above (see Fig. 1), the PLNA is very probably capable of detecting the induction phase of all types of sensitization, including the type-IV reactions involved in contact dermatitis. In fact, the capacity of the PLNA to detect contact sensitizers has been demonstrated (Kammüller *et al.*, 1989). The ALNA, by contrast, is deliberately restricted to the detection of contact sensitizers. Whether or not the ALNA is superior to the PLNA in this respect has not been studied. Until now, no secondary immune response to contact sensitizers has been described using the ALNA. It is also unknown whether or not the ALNA lends itself to detection of sensitizing metabolites, as described above for the adoptive transfer PLNA.

The mouse has been employed not only in the PLNA and ALNA, but also in other attempts to develop methods for identifying contact allergens; in these assays, reactivity is measured as challenge-induced increases in ear thickness (Gad *et al.*, 1986; Maisey & Miller, 1986). In a comprehensive study by Gad *et al.* (1986), the mouse ear swelling test was optimized and used to examine a variety of skin-sensitizing and nonsensitizing chemicals, including a number of those tested by Kimber and Weisenberger (1989) in the ALNA. Among the chemicals that elicited the strongest response in the mouse ear swelling test were oxazolone, picryl chloride, dinitrofluorobenzene, dinitrochlorobenzene, *para*-nitrosodimethylaniline and *para*-phenylenedi-amine (Gad *et al.*, 1986). At the concentrations examined, all of these agents caused very substantial (> 15-fold) increases in lymphocyte proliferation in the ALNA. Some of the chemicals that resulted in less marked net increases in ear thickness, such as eugenol (19%) and formalin (15%), also gave positive results in the ALNA.

Other chemicals examined in the ALNA have also been evaluated in an ear thickness assay described by Maisey and Miller (1986), in which mice were maintained on a diet supplemented with vitamin A. In their study, reactions were recorded for individual animals. Thus, for instance, exposure to cinnamic aldehyde resulted in a greater than 50% increase in ear thickness in six of ten mice tested. Dihydrocoumarin and benzocaine caused a greater than 50% increase in two of ten and in seven of ten animals, respectively (Maisey & Miller, 1986). All of these chemicals gave positive results in the ALNA, too (Kimber & Weisenberger, 1989).

TESTS FOR PREDICTING SENSITIZATION IN MAN

In man, tests to detect adverse immunological reactions to chemicals are performed *a posteriori*, i.e., after a presumed sensitization to a xeno-biotic. At the antibody level, a variety of serological tests to detect specific antibodies to the suspected drugs can be performed *in vitro*. *In vivo*, the scratch test and the prick test are frequently used, both of which involve topical application of the suspected drug into the dermis. Both tests preferentially detect preformed antibodies against the test compound, in particular those of the IgE isotype (type-I reaction). At the T-cell level, chemical compounds are tested for their capacity to elicit contact dermatitis (type-IV reaction) by using the patch test (epicutaneous application).

In-vivo testing of humans harbours the risk of de-novo sensitization and enhancement of existing sensitization. What is needed, therefore, is a test method that demonstrates specific sensitization of human T helper cells to small chemicals *in vitro*. In principle, such sensitization can be demonstrated by the lymphocyte transformation test, in which peripheral blood lymphocytes (essentially T cells) are obtained from a sensitized patient and cultured in the presence of the suspected drug. A problem with this test in its present form is, however, that it has produced many 'false' negative, and also some 'false' positive results. Therefore, its accuracy must be improved (Stejskal *et al.*, 1986), and, in particular, the conditions required for properly 'presenting' the test compound to the responder T cell must be elaborated. Here, too, the question arises of whether the sensitized T cells of a given patient 'see' the parent compound or a metabolite. With certain drugs, evidence in favour of metabolites has been presented (Victorino & Maria, 1985; Merk *et al.*, 1988). While Merk and colleagues failed to detect T-cell transformation in response to parent compounds, they did observe T-cell transformation in response to drugs that were preincubated with liver microsomes as a source of cytochrome P450.

The microsomal cytochrome P450 monooxyqenase enzyme system is involved in the metabolism of a wide variety of structurally unrelated pharmaceutical and environmental agents. In addition to the fact that the P450 system consists of several distinct enzymes coded for by different genes, several genetically determined polymorphisms of P450-mediated drug oxidation have been discovered (Skoda *et al.*, 1988). Monooxygenases may transform xenobiotics into highly reactive metabolites that are capable of covalent binding and thus may exert various biological activities. There is indirect evidence that this includes the induction of autoimmune reactions to proteins of the P450 system. Beaune *et al.* (1987) showed that patients who developed a nonviral hepatitis after treatment with tienilic acid had IgG autoantibodies directed against the isoform P450-8 and that these autoantibodies specifically inhibited the hydroxylation of tienilic acid by human liver microsomes. The authors suggested that cytochrome P450, originally present in the endoplasmic reticulum of the hepatocyte, could be alkylated by a reactive metabolite and migrate onto the hepatocyte membrane surface. At this level, the modified protein could be recognized by specific T helper cells that react to that part of the molecule derived from the reactive metabolite. These functionally active T helper cells would, in turn, allow formation of IgG autoantibodies that recognize the native protein (see Gleichmann *et al.*, 1989a).

While in the system described by Beaune *et al.* (1987) the etiological agent, tienilic acid, is known, it is unknown whether or not genetic polymorphism is involved, i.e., whether their patients were extensive or poor metabolizers of the etiological agent. It is noteworthy in this context that, at least for certain cytochrome P450 genes, it is now possible to distinguish different alleles by means of restriction fragment length polymorphism, using the proband's genomic DNA isolated from peripheral leukocytes. Thus, two alleles of the P450*dbl* gene can be distinguished, which allows phenotyping of 'extensive' and 'poor' metabolizers (Skoda *et al.*, 1988). The P450*dbl* gene affects the metabolism of more than 20 drugs, including β-adrenergic blocking agents, antidepressants, antiarrhythmics and other drugs widely used in clinical medicine.

Whether or not the differential drug metabolism determined by the two alleles of P450*dbl* is responsible for generating metabolites of different immunogenicity is not known at present, but it is not an unlikely possibility. Interestingly, certain patients with idiopathic autoimmune hepatitis produce IgG autoantibodies to P450*dbl* (Manns *et al.*, 1989), and all of these were extensive metabolizers (M. Manns, personal communication). It is conceivable, therefore, that an environmentally altered form of this P450 is rendered immunogenic and thus induces autoimmune hepatitis. In any event, identification of poor and extensive metabolizers before administration of any of the drugs mentioned above will be of great predictive value for the physician, and it is likely that this is also relevant for the prediction of adverse immune reactions to these agents.

ACKNOWLEDGEMENTS

Supported in part by grants 01VM8614 from the programme on rheumatic diseases and 07ALL050 from the programme on allergy and environment from the Federal Ministry of Research and Technology, Bonn, Federal Republic of Germany

REFERENCES

Amos, H.E. (1983) Drugs acting on the cardiovascular system. In: De Weck, A.L. & Bundgaard, H., eds, *Allergic Reactions to Drugs,* Berlin (West), Springer, pp. 391-422

Andersen, K.E. & Maibach, H.I. (1985) Guinea pig sensitization assay. An overview. *Curr. Probl. Dermatol.*, **14**: 263-290

Anon. (1986) Withdrawal of nomifensine. *Lancet* , **i**, 281

Ayesh, R., Mitchell, S.C. & Waring, R.H. (1987) Sodium aurothiomalate toxicity and sulphoxidation capacity in rheumatoid arthritis patients. *Br. J. Rheumatol.*, **26**: 197-201

Bärtsch A. & Schlatter, C. (1988) [Platinum emmissions from automobile catalysts. Literature research of the Institut für Toxikologie der Eidgenössischen Technischen Hochschule and the Universität Zürich.] (in German) (*Schriftenreihe Umweltschutz No. 95.*), Bern, Schweizerischen Bundesamt für Umweltschutz

Beaune, P.H., Dansette, P.M., Mansuy, D., Kiffel, L., Finck, M., Amar, C., Leroux, J.P. & Homberg, J.C. (1987) Human antiendoplasmatic reticulum autoantibodies appearing in a drug-induced hepatitis are directed against a human liver cytochrome P-450 that hydroxylates the drug. *Proc. natl Acad. Sci. USA*, **84**: 551-555

Biagini, R.E., Bernstein, I.L., Gallagher, J.S., Moorman, W.J., Brooks, S. & Gann, P.H. (1985) The diversity of reaginic immune responses to platinum and palladium metallic salts. *J. Allergy clin. Immunol.*, **76**: 794-802

Bradford, C.W. (1987) Platinum. In: Seiler, H.G. & Sigel, H., eds, *Handbook of Toxicity of Inorganic Compounds*, New York, Marcel Dekker, pp. 533-539

Cleare, M.J., Hughes, E.G., Jacoby, B. & Pepys, J. (1976) Immediate (type I) allergic responses to platinum compounds. *Clin Allergy*, **6**: 183-195

Cohnen, G. (1985) [Drug-induced lupus erythematodsus-like syndrome.](in German) *Allergologie*, **8**: 282-292

Davis, P. (1979) Undesirable effects of gold. *J. Rheumatol.*, **6** (Suppl. 5): 18-23

Denman, E.F. & Denman, A.M. (1969) The lymphocyte transformation test and gold hypersensitivity. *Ann. rheum. Dis.*, **27**: 582-589

Freedman, S.O. & Krupey, J. (1968) Respiratory allergy caused by platinum salts. *J. Allergy*, **42**: 233-237

Gad, S.C., Dunn, B.J., Dobbs, D.W., Reilly, C. & Walsh, R.D. (1986) Development and validation of an alternative dermal sensitization test: the mouse ear swelling test (MEST). *Toxicol. appl. Pharmacol.*, **84**: 93-114

Gell, P.G.H. & Coombs, R.R.A. (1963) *Clinical Aspects of Immunology*, Oxford, Blackwell

Gleichmann, E. & Gleichmann, H. (1989) [The popliteal lymph node (PLN) test in rodents, a simple functional test for the detection of sensitizing chemicals.] (in German) In: Grosdanoff, P., Kraupp, O. & Schulte-Hermann, R., eds [Toxicological and clinical studies in the framework of public health.] (*Proceedings of a Symposium held in Salzburg, Oct. 16-18, 1988*), Berlin (West), Walter de Gruyter, pp. 259-280

Gleichmann, E., Pals, S.T., Rolink, A.G., Radszkiewicz, T. & Gleichmann, H. (1984) Graft-versus-host reactions (GVHR): clues to the etiopathology of a spectrum of immunological diseases. *Immunol. Today*, **5**: 324-332

Gleichmann, E., Kimber, I. & Purchase, I.F.H. (1989a) Immunotoxicology: suppressive and stimulatory efects of drugs and environmental chemicals on the immune system. *Arch. Toxicol.*, **63**: 257-273

Gleichmann, E., Vohr, H.-W., Stringer, C., Nuyens, J. & Gleichmann, H. (1989b) Testing the sensitization of T cells to chemicals. From murine graft-versus-host reactions (GVHRs) to chemical-induced GVH-like immunological diseases. In: Kämmuller, M.E., Bloksma, N. & Seinen, W., eds, *Autoimmunity and Toxicology. Immunedysregulation Induced by Drugs and Chemicals*, Amsterdam, Elsevier, pp. 363-390

Gleichmann, H. (1981) Studies on the mechanism of drug sensitization: T cell dependent popliteal lymph node reaction to diphenylhydantoin. *Clin. Immunol. Immunopathol.*, **18**: 203-211

Gleichmann, H., Pals, S.T. & Radaszkiewcs, T. (1983) The T-cell-dependent B-cell proliferation and activation induced by administration of the drug diphenylhydantoin (DPH) to mice. *Hematol. Oncol.*, **1**: 165-176

Hallauer, J., Spix, C., Dolgner, R., Stiller-Winkler, R., Gleichmann, E. & Schlipköter, H.-W. (1989) Correlation between air pollution and total IgE serum levels in humans, and studies on the IgE-enhancing and autoimmunizing effects of mercuric chloride in mice. In: Pichler, W.J., Stadler, B.M., Dahinden, C.A., Pecoud, A.R., Frei, P., Schneider, C.H. & De Weck, A.L., eds, *Progress in Allergy and Clinical Immunology*, Toronto, Hogrefe & Huber, pp. 271-274

Hurtenbach, U., Gleichmann, H., Nagata, N. & Gleichmann, E. (1987) Immunity to D-penicillamine: genetic, cellular and chemical requirements for induction of popliteal lymph node enlargement in the mouse. *J. Immunol.*, **139**: 411-416

Kammüller, M.E. & Seinen, W. (1988) Structural requirements for hydantoins and 2-thiohydantoins to induce lymphoproliferative popliteal lymph node reactions in the mouse. *Int. J. Immunopharmacol.*, **10**: 997-1010

Kammüller, M. E., Thomas, C., De Bakker, J.M., Bloksma, N. & Seinen, W. (1989) The popliteal lymph node assay in mice to screen for the immune disregulating potential of chemicals. A preliminary study. *Int. J. Immunopharmacol.*, **11**: 293-300

Kimber, I. & Weisenberger, C. (1989) A murine local lymph node assay for the identification of contact allergens: assay development and results of an initial validation study. *Arch. Toxicol.*, **63**: 274-282

Klinkhammer, C., Popowa, P. & Gleichmann, H. (1988) Specific immunity to the diabetogen streptozotocin: cellular requirements for induction of lymphoproliferation. *Diabetes*, **37**: 74-80

Kristofferson, A. & Nilsson, B.B. (1989) Zimeldine: febrile reactions and peripehral neuropathy. In: Kammüller, M.E., Bloksma, N. & Seinen, W.E., eds, *Autoimmunity and Toxicology. Immune Disregulation Induced by Drugs and Chemicals*, Amsterdam, Elsevier, pp. 183-214

Lockie, L.M. & Smith, D.M. (1985) Forty-seven years experience with gold therapy in 1,019 rheumatoid arthritis patients. *Sem. Arthr. Rheum.*, **14**: 238-246

Louyot, P., Grilliat, J.P., Monneret-Vautron, D., Pourel, J. & Pupil, P. (1974) [Immunological study of intolerance to chrysotherapy.] (in French) *Rev. Rhum.*, **41**: 1-6

Magnusson, B. & Kligman, A.M. (1969) The identification of contact allergens by animal assay, the guinea pig maximization test method. *J. invest. Dermatol.*, **52**: 268-276

Maisey, J. & Miller, K. (1986) Assessment of the ability of mice fed on vitamin A supplemented diet to respond to a variety of potential contact sensitizers. *Contact Dermatitis*, **15**: 17-23

Manns, M.P., Johnson, E.F., Griffin, K.J., Tan, E.M. & Sullivan, K.F. (1989) Major antigen of liver kidney microsomal autoantibodies in idiopathic autoimmune hepatitis is cytochrome P450dbl. *J. clin. Invest.*, **83**: 1066-1072

Merget, R., Schultze-Werninghaus, G., Muthorst, T., Friedrich, W. & Meier-Sydow, J. (1988) Asthma due to the complex salts of platinum - a cross-sectional survey of workers in a platinum refinery. *Clin Allergy*, **18**: 569-580

Merk, H., Schneider, R. & Scholl, P. (1988) Lymphocyte stimulation by drug-modified microsomes. In: Estarbrook, R.W., Lindenlaub, E., Oesch, F. & De Weck, A.L., eds, *Toxicological and Immunological Aspects of Drug Metabolism and Environmental Chemicals (Symposia Medica Hoechst 22)*, Stuttgart, Schattauer, pp. 211-219

Miyamoto, T., Takafuji, S., Suzuki, S., Tadokoro, K. & Muranaka, M. (1989) Allergy and changing environments - industrial/urban pollution. In: Pichler, W.J., Stadler, B.M., Dahinden, P., Pecoud, A.R., Frei, P., Schneider, C.H. & De Weck, A.L., eds, *Progress in Allergy and Clinical Immunology*, Toronto, Hogrefe & Huber, pp. 265-270

Mosmann, T.R. & Coffman, R.L. (1987) Two types of mouse helper T-cell clone. *Immunol. Today*, **8**: 223-227

Murdoch, R.D., Pepys, J. & Hughes, E.G. (1986) IgE antibody responses to platinum group metal salts. A large scale refinery survey. *Br. J. ind. Med.*, **43**: 37-43

Pietsch, P., Vohr, H.-W., Degitz, K. & Gleichmann, E. (1989) Immunological alterations inducible by mercury compounds. II. $HgCl_2$ and gold sodium thiomalate enhance serum IgE and IgG concentrations in susceptible mouse strains. *Int. Arch. Allergy appl. Immunol.*, **90**: 47-53

Roberts, H.E. (1951) Platinosis. A five-year study of the effects of soluble platinum salts on employees in a platinum laboratory and refinery. *Arch. ind. Hyg.*, **4**: 549-559

Robinson, C.J.G., Balazs, T. & Egorov, I.K. (1986) Mercuric chloride-, gold sodium thiomalate- and D-penicillamine-induced anti-nuclear antibodies in mice. *Toxicol. appl. Pharmacol.*, **86**: 159-169

Rosner, G. & Hertel, R.F. (1986) [Risk potential of platinum emissions from automobile catalysts.] (in German) *Staub Reinhalt Luft*, **46**: 281-285

Rothschild, B. & Marshall, H. (1986) Lymphadenopathy and lymph node infarction in the course of gold therapy. *Am. J. Med.*, **80**: 537-540

Rotmensch, H.H., Leiser, M., Dan, M., Klejman, A., Livni, E., Illie, B., Messer, G., Kadish, U. & Liran, M. (1981) Evaluation of prajmalium-induced cholestasis by immunologic tests. *Ann. intern. Med.*, **141**: 1797-1802

Rubin, R.L. & Curnutte, J.T. (1989) Metabolism of procainamide to the cytotoxic hydroxylamine by neutrophils activated in vitro. *J. clin. Invest.*, **83**: 1336-1343

Scherak, O., Smolen, J.S., Mayr, R., Mayhofer, G., Kolarz, G. & Thumb, N.J. (1984) HLA-antigens and toxicity to gold and penicillamine in rheumatoid arthritis. *J. Rheumatol.*, **11**: 610-615

Schöpf, E., Wex, O. & Schulz, K.H. (1970) [Allergic contact stomatitis with specific lympho-cyte stimulation by gold.] (in German) *Hautarzt*, **21**: 422-424

Schuhmann, D., Kubicka-Muranyi, M., Mirtschewa, J., Kind, P. & Gleichmann, E. (1989) Adverse immune reactions to gold. I. Chronic treatment with an Au[I] drug sensitizes mouse spleen cells not to Au[I], but to Au[III] and induces autoantibody formation. (Submitted)

Skoda, R.C., Gonzales, F.J., Demierre, A. & Meyer, U.A. (1988) Two mutant alleles of the human cytochrome P-450dbl gene (*P450C2D*) associated with genetically deficient metabolism of debrisoquine and other drugs. *Proc. natl Acad. Sci. USA*, **85**: 5240-5243

Stark, M., Zaidi, S., Hilscher, B., Hilscher, W. & Gleichmann, E. (1988) High- and low-responder mouse strains with respect to silica-induced fibrosis (Abstract). *Immunbiology*, **178**: 100-101

Stejskal, V.D.M., Olin, R. & Forsbeck, M. (1986) The lymphocyte transformation test for diagnosis of drug-induced occupational allergy. *J. Allergy clin. Immunol.*, **77**: 411-426

Stiller-Winkler, R., Radaszkiewicz, T. & Gleichmann, E. (1988) Immunopathological signs in mice treated with mercury compounds. I. Popliteal lymph node reactions to mercury compounds: responder and non-responder mouse strains to HgCl₂. *Int. J. Immuno-pharmacol.*, **10**: 475-484

Stollenwerk, R., Annefeld, M., Schilling, F. & Dreher, R. (1986) [Rare adverse effects of gold.] (in German) *Z. Rheumatol.*, **45**: 107-110

Victorino, R.M.M. & Maria, V.A. (1985) Modifications of the lymphocyte transformation test in a case of drug-induced cholestatic hepatitis. *Diagn. Immunol.*, **3**: 177-183

Vohr, H.-W., Kubicka-Muranyi, M. & Gleichmann, E. (1989) [Development of the popliteal lymph node test: a simple functional test for detection of sensitizing chemicals.] (in German) In: *Umwelthygiene*, Vol. 21, Düsseldorf, Gesellschaft zur Förderung der Lufthygiene und Silikoseforschung, pp. 203-227

IMMUNOTOXICITY OF METALS

IMMUNOLOGICAL AND IMMUNE-MEDIATED TOXIC EFFECTS OF GOLD COMPOUNDS USED IN THE TREATMENT OF RHEUMATOID ARTHRITIS

G.S. Panayi

Rheumatology Unit, Division of Medicine
United Medical and Dental Schools of Guy's and St Thomas' Hospitals
Guy's Hospital, London SE1 9RT, UK

ABSTRACT

A variety of immune-mediated side-effects can follow treatment of patients with rheumatoid arthritis with gold salts. The two commonest are gold-induced glomerulonephritis and thrombocytopenia; both are strongly linked to two genetic markers, HLA-DR3 and poor sulfoxidation. These side-effects may come about as a result of hapten formation and inhibition of macrophage function. It is of interest to note that patients who respond best to gold treatment are those likely to develop side-effects. It may be concluded that the two manifestations are due to the same underlying mechanism.

INTRODUCTION

Gold salts have been used for the treatment of rheumatoid arthritis and other inflammatory arthritides for some 60 years. Their anti-inflammatory potency was discovered empirically, and even today there is no clear understanding as to their mode of action. Despite their effectiveness, their use is restricted by toxic side-effects; thus, only some 15% of patients are still on treatment after five years. The side-effects include skin rashes, blood dyscrasias, mouth ulcers, proteinuria, colitis (Langer *et al.*, 1987), hepatitis (Edelman *et al.*, 1983) and pneumonitis (Hakala *et al.*, 1986) (Table 1). They usually occur early during the course of treatment, after three or four months, when the gold is beginning to have a suppressive effect on disease activity. Indeed, recent studies have shown, what has long been suspected, that those patients who respond best are those most likely to develop side-effects. This phenomenon of the concurrence of response and toxicity needs to be explained by any proposed mechanism of the action of gold salts but may be linked by the fact that such patients are often HLA-DR3-positive (van Riel *et al.*, 1983; Speerstra *et al.*, 1986; Caspi *et al.*, 1989).

Many of the side effects are immunological. Thus, the thrombocytopenia is usually very rapid and is associated with normal bone-marrow cytology (Madhok *et al.*, 1985) and usually responds promptly to steroids. Antiplatelet antibodies have been described (Armstrong *et al.*, 1983; Adachi *et al.*, 1987). The proteinuria is caused by a glomerulonephritis indistinguishable from that of idiopathic glomerulonephritis. It is characterized by the presence of lumpy deposits of immunoglobulin and complement within the glomerulus. The skin rash has all of the characteristics of a fixed drug eruption, although no distinctive pathology has been described. The immunological features of the lesions, their sudden appearance early in the course of therapy and their reappearance on drug challenge led to the hypothesis that a genetic factor may be linked to the major histocompatibility complex, which regulates immune responsiveness (Panayi *et al.*, 1978). It was soon established in our laboratory and in others that the glomerulonephritis (Wooley *et al.*, 1980)

Table 1. Gold preparations used in the treatment of rheumatoid arthritis, their toxic side-effects and HLA associations

Preparation	Toxicity	HLA	Reference
Aurothiopropanol sulfate	Proteinuria	nil	Dequeker et al. (1984)
	Blood	nil	
Gold thioglucose	Proteinuria	DR3	Speerstra et al. (1983)
Gold thioglucose	All	nil	Speerstra et al. (1986)
Gold thiomalate	Proteinuria	DR3	Panayi et al. (1978)
	Mouth ulcers	DR2	
Gold thiomalate	Proteinuria	DR3	Wooley et al. (1980)
Gold thiomalate	Thrombocytopenia	DR3	Coblyn et al. (1981)
Gold thiomalate	Hepatitis	Not done	Edelman et al. (1983)
Gold thiomalate	Proteinuria	DR3	Gran et al. (1983)
	Skin	nil	
	Leukopenia	nil	
Gold thiomalate	Proteinuria	DR3	van Riel et al. (1983)
Gold thiomalate	Proteinuria	DR3	Barger et al. (1984)
Gold thiomalate	All	DR3	Bensen et al. (1984)
Gold thiomalate	Proteinuria	DR3	Scherak et al. (1984)
	Skin rash	B7	
Gold thiomalate	Skin rash	Bw35	Alarcon et al. (1985)
Gold thiomalate	All	DR3	Dahlqvist et al. (1985)
Gold thiomalate	Thrombocytopenia	DR3	Madhok et al. (1985)
Gold thiomalate	Proteinuria	nil (blacks)	Alarcon et al. (1986)
	Skin rash	nil	
Gold thiomalate	All	nil	Nuotio et al. (1986)
Gold thiomalate	Proteinuria	DR3 (Greeks)	Pachoula-Papasteriades
	Skin rash	DRw6	et al. (1986)
Gold thiomalate	Thrombocytopenia	DR3	Adachi et al. (1987)
Gold thiosulfate	Skin rash	B35	Ferracciolo et al. (1986)
Not given	All	nil	Gladman & Anhorn (1986)
Not given	Pneumonitis	B40, Dwl	Hakala et al. (1986)
	Proteinuria	DR3	
	Skin rash	B7	

and the thrombocytopenia (Coblyn et al., 1981) were linked to HLA-DR3 and mouth ulcers to HLA-DR2 (Panayi et al., 1978). To date, only a weak association has been discovered between HLA-B35 and skin rash (Ferraccioli et al., 1986), but to my knowledge no study has been undertaken to investigate any possible involvement of the HLAD-DQ or -DP loci of the major histocompatibility complex. Most studies have been in agreement about these associations, but some have not, especially with regard to HLA-DR3 and proteinuria. Part of this discrepancy may be explained by differences in selection criteria, part by the racial composition of the patients studied (Alarcon et al., 1986) and part by the nature of the gold preparation used, such as aurothiopropanol sulfate (Dequeker et al., 1984). The observation that the gold preparation is important is supported by the fact that proteinuria and other side-effects are uncommon in patients taking the oral preparation of gold (triethylphosphine gold) (Tozman & Gottlieb, 1987) and are not linked to HLA-DR3 (van Riel et al., 1983), and by studies in which different gold preparations were used to induce antinucleolar antibodies in A.SW mice (Goter Robinson, 1989).

There has been prolonged discussion as to whether gold or thiomalate is the active moiety of sodium aurothiomalate (SAT). A recent controlled study has shown that thiomalate has no clinical benefit (Rudge et al., 1988). It may be concluded that gold is directly or indirectly involved in the genesis of the clinical benefit and of the toxic side-effects in humans. Possible mechanisms will be discussed below, but the failure to show any correlation between serum gold levels and toxicity adds further weight to the concept that this is immunologically mediated. In many tissues, the gold is found within macrophages, sequestered within aurosomes, which are gold-laden lysosomes. Since macrophages are important accessory cells in the immune response, it is of some interest to note that panhypogamma-globulinaemia following SAT therapy has been described in a few patients (Burns et al., 1987). This observation supports the finding of Lipsky (1983) that gold inhibits lymphocyte function *in vitro* by an effect on macrophages, and by the work of Littman and Hall (1985), who showed that SAT inhibits monocyte-macrophage maturation and differentiation. Macrophages within the synovial membrane are particularly rich in aurosomes. In the human kidney, gold has been detected in the proximal tubules but not in the glomerulus. More recently, it has been proposed that gold may produce some of its effects by nonimmunological means, such as by inhibition of endothelial cell proliferation (Matsubara & Ziff, 1987) and of the production of macrophage-derived angiogenic activity (Koch et al., 1988).

Nevertheless, the thiomalate component of SAT may still have a role to play in toxicity. First, patients taking sodium thiomalate can develop skin rashes that are sufficiently severe to necessitate withdrawal of the substance (Rudge et al., 1988). Second, it has been shown that oxidation of the sulfur in thiol groups is under genetic control and that deficient sulfoxidation may be an important factor in the predisposition to develop D-penicillamine toxicity (Emery et al., 1984). Ayesh and colleagues (1987) have shown that 81% (van Riel et al., 1983; Langer et al., 1987) of patients who developed side-effects to SAT were poor sulfoxidizers compared to 32% (Burns et al., 1987; Matsubara & Ziff, 1987) of those not displaying adverse effects. They calculated that a patient with poor sulfoxidation had a nine-fold greater risk of developing toxicity. Acetylator phenotype is not a risk factor (Rantapaa-Dahlqvist & Mjorndal, 1987).

IMMUNE FUNCTION IN HLA-DR3-POSITIVE INDIVIDUALS

In addition to being linked to idiopathic and SAT-induced glomerulonephritis and to thrombocytopenia, HLA-DR3 is linked to a number of organ-specific autoimmune diseases (such as Graves' disease, myasthenia gravis and type-I diabetes mellitus) and to non-organ-specific autoimmune diseases such as systemic lupus erythematosus and Sjogren's syndrome. All these conditions are characteried by the presence of a wide variety of autoantibodies in the serum. Clearly, additional factors, both genetic and environmental, must be operating in order to explain the expression of one disease rather than another in a particular individual. Nevertheless, the striking association of HLA-DR3 with spontaneous autoimmune disease and with SAT-induced immune-mediated toxic effects suggests that individuals with this genetic make-up are particularly prone to perturbation of their immune system.

There is considerable experimental evidence to support this hypothesis. Patients with systemic lupus erythematosus have B-cell hyperactivity resulting in a polyclonal hypergammaglobulinaemia. *In vitro*, B cells from lupus patients required 75 times as much anti-IgG to inhibit pokeweed mitogen-induced activation as normal controls (Salata et al., 1988). Interestingly, a similar abnormality was found in healthy HLA-DR3-positive controls. The genetic control of the immunoglobulin and lymphocyte immune response to α-*Helix pomatia* haemocyanin in healthy subjects was found to be dependent on the presence of HLA-DR3 and certain Gm allotypes (Kallenberg et al., 1988). Patients with Sjogren's syndrome who have anti-Ia antibodies in their serum are DR3-positive. In normal healthy individuals, pokeweed mitogen induced production of anti-Ia antibodies but not of anti-DNA or anti-RNP/Sm antibodies occurred only in DR3-positive subjects (Venables et al., 1988).

Healthy HLA-DR3-positive individuals show increased spontaneous and mumps virus-induced immunoglobulin production *in vitro* (Ilonen et al., 1986). There is increased natural killer cytotoxicity in persons positive for HLA-B8 and -DR3 (Jakobisiak et al., 1986), and this may be of some relevance as natural killer cells may be involved as accessory cells in immunoglobulin production (Abruzzo & Rowley, 1983). Peripheral blood monocytes from DR3-positive individuals show decreased phagocytosis of IgG-sensitized erythrocytes *in vitro* but not of neuraminidase-treated erythrocytes (Salmon et al., 1986), and it has been speculated that this defect may contribute to the autoimmune predisposition of such individuals. In the circulation of HLA-B8-positive individuals, there are increased numbers of IgM-containing B cells, a significantly increased CD4:CD8 T-cell ratio, increased Ig production to pokeweed mitogen by B cells and decreased conconavalin A-induced T-cell suppression (McCombs et al., 1986). Furthermore, these individuals show decreased T-lymphocyte proliferation in the autologous mixed lymphocyte reaction (Davey et al., 1984), which may be of relevance in this context since, during this reaction, suppressor T cells may be generated. Finally, it is of particular interest that high antibody responses to two non-cross-reacting components of

Lolium perenne (rye grass) pollen extract, Lol p I (Rye I) and Lol p II (Rye), were found in HLA-DR3-positive individuals (Freidhoff *et al.*, 1988). These findings may be of biological relevance (Granoff *et al.*, 1984), as shown by the increased prevalence of *Haemophilus* meningitis or epiglottitis in HLA-DR3-positive individuals with the Gm allotype (Ilonen *et al.*, 1986; McCombs *et al.*, 1986; Adachi *et al.*, 1987; Balazs, 1987; Salata *et al.*, 1988; Venables *et al.*, 1988). Taken together, these findings strongly support the hypothesis that HLA-DR3-positive people have a hyperactive immune system, which, when perturbed in an appropriate manner, can lead to autoimmune disease.

STUDIES IN EXPERIMENTAL ANIMALS

Mercuric chloride can induce autoimmune glomerulonephritis in Brown Norway rats and ASW mice but not in other strains of rats or mice; susceptibility is determined by an interaction of the major histocompatibility complex with background genes (Balazs, 1987). Gold salts can induce glomerulophritis in Brown Norway rats, and the antiglomerular basement membrane antibodies (anti-laminin) found transiently in their serum share a cross-reactivity idiotype with anti-laminin antibodies produced during toxicity due to mercuric chloride. Antibodies with this idiotype have been found both in the circulation and in the kidney of Brown Norway rats with nephritis induced by mercuric chloride or gold salts (Guerry *et al.*, 1989). It is of interest to note that Lewis rats, which are particularly susceptible to the induction of adjuvant arthritis, are resistant to the induction of glomeruloneprhitis by gold salts (Tournade *et al.*, 1989). The link with the major histocompatibility complex strongly suggests that T cells are involved, and it remains to be seen what disturbances in immune regulation are induced by gold. A likely mechanism may be interference with peripheral tolerance. In BALB/c mice, interstitial nephritis can be induced by injecting them with tubular basement membrane antigen in Freund's complete adjuvant. The nephritis can be transferred by splenic T cells. If BALB/c mice are injected with the antigen alone they do not develop interstitial nephritis, and their thymus T cells can suppress interstitial nephritis in other mice. Pretreatment of animals with gold salts before immunization with tubular basement membrane antigen decreases the nephritogenicity of splenic T cells and increases the suppressive effect of thymic T cells (Azemoto *et al.*, 1989). Hence, gold salts can have effects that depend on the state of the immune system (immunization with or without Freund's complete adjuvant) and on the cellular population being studied. Wakashin and colleagues (1989) have demonstrated that peripheral blood T cells from patients with rheumatoid arthritis who have developed gold-induced nephropathy will proliferate in response to tubular basement membrane antigen only after adherent cells have been removed by passage over a nylon-wool column. This is a very important finding, which suggests that a peptide from the antigen is presented by the HLA-DR3 molecule to appropriate T cells, which then provide help to B cells for an antibody response that causes glomerulonephritis.

PATHOGENESIS OF GOLD-INDUCED TOXICITY IN HUMANS

At least two genetic factors would appear to be involved in the pathogenesis of gold-induced toxicity in humans: HLA-DR3 and decreased sulfoxidation; but others are undoubtedly involved, as suggested by a study in two pairs of monozygotic twins (van de Putte *et al.*, 1986) and by a failure to find any of the known HLA associations in American blacks (Alarcon *et al.*, 1986).

The autoimmune thrombocytopenia could best be explained by the formation of haptenic groups on the platelet surface, which would initiate the autoimmune process by breaking tolerance. Individuals who are HLA-DR3-positive may be particularly prone to the development of anti-platelet antibodies, since the immune response to the human platelet antigens Zwa (Mueller-Eckhardt *et al.*, 1985) and PLA1 (Muller *et al.*, 1983) during pregnancy is strongly linked to that HLA antigen. Indeed, 20/21 mothers who developed anti-PLA1 antibodies were HLA-DR3-positive. A similar hypothesis has been proposed for the pathogenesis of the glomerulonephritis: gold hapten-antibody complexes would be deposited in the glomerulus (Duke *et al.*, 1982); however, electron microprobe analysis failed to reveal gold in the subepithelial deposits of patients (Strunk & Ziff, 1970), making this an unlikely mechanism. An alternative hypothesis (Duke *et al.*, 1982) is that renal tubular antigen(s) are released during chrysotherapy and that antibodies are made to this antigen, in keeping with the general immune hyperactivity of HLA-DR3-positive individuals (*vide supra*). Immune complexes of antibody and renal tubular antigen would then be deposited in the glomerulus, as in Heymann nephritis. Renal tubular damage following therapy with gold thiomalate has not, however, been found in patients; but the indicators used were rather insensitive (Crisp *et al.*, 1983), and a search for renal tubular antigen in the urine and serum of treated patients is urgently indicated. The situation may be exacerbated by the fact that patients with rheumatoid arthritis have poor reticuloendothelial clearance (Williams *et al.*, 1979), which may be depressed even further by gold salts, which have been shown to reduce the phagotytic ability of macrophages *in vitro* and *in vivo* (Jessop *et al.*, 1973; Davis *et al.*, 1979).

Thus, further work is needed in order to elucidate fully the mechanisms leading to gold toxicity but they provide an interesting example of the interplay of genetic and environmental factors *via* the medium of the immune system.

REFERENCES

Abruzzo, L.V. & Rowley, D.A. (1983) Homeostasis of the immune response: immunoregulation by NK cells. *Science*, **222**: 581-584

Adachi, J.D., Bensen, W.G., Kassam, Y., Powers, P.J., Bianchi, F.A., Cividino, A., Kean, W.F., Rooney, P.J., Craig, G.L., Buchanan, W.W. *et al.* (1987) Gold induced thrombocytopenia: 12 cases and a review of the literature. *Semin. Arthritis Rheum.*, **16**: 287-293

Alarcon, G.S., Koopman, W.J., Acton, R.T. & Barger, B.O. (1985) HLA-Bw35 and gold toxicity in rheumatoid arthritis (Letter). *Arthritis Rheum.*, **28**: 236-237

Alarcon, G.S., Barger, B.O., Acton, R.T. & Koopman, W.J. (1986) HLA antigens and gold toxicity in American blacks with rheumatoid arthritis. *Rheumatol. int.*, **6**: 13-17

Armstrong, R.D., Faith, A., Panayi, G.S. & Batchelor, J.R. (1983) Gold-induced thrombocytopenia: detection of anti-platelet antibody. *Clin. Rheum.*, **2**: 183-276

Ayesh, R., Mitchell, S.C., Waring, R.H., Withrington, R.H., Seifert, M.H. & Smith, R.L. (1987) Sodium aurothiomalate toxicity and sulphoxidation capacity in rheumatoid arthritis patients. *Br. J. Rheumatol.*, **26**: 197-201

Azemoto, R., Ueda, S., Wakashin, Y., Ogawa, M., Yoshida, H., Mori, Y. & Wakashin, M. (1989) Immunosuppressive and immunoenhancing effects of gold. In: *Seventh International Congress of Immunology*, Abstract WH90-4, p. 581

Balazs, T. (1987) Immunogenetically controlled autoimmune reactions induced by mercury, gold and D-penicillamine in laboratory animals: a review from the vantage point of premarketing safety studies. *Toxicol. ind. Health*, **3**: 331-336

Barger, B.O., Acton, R.T., Koopman, W.J. & Alarcon, G.S. (1984) DR antigens and gold toxicity in white rheumatoid arthritis patients. *Arthritis Rheum.*, **27**: 601-605

Bensen, W.G., Moore, N., Tugwell, P., D'Souza, M. & Singal, D.P. (1984) HLA antigens and toxic reactions to sodium aurothiomalate in patients with rheumatois arthritis. *J. Rheumatol.*, **11**: 358-361

Burns, H.J., Klimiuk, P.S., Hilton, R.C. & Haeney, M. (1987) Gold-induced hypogammaglobulinaemia. *Br. J. Rheumatol.*, **26**: 53-55

Caspi, D., Tishler, M. & Yaron, M. (1989) Association between gold induced skin rash and remission in patients with rheumatois arthritis. *Ann. rheum. Dis.*, **48**: 730-732

Coblyn, J.S., Weinblatt, M., Hodsworth, D. & Glass, D. (1981) Gold-induced thrombocytopenia. *Ann. intern. Med.*, **95**: 178-181

Crisp, A.J., Coughlan, R.J., Clark, B., Mackintosh, D., Panayi, G.S., Sweny, P., Hopper, J. & Varghese, Z. (1983) Failure of sodium aurothiomalate and triethyl phosphine gold to cause renal tubular injury in rheumatoid arthritis. *Clin. Rheum.*, **2**: 273-276

Dahlqvist, S.R., Strom, H., Bjelle, A. & Moller, E. (1985) HLA antigens and adverse drug reactions to sodium aurothiomalate and D-penicillamine in patients with rheumatoid arthritis. *Clin. Rheumatol.*, **4**: 55-61

Davey, F.R., Kurec, A.S., Dock, N.L., Hubbell, C. & Falen, S.W. (1984) Association of HLA-DR antigens with the autologous mixed lymphocyte reaction. *Tissue Antigens*, **24**: 98-106

Davis, P., Miller, C.L. & Johnston, C.A. (1979) Effect of gold salts on adherent mononuclear cells in tissue culture. *J. Rheumatol.*, **6** (Suppl. 5): 98-102

Dequeker, J., Van Wanghe, P. & Verdikt, W.A. (1984) Systematic survey of HLA-A, -B, -C and -D antigens and drug toxicity in rheumatoid arthritis. *J. Rheumatol.*, **11**: 282-290

Duke, O., Richter, M. & Panayi, G.S. (1982) Gold related nephropathy. In: Bach, P.H., Bonner, F.W., Bridges, J.W. & Lock, E.A., eds, *Nephrotoxicity: Assessment and Pathogenesis*, Chichester, John Wiley & Sons, pp. 349-355

Edelman, J., Donnelly, R., Graham, D.N. & Percy, J.S. (1983) Liver dysfunction associated with gold therapy for rheumatoid arthritis. *J. Rheumatol.*, **10**: 510-511

Emery, P., Panayi, G.S., Huston, G., Welsh, K.I., Mitchell, S.C., Shah, R.S., Idle, J.R., Smith, R.L. & Waring, R.H. (1984) D-Penicillamine induced toxicity in rheumatoid arthritis: the role of sulphoxidation status and HLA-DR3. *J. Rheumatol.*, **11**: 626-632

Ferraccioli, G., Peri, F., Nervetti, A., Ambanelli, U. & Savi, M. (1986) Toxicity due to remission inducing drugs in rheumatoid arthritis. Association with HLA-B35 and Cw4 antigens. *J. Rheumatol.*, **13**: 65-68

Freidhoff, L.R., Ehrlich-Kautzky, E., Meyers, D.A., Ansari, A.A., Bias, W.B. & Marsh, D.G. (1988) Association of HLA-DR3 with human response to Lol p I and Lol p II allergens in allergic subjects. *Tissue Antigens*, **31**: 211-219

Gladman, D.D. & Anhorn, K.A. (1986) HLA and disease manifestations in rheumatoid arthritis - a Canadian experience. *J. Rheumatol.*, **13**: 274-276

Goter Robinson, C.J. (1989) Induction of anti-nucleolar antibodies by gold compounds in ASW mice. In: *Seventh International Congress of Immunology*, Abstract WH90-10, p. 582

Gran, J.T., Husby, G. & Thornsby, E. (1983) HLA-DR antigens and gold toxicity. *Ann. rheum. Dis.*, **42**: 63-66

Granoff, D.M., Boies, E., Squires, J., Pandey, J.P., Suarez, B., Oldfather, J. & Rodey, G.E. (1984) Interactive effect of genes associated with immunoglobulin allotypes and HLA specificities on susceptibility to *Haemophilus influenzae* disease. *J. Immunogenet.*, **11**: 181-188

Guerry, J.C., Tournade, H. & Druet, P. (1989) Cross-reactive idiotype of anti-glomerular basement membrane antibodies in drug and toxic-induced glomerulonephritis. In: *Seventh International Congress of Immunology*, Abstract WH90-10, p. 582

Hakala, M., van Assendelft, A.H., Ilonen, J., Jalava, S. & Tiilikainen, A. (1986) Association of different HLA antigens with various toxic effects of gold salts in rheumatoid arthritis. *Ann. rheum. Dis.*, **45**: 177-182

Ilonen, J., Salonen, R., Hyypia, T., Lankinen, K., Karttunen, R. & Salmi, A. (1986) Immune functions in healthy blood donors with HLA-DW2 and -DW3 antigens. *Immunobiology*, **171**: 388-389

Jakobisiak, M., Saidman, S., Schlaut, J., Pazderka, F. & Dossetor, J.B. (1986) Elevated natural killer cytotoxicity in HLA-B8 and HLA-DR3-positive individuals. *Immunol. Lett.*, **12**: 61-63

Jessop, J.D., Vernon-Roberts, B. & Harris, J. (1973) Effects of gold salts and prednisolone on inflammatory cells. *Ann. rheum. Dis.*, **32**: 294-307

Kallenberg, C.G., Klaassen, R.J., Westra, J., Beelen, J.M. & Ockhuizen, T. (1988) Immunoglobulin genes, HLA-B8/DR3, and immune responsiveness to primary immunogen and mitogens in normal subjects. *Clin. Immunol. Immunopathol.*, **47**: 333-342

Koch, A.E., Cho, M., Burrows, J., Leibovich, S.J. & Polverini, P.J. (1988) Inhibition of production of macrophage-derived angiogenic activity by the anti-rheumatic agents gold sodium thiomalate and auranofin. *Biochem. biophys. Res. Commun.*, **154**: 205-212

Langer, H.E., Hartmann, G., Heinemann, G. & Richter, K. (1987) Gold colitis induced by auranofin treatment of rheumatoid arthritis: case report and review of the literature. *Ann. rheum. Dis.*, **46**: 787-792

Lipsky, P.E. (1983) Remission-inducing therapy in rheumatoid arthritis. *Am. J. Med.*, **75**: 40-49

Littman, B.H. & Hall, R.E. (1985) Effects of gold sodium thiomalate on functional correlates of human monocyte maturation. *Arthritis Rheum.*, **28**: 1384-1392

Madhok, R., Pullar, T., Capell, H.A., Dawood, F., Sturrock, R.D. & Dick, H.M. (1985) Chrysotherapy and thrombocytopenia. *Ann. rheum. Dis.*, **44**: 589-591

Matsubara, T. & Ziff, M. (1987) Inhibition of human endothelial cell proliferation by gold compounds. *J. clin. Invest.*, **79**: 1440-1446

McCombs, C.C., Michalski, J.P., deShazo, R., Bozelka, B. & Lane, J.T. (1986) Immune abnormalities associated with HLA-B8: lymphocyte subsets and functional correlates. *Clin. Immunol. Immunopathol.*, **39**: 112-120

Mueller-Eckhardt, C., Mueller-Eckhardt, G., Willen-Ohff, H., Horz, A., Kuenzlen, E., O'Neill, G.J. & Schendel, D.J. (1985) Immunogenicity of and immune response to the human platelet antigen Zwa is strongly associated with HLA-B8 and DR3. *Tissue Antigens*, **26**: 71-76

Muller, J.Y., Reznikoff-Etievant, M.F., Patereau, C. & Julien, F. (1983) [Neonatal thrombopenia caused by antiPLA1 and HLA-DR3 antigen alloimmunization.] (in French) *C.R. Seances Acad. Sci. [III]*, **296**: 953-956

Nuotio, P., Nissila, M. & Ilonen, J. (1986) HLA-D antigens in rheumatoid arthritis and toxicity to gold and penicillamine. *Scand. J. Rheumatol.*, **15**: 255-258

Pachoula-Papasteriades, C., Boki, K., Varla-Leftherioti, M., Kappos-Rigatou, I., Fostiropoulos, G. & Economidou, J. (1986) HLA-A, -B, and -DR antigens in relation to gold and D-penicillamine toxicity in Greek patients with RA. *Dis. Markers*, **4**: 35-41

Panayi, G.S., Wooley, P. & Batchelor, J.R. (1978) Genetic basis of rhematoid disease: HLA antigen, disease manifestations and toxic reactions to drugs. *Br. med. J.*, **ii**: 1326-1328

van de Putte, L.B., Speerstra, F., van Riel, P.L., Boerbooms, A.M., van't Pad Bosch, P.J. & Reekers, P. (1986) Remarkably similar response to gold therapy in HLA identical sibs with rheumatoid arthritis. *Ann. rheum. Dis.*, **45**: 1004-1006

160

Rantapaa-Dahlqvist, S. & Mjorndal, T. (1987) Acetylator phenotypes in rheumatoid arthritis patients with or without adverse drug reactions to sodium-aurothiomalate or d-penicillamine. *Scand. J. Rheumatol.*, **16**: 235-239

van Riel, P.L., Reekers, P., van de Putte, L.B. & Gribnau, F.W. (1983) Association of HLA antigens, toxic reactions and therapeutic response to auranofin and aurothioglucose in patients with rheumatoid arthritis. *Tissue Antigens*, **22**: 194-199

Rudge, S.R., Perrett, D. & Kelly, M. (1988) Failure of oral thiomalate to act as an alternative to intramuscular gold in rheumatoid arthritis. *Ann. rheum. Dis.*, **47**: 224-227

Salata, M., Golbus, J. & Richardson, B.C. (1988) Diminished response to an inhibitory signal in lymphocytes from patients with sytemic lupus erythematosus. *Clin. exp. Immunol.*, **71**: 439-444

Salmon, J.E., Kimberly, R.P., Gibofsky, A. & Fotino, M. (1986) Altered phagocytosis by monocytes from HLA-DR22 and DR3-positive healthy adults is Fc gamma receptor positive. *J. Immunol.*, **136**: 3625-3630

Scherak, O., Smolen, J.S., Mayr, W.R., Mayrhofer, F., Kolarz, G. & Thumb, N.J. (1984) HLA antigens and toxicity to gold and penicillamine in rheumatoid arthritis. *J. Rheumatol.*, **11**: 610-614

Speerstra, F., Reekers, P., van de Putte, L.B., Vandenbroucke, J.P., Rasker, J.J. & de Rooij, D.J. (1983) HLA-DR antigends and proteinuria induced by aurothioglucose and D-penicillamine in patients with rheumatoid arthritis. *J. Rheumatol.*, **10**: 948-953

Speerstra, F., van Riel, P.L., Reekers, P., van de Putte, L.B. & Vandenbroucke, J.P. (1986) The influence of HLA phenotypes on the response to parenteral gold in rheumatoid arthritis. *Tissue Antigens*, **28**: 1-7

Strunk, S.W. & Ziff, M. (1970) Ultrastructural studies of the passage of gold thiomalate across the renal glomerular capillary wall. *Arthritis Rheum.*, **13**: 39-52

Tournade, H., Pasquier, R., Vial, M.-C. & Druet, P. (1989) Gold salt-induced autoimmunity in BN rats. In: *Seventh International Congress of Immunology*, Abstract WH90-36, p. 586

Tozman, E.C. & Gottlieb, N.L. (1987) Adverse reactions with oral and parenteral gold preparations. *Med. Toxicol.*, **2**: 177-189

Venables, P.J., Rigby, S., Mumford, P.A., Markwick, J. & Maini, R.N. (1988) Autoimmunity to La (SS-B) in vitro is related to HLA-DR3 in healthy subjects. *Ann. rheum. Dis.*, **47**: 22-27

Wakashin, Y., Ueda, S., Yoshida, H., Iesato, K., Azemoto, R., Mori, Y., Mori, T., Ogawa, M. & Wakashin, M. (1989) Cellular recognition of the TBM antigen in gold nephropathy. In: *Seventh International Congress of Immunology*, Abstract WH90-39, p. 587

Williams, B.D., Russell, B.A., Lockwood, C.M. & Cotton, C. (1979) Defective reticuloendothelial system function in rheumatoid arthritis. *Lancet*, **ii**: 1311-1314

Wooley, P.H., Griffin, J., Panayi, G.S., Batchelor, J.R., Welsh, K.I. & Gibson, T.J. (1980) HLA-DR antigens and toxic reaction to sodium aurothiomalate and D-penicillamine in patients with rheumatoid arthritis. *New Engl. J. Med.*, **303**: 300-302

TOXICOLOGY OF INORGANIC MERCURY

L. Friberg[1] & S. Eneström[2]

[1]Department of Environmental Hygiene and Institute of Environmental Medicine, Karolinska Institutet, 10401 Stockholm; and [2]Department of Pathology, Faculty of Health Sciences, 58185 Linköping, Sweden

ABSTRACT

Exposure, biokinetics, effects and dose-response for different forms of inorganic mercury are reviewed. The emphasis is laid on immunological and allergic manifestations in experimental animals and humans. The central nervous system is usually the critical organ for the toxic effects of mercury vapour. We discuss minor effects at concentrations that were previously considered to be harmless. In susceptible individuals, the immune system and the kidneys are the critical organs for the effects of exposure to mercury vapour or inorganic mercury compounds. Data from experiments in animals show that differences in susceptibility are regulated partly by genetic factors. Exposure to mercury vapour constitutes a potential risk for the fetus. The predominant exposure of the general population to mercury vapour is from dental amalgams. Recent data on the release of mercury from amalgams as well as information on uptake, accumulation, excretion and possible adverse effects are reviewed and discussed. An estimation of risk from exposure to low doses of mercury is presented.

INTRODUCTION

Differences in toxicity and metabolism between different mercury species are well recognized (see, e.g., World Health Organization, 1976; Berlin, 1986; Clarkson et al., 1988a; Elinder et al., 1988; World Health Organization, 1990). Short-chain organic mercury compounds, like methylmercury, are considered to be the most toxic, but immunological effects have so far been related mostly to inorganic mercury.

EXPOSURE AND BIOKINETICS

Inorganic mercury exists in three oxidation states: Hg° (metallic), Hg_2^{++} (mercurous) and Hg^{++} (mercuric) mercury. Exposure to inorganic mercury occurs in various occupations, such as in chloralkali plants, in the production of lamps and batteries, in gold mining, and in dentistry. The predominant exposure of the general population is to metallic mercury vapour from dental amalgams (Elinder et al., 1988; World Health Organization, 1990). Use of skin-lightening soaps and creams can result in substantial exposure to mercury.

Absorption of mercury vapour by the alveoli is nearly complete, which means that about 80% of inhaled mercury is absorbed; only about 5-10% of ingested mercuric mercury is absorbed. After absorption, metallic mercury easily penetrates the blood-brain barrier and the placental barrier; this is not the case for divalent inorganic mercury (Berlin, 1986; Clarkson et al., 1988a). In studies on rats and monkeys, only a fraction of a per cent of the absorbed dose of mercury penetrated the blood-brain barrier (Friberg, 1956; Friberg & Mottet, 1989).

Metallic mercury is rapidly oxidized to ionic mercury in the body, but it remains in the blood in the elementary form long enough for some of it to penetrate the blood-brain barrier and then, after oxidation, accumulate in the brain. In animals and man, inorganic mercury accumulates in the thyroid, pituitary, brain, kidney, liver, pancreas, testes, ovaries and prostate, but within these organs the distribution is not uniform. The kidney is the chief depository of mercury after exposure to elemental mercury vapour or inorganic salts. In animals, 50-90% of the body burden is in the kidneys (World Health Organization, 1976, 1990).

Tracer studies on volunteers (Nakaaki *et al.*, 1975; Hursh *et al.*, 1976; Cherian *et al.*, 1978; Nakaaki *et al.*, 1978; Newton & Fry, 1978; Hursh *et al.*, 1980) and animals (Berlin *et al.*, 1975) indicate that the kinetics of inorganic mercury during the first months after exposure follow a complicated pattern, with biological half-lives that differ for different tissues and for different times after exposure. After short-term exposure to mercury vapour, the first elimination phase from blood has a half-life of approximately two to four days and accounts for about 90% of the mercury. This is followed by a second phase with a half-life of 15-30 days.

The half-life of mercury in the brain seems to be approximately 20 days during the first 1-1.5 months. A study lasting several years in *Macaca fascicularis* monkeys provided evidence that a fraction of the inorganic mercury has a very long biological half-life - years - in several organs, including brain and kidney. This is in accord with the finding in occupationally exposed persons of very high concentrations of mercury in brain, thyroid, pituitary and kidneys many years after the end of exposure to metallic mercury vapour (Kosta *et al.*, 1975; Nylander *et al.*, 1989).

EFFECTS AND DOSE-RESPONSE RELATIONSHIPS

Acute exposure

Acute exposure to high concentrations of metallic mercury vapour may lead to pneumonitis or metal fume fever. Acute poisoning with mercuric salts gives rise to gastrointestinal disturbances and renal damage and, in severe cases, tubular necrosis. The lethal dose in man is about 1 g of mercuric salt. In cases of fatal poisoning, concentrations of 10-70 mg/kg wet weight mercury have been found in the kidneys (Berlin, 1986).

Effects on the central nervous system

After long-term exposure to metallic mercury vapour, the critical organ in the vast majority of people is the central nervous system. At low exposure levels, nonspecific asthenic and vegetative symptoms (often called micromercurialism) are seen, but at higher exposure levels tremor and/or severe behavioural and personality changes dominate. Prolonged exposure to mercury levels in air of 100 μg/m³, corresponding to a urinary excretion of mercury at 100 μg/g creatinine, confers a high probability of developing the classical signs of mercurial poisoning (tremor and erethism) and proteinuria. At lower levels of exposure, the effects are less frequent and less severe. Subtle effects have been reported in a few studies after long-term exposure to concentrations as low as 25-35 μg/m³ (or μg/g creatinine). There is no evidence that a no-effect threshold level exists. Recently, the World Health Organization (1990) published a review of available information on the subject in an Environmental Health Criteria Document on inorganic mercury.

Renal and immunological effects

The critical effect after chronic exposure to mercuric mercury is usually considered to be renal damage, as demonstrated in several animal species; information on effects after chronic human exposure is lacking. A nephrotic syndrome has been associated with occupational exposure to metallic mercury vapour, in some cases in association with simultaneous exposure to mercuric mercury, as in the chloralkali industry.

Neal and Jones (1938) reported an increased occurrence of proteinuria in workers exposed to mercury vapour in the felt-hat industry. The nephrotic syndrome, with massive albuminuria, hypoproteinaemia and oedema was first described by Riva (1945) and Jordi (1947) in workers exposed to mercury in an ammunition factory. The symptons were explained as 'hypersenstivity' to mercury. Similar findings were published by several other authors, including Ledergerber (1949), Friberg *et al.* (1953) and Kazantzis *et al.* (1962).

The nephrotic syndrome seems to occur only occasionally and may have an immunological basis. Kazantzis (1978) and, more recently, Fillastre et al. (1984) reviewed the role of hypersensitivity and the immune response in influencing susceptibility to metal toxicity and reported several case histories of clinical kidney disease in persons exposed to mercury, occupationally as well as among the general population.

Of 60 adult Africans with the nephrotic syndrome, 53% were using skin-lightening creams containing inorganic mercury; in a control group, about 11% showed the same effects (Barr et al., 1972). Kibukamusoke et al. (1974) reported one case of membranous nephropathy due to the use of skin-lightening cream, in which immunofluorescence showed finely granular IgG, IgM and C3 complement deposits. IgG and C3 complement deposits were also reported by Lindqvist et al. (1974) in eight cases of nephrotic syndrome. Agner and Jans (1978) reported two cases of mercury poisoning and nephrotic syndrome in two young siblings, aged two and three years. Urinary mercury concentrations in the two sisters were 135 and 250 µg/l, respectively. Mercury from a measuring instrument had been spilled in the girls' bedroom a few weeks earlier.

Another form of renal injury is tubular damage. In one Belgian study of workers exposed to metallic mercury vapour in different industries (Roels et al., 1985), slight tubular effects were detected in both men and women in the form of increased urinary ß-galactosidase activity and increased urinary excretion of retinol-binding proteins. The effects were dose-related. Rosenman et al. (1986) similarly reported that urinary N-acetyl-ß-glucosaminidase (NAG) enzyme levels increased with increasing mercury levels of 100-250 µg/l. In a recent Swedish study of workers in the chloralkali industry (Langworth, 1987), there was a slight increase in the urinary concentration of this enzyme among exposed workers (average, 50 µg Hg/l urine) compared with a control group.

Eight of 62 exposed workers in chloralkali plants developed antibodies against a component of basal membranes (laminin) (Lauwerys et al., 1983). Circulating immune complexes have also been found in a mercury-exposed group, but there was no correlation with renal disturbances and there were no anti-glomerular basement membrane antibodies in the serum (Stonard et al., 1983).

Brown-Norway and MAXX rats and New Zealand rabbits exposed to mercuric chloride developed immune-mediated glomerulonephritis, with an initial phase of antiglomerular basement reactivity followed by mesangial deposits (Sapin et al., 1977; Druet et al., 1978; Roman-Franco et al., 1978; Bellon et al., 1982; Bowman et al., 1983; Michaelson et al., 1985). These animals demonstrated proteinuria, sometimes including a nephrotic syndrome. Transiently raised concentrations of circulating immune complexes may appear in such animals, involving an unknown antigen or antigens (Hirsch et al., 1982; Houssin et al., 1983; Henry et al., 1988).

Certain strains of mice developed circulating immune complexes about ten days after mercury treatment, which formed deposits in the glomerular mesangial areas as well as in vessel walls (Hultman et al., 1989). This finding parallels a hyperimmunoglobulinaemia with the occurrence of anti-nucleolar reactivity (Hultman & Eneström, 1988). Elution studies have shown that the antibodies that form part of the glomerular mesangial deposits are specific against a nucleolar protein, which has been identified as fibrillarin (Hultman et al., 1990). Similar results have been reported recently by Reuter et al. (1989).

All species of animals tested so far have shown immunological effects; however, some strains are resistant. Rats with certain major histocompatibility haplotypes, such as Lewis rats, are resistant, whatever the dose used. It has been shown that susceptibility depends on three to four genes (Pelletier et al., this volume). A similar resistance is found in strains of mice in which the susceptibility for developing antinuclear antibodies and immune complexes is very low: C57Bl/6J[b], C57Bl/10J[b], A/J[a] and CBA[k]; in comparison to SJL[a], which are high responders (P. Hultman & S. Eneström, in preparation).

The lowest dose of mercuric chloride that resulted in autoimmune effects on the glomerular basement membrane in rats was 50 µg/kg bw thrice weekly (Druet et al., 1978). When recalculated as ionic mercury, this dose corresponds to 16 µg/kg bw. Table 1 gives

Table 1. Studies in experimental animals on mercuric chloride resulting in autoimmune effects on the glomerular basement membrane (from World Health Organization, 1990)

Study	Animal	Route	Duration	Adverse effect level (mg/kg per day)
Bernaudin et al. (1981)	BN rat	Oral	60 days	0.32
Andres (1984)	BN rat	Oral	60 days	0.63
Druet et al. (1978)	BN rat	Subcutaneous	12 weeks	0.016
Druet et al. (1978)	BN rat	Subcutaneous	8 weeks	0.032[a]
Roman-Franco et al. (1978)	Rabbit	Intramuscular	1-17 weeks	0.633

[a]Proteinuria was observed in addition to autoimmune glomerulonephritis.

the results of a number of studies on rats and rabbits treated by different routes of exposure and at different doses. Similar effects are seen in the two species after parenteral and oral administration of mercuric chloride.

Results of recent studies in mice by S. Eneström and P. Hultman (in preparation) demonstrated dose-response relationships between oral exposure to mercuric chloride and nucleolar antinuclear antibody titres. Groups of SJL mice (high responders), ten weeks old, were given drinking-water *ad libitum* containing mercuric chloride at 0-5000 µg/l. An additional group of mice (three days old) was given 0.1 g amalgam intraperitoneally. The response was assessed after 12 weeks by testing serum for the presence of antinuclear antibodies using human epithelial (HEp-2) cells as substrate. The animals responded by making antibodies against a nucleolar antigen that was characterized earlier as fibrillarin (Hultman et al., 1990).

The results of the studies are presented in Figure 1, which shows significant effects (Wilcoxon's rank sum test) at concentrations of mercuric chloride of 2500 µg/l drinking-water and higher, as well as for amalgam. A tendency for an effect is seen even at 1250 µg/l.

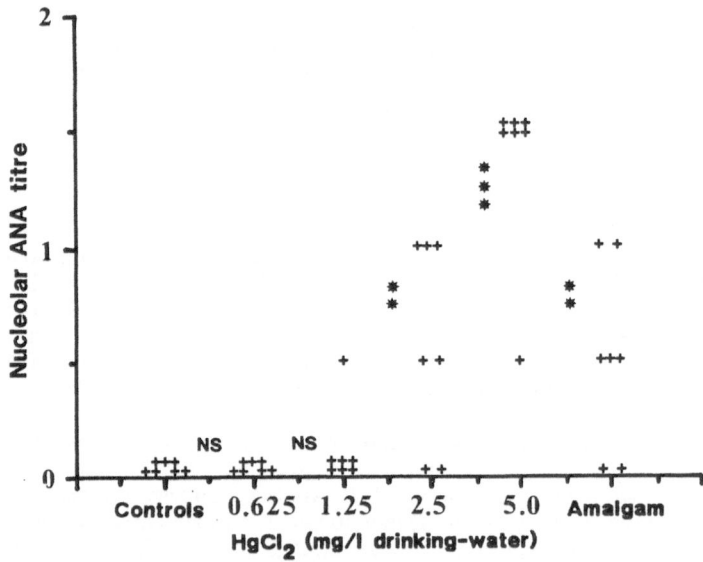

Fig. 1. Nucleolar antinuclear antibody (ANA) titre after 12 weeks of oral exposure to mercuric chloride or intraperitoneal exposure to amalgam at 100 mg (from S. Eneström & P. Hultman, in preparation). ANA titre measured by fluorescence intensity: 0.5, very weak; 1.0, moderate; 1.5, strong; 2.0, very strong. +, individual mice. Significance estimated on the basis of Wilcoxon's rank sum test: NS, not significant; *, p < 0.05; **, p < 0.02; ***, p < 0.01.

A no-effect level could not be determined owing to the small number of animals. The concentrations of mercury in body organs (Figure 2) also showed a dose-response relationship. The average level of mercury in the kidneys corresponding to the 'lowest observed adverse effect level' was about 5000 µg/kg wet weight.

As the mice in these studies had an average weight of 35 g and consumed an average of about 3.5 ml drinking-water per day, the daily exposure to mercury of mice receiving 2500 µg/l would be:

$$2.5 \ (\mu g/ml) \times 3.5 \ (ml) \ / \ 0.035 \ (weight, kg) = 250 \ \mu g/kg.$$

With 7% absorption of mercury, the uptake would be 17.5 µg/kg bw. With an assumed 100% absorption *via* the subcutaneous route, the 'lowest observed adverse effect level' of mercury in the studies of Druet *et al.* (1978) is 16 µg/kg bw. The results of Druet *et al.* and of Eneström and Hultman are thus in close agreement.

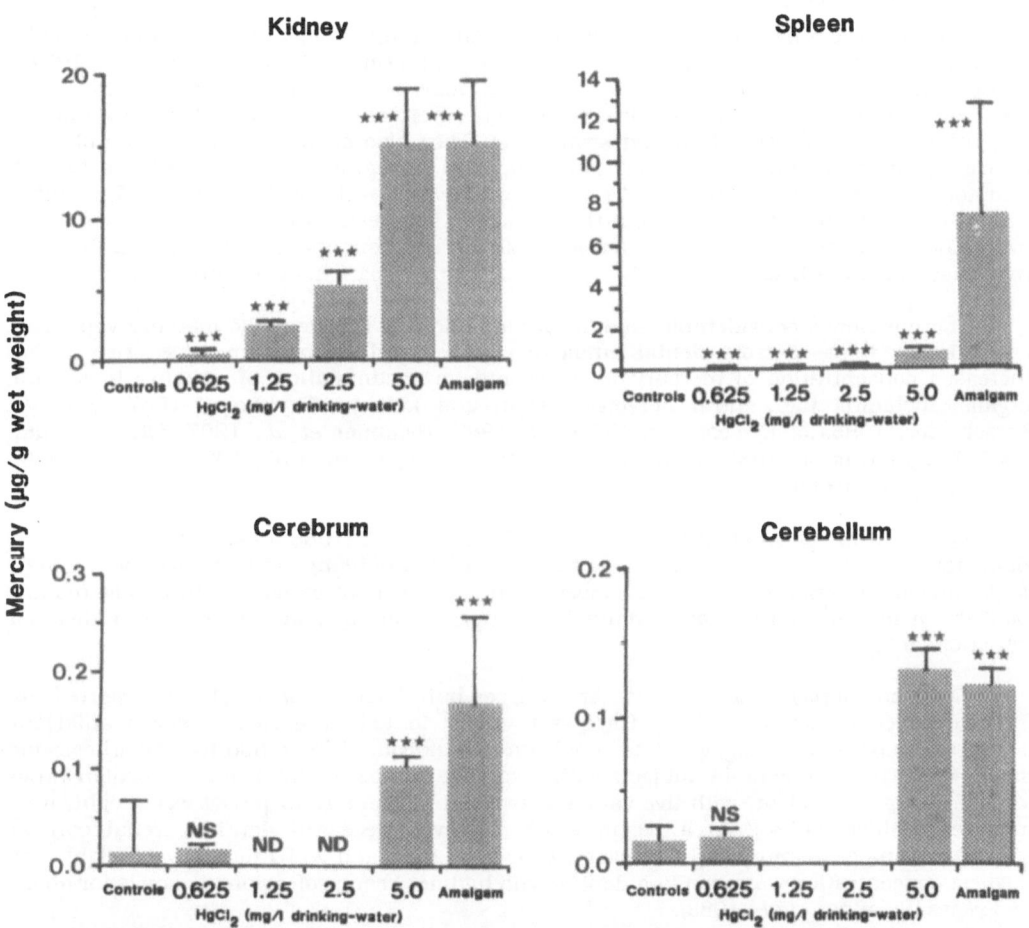

Fig. 2. Mercury concentrations in mouse tissues after 12 weeks' oral exposure to mercuric chloride or intraperitoneal exposure to 100 mg amalgam (from S. Eneström and P. Hultman, in preparation).

Allergic skin reactions

Finne *et al.* (1982) performed patch tests on 29 patients with amalgam fillings and oral lichen planus: contact allergy was found in 62% of subjects compared wth 3.2% in a control group. When the amalgam restorations were removed from four patients and replaced by gold and composite materials, the lesions healed completely in three patients after an observation period of one year; in the remaining case there was considerable improvement.

Primary hypersensitivity to metallic mercury is considered to be rare (Burrows, 1986). A few cases of allergic dermatitis have been seen among dental personnel (White & Brandt, 1976; Rudzki, 1979; Ancona *et al.*, 1982), and, on the basis of patch testing of dental students (White & Brandt, 1976), the rate of mercury hypersensitivity was found to increase by class, from pre-freshmen to seniors, from 2.0 to 10.8%. In a later study (Miller *et al.*, 1987), these results were not confirmed, but positive results on patch testing increased in relation to the number of amalgam restorations in the students.

Occasionally, symptoms have been reported in relation to amalgam fillings (Frykholm, 1957; Thomson & Russell, 1970; Duxbury *et al.*, 1982). In most cases, the main symptoms were facial dermatitis; symptoms in the mouth (oral lichen) also occurred. Nakayama *et al.* (1983) reported 15 cases of generalized dermatitis caused by exposure to broken thermometers or dental treatment.

Dental amalgam and general health

Recently, there has been intense debate in some countries (e.g., Sweden and the USA) about the possible health hazards of dental amalgams (Ziff, 1984; Socialstyrelsen, 1987). Those who claim that mercury from amalgam may be a severe health hazard base themselves on information on the release of mercury from amalgam and subsequent uptake into the body due to inhalation and swallowing. They also claim that a large number of people suffer from diseases with an immunological background and exhibit the typical symptoms of mercury sensitization. Those who deny a causal relationship between dental amalgams and health effects point out that amalgam has been used for many years with no proven health effect. Furthermore, the uptake of mercury from amalgam is considerably less than that which has been associated with effects after occupational exposure (Fan, 1987).

There is now a considerable amount of data showing that metallic mercury vapour is continuously released from dental amalgams and that this exposure gives rise to an increased concentration of mercury in urine and an accumulation of mercury in several organs, including the central nervous system and kidneys (Frykholm, 1957; Vimy & Lorscheider, 1985a,b; Eggleston & Nylander, 1987; Nylander *et al.*, 1987; Olstad *et al.*, 1987; Berglund *et al.*, 1988; Clarkson *et al.*, 1988b; Langworth *et al.*, 1988; Schiele, 1988; Aronsson *et al.*, 1989).

On the basis of published information, Clarkson *et al.* (1988b) estimated the average daily uptake of mercury vapour from a moderate number of fillings to be 8 µg/day, but with large individual variations. Average concentrations in urine of persons with amalgams are similarly a few micrograms of mercury to 10 µg/g creatinine, also with large individual variations (Fig. 3).

Data on kidney concentrations are scarce, but Nylander *et al.* (1987) reported an average concentration of 433 ng Hg/g wet weight in kidney cortex of seven amalgam carriers, compared to 49 ng/g in four amalgam-free individuals who had had prostheses for many years. In a study of 44 subjects with a varying number of amalgams, a median value of 187 µg/kg wet weight, with five values between 1000 and 1500 µg/kg wet weight, were reported (Schiele, 1988). In a recent study of seven deceased dentists, renal cortical concentrations of mercury in three cases were 945, 1545 and 2110 µg/kg wet weight. The highest concentration was seen in a dentist who had not been professionally active for about ten years (Nylander *et al.*, 1989).

Many individuals claim to be suffering from a variety of invalidating symptoms which they associate with exposure to mercury from amalgam. It has also been claimed that improvement has occurred after the replacement of amalgam fillings with other materials

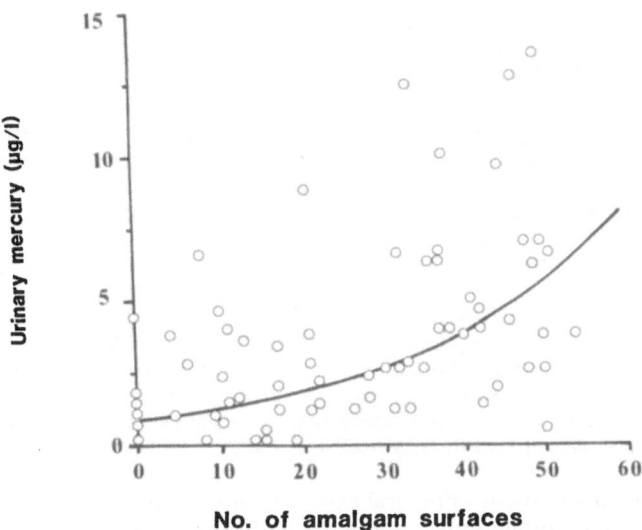

Fig. 3. Mercury concentrations in urine in relation to number of amalgam surfaces (from Langworth *et al.*, 1988).

(Socialstyrelsen, 1987). In one questionnaire study (Hansson, 1986) of members of a Swedish society of patients who consider themselves to have been affected by amalgam, very diverse symptoms were reported, including pains in joints and muscles (50%), fatigue (40%), dizziness (40%), headache (40%), gastrointestinal symptoms (30%), symptoms related to the heart and circulation (20%), nervousness (15%), insomnia (15%), tremor (10%), irritability (10%) and allergic reactions (10%). Similar results were reported from Colorado by Siblerud (1988), who examined volunteers in a college. None of the studies provides conclusions about the cause of the symptoms.

Very few epidemiological studies have addressed the possible relationship between amalgam and health. Ahlqwist *et al.* (1988) reported a study in which data collection was carried out during 1968-69 and 1980-81, i.e., before the issue of a possible causal association between amalgam and symptoms became acute in mass media. Most of the participants (85%) were women who had participated in a longitudinal descriptive study of different diseases in the city of Gothenburg, Sweden. Altogether, 1024 women (aged 38-72 years) participated in the study, which included a dental examination as well as a medical examination and a standardized, self-administered questionnaire. No significant positive correlation was found between number of amalgalm fillings and symptoms or signs. On the other hand, risk ratios and 95% confidence limits for women with 20 fillings or more compared with women with 0-4 fillings were well above one. Even if the results do not support a correlation between numbers of surfaces with amalgam and symptoms, as studied on the population level, they do not exclude the possibility of an association between amalgam fillings and symptoms and complaints on the individual level. Largely similar outcomes were reported from another epidemiological study based on observations in a population in the Stockholm area of Sweden in 1970 (Lavstedt & Sundberg, 1989).

RISK ESTIMATION

It is well documented that prolonged exposure to metallic mercury vapour at about 100 µg/m³, corresponding to a urinary excretion of about 100 µg/g creatinine, increases the probability of developing the classical neurological signs of mercurial intoxication - tremor, erethism and proteinuria.

More recent studies have shown subtle but clear effects on the central nervous system and kidneys after exposure to elemental mercury vapour corresponding to average urinary concentrations of about 50 µg Hg/g creatinine. In some studies, effects have been noted at an exposure corresponding to average urinary levels of 25-35 µg/g creatinine. Whether effects occur at still lower concentrations is unknown, but effects may occur, even if the association between the degree of exposure and effects and response is not known.

On the basis of urinary concentrations of mercury (Fig. 2), the average exposure of the general population from dental amalgam fillings is below the average exposure levels associated with effects among occupationally exposed individuals. The individual spread is considerable, however, and the safety margin is small, if existent.

A particular problem in the risk assessment of mercury is that it can give rise to allergic and immunotoxic reactions, which are partially genetically regulated. A fraction of the population may be particularly sensitive, as has been observed among experimental animals. A consequence of an immunological etiology is that, on the basis of present knowledge, it is not possible scientifically to set a level for mercury in, e.g., blood or urine, below which mercury-related symptoms will not occur in an individual. In order to do so, it will be necessary to have the results of dose-response studies on groups of immunologically sensitive individuals (World Health Organization, 1990).

In studies of subcutaneous and oral exposure of susceptible rats and mice to mercuric chloride, well-defined autoimmune effects have been observed within a few weeks of exposure after an uptake (absorbed dose) of mercury of about 15 µg/kg bw per day, equivalent to about 1000 µg for a 70-kg human. A 'no observed adverse effect level' could not be established for either animals or humans.

If kidney mercury levels are taken as the endpoint, average concentrations of about 5000 µg/kg wet weight have been associated with a lowest observed adverse effect level in mice. In humans, several cases have been reported in which concentrations of mercury of 1000-1500 µg/g wet weight were measured in individuals with a large number of dental amalgams and no other source of exposure to mercury.

Some papers have described miscarriages and spontaneous abortions after occupational exposure to mercury, but this was not confirmed in other reports. Until additional data have been acquired, the World Health Organization (1990) considered that the prudent statement of a previous World Health Organization study group (1980) still held: 'The exposure of women of child-bearing age to mercury vapour should be as low as possible. The Group was not in a position to recommend a specific value.'

REFERENCES

Agner, E. & Jans, H. (1978) Mercury poisoning and nephrotic syndrome in two young siblings. *Lancet,* **ii:** 951

Ahlqvist, M., Bengtsson, C., Furunes, B., Hollender, L. & Lapidus, L. (1988) Number of amalgam tooth fillings in relation to subjectively experienced symptoms in a study of Swedish women. *Community dent. oral Epidemiol.,* **16:** 227-231

Ancona, A., Ramos, M., Suarez, R. & Macotela, E. (1982) Mercury sensitivity in a dentist. *Contact Dermatitis,* **8:** 218

Andres, P. (1984) IgA-IgG disease in the intestine of Brown-Norway rats ingesting mercuric chloride. *Clin. Immunol. Immunopathol.,* **30:** 488-494

Aronsson, A.M., Lind, B., Nylander, M. & Nordberg, M. (1989) Dental amalgam and mercury. *Biol. Metals,* **2:** 25-30

Barr, R.D., Rees, P.H., Cordy, P.E., Kungu, A., Woodger, B.A. & Cameron, H.M. (1972) Nephrotic syndrome in adult Africans in Nairobi. *Br. med. J.,* **ii:** 131-134

Bellon, B., Capron, M., Druet, E., Verroust, P., Vial, M.C., Sapin, C., Girard, J.F., Foidart, J.M., Mahieu, P. & Druet, P. (1982) Mercuric chloride induced autoimmune disease in Brown-Norway rats: sequential search for anti-basement membrane antibodies and circulating immune complexes. *Eur. J. clin. Invest.,* **12:** 127-133

Berglund, A., Pohl, L., Olsson, S. & Bergman, M. (1988) Determination of the rate of release of inter-oral mercury vapour from amalgam. *J. dent. Res.,* **62:**1235-1242

Berlin, M. (1986) Mercury. In: Friberg, L., Nordberg, G.F. & Vouk, V., eds, *Handbook on the Toxicology of Metals,* Vol. II, Amsterdam, Elsevier, pp. 387-445

Berlin, M., Carlson, J. & Norseth, T. (1975) Dose-dependence of methylmercury metabolism. *Arch. environ. Health,* **30:** 307-313

Bernaudin, J.F., Druet, E., Druet, P. & Masse, R. (1981) Inhalation or ingestion of organic or inorganic mercurials produces auto-immune disease in rats. *Clin. Immunol. Immunopathol.*, **20**: 129-135

Bowman, C., Mason, D.W., Pusey, C.D. & Lockwood, C.M. (1983) Autoregulation of autoantibody synthesis in mercuric chloride nephritis in the Brown-Norway rat. I. A role for T suppressor cells. *Eur. J. Immunol.*, **14**: 464-470

Burrows, D. (1986) Hypersensitivity to mercury, nickel and chromium in relation to dental materials. *Int. dent. J.*, **36**: 30-34

Cherian, M.G., Hursh, J.B., Clarkson, T.W. & Allen, J. (1978) Radioactive mercury distribution in biological fluids and excretion in human subjects after inhalation of mercury vapor. *Arch. environ. Health.*, **33**: 109-114

Clarkson, T.W., Hursh, J.B., Sager, P.R. & Syversen, T.L.M. (1988a) Mercury. In: Clarkson, T.W., Friberg, L., Nordberg, G.F. & Sager, P., eds, *Biological Monitoring of Metals*, New York, Plenum Press, pp. 199-246

Clarkson, T.W., Friberg, L., Hursh, J.B. & Nylander, M. (1988b) The prediction of intake of mercury vapor from amalgams. In: Clarkson, T.W., Friberg, L., Nordberg, G.F. & Sager, P., eds, *Biological Monitoring of Metals*, New York, Plenum Press, pp. 247-264

Druet, P., Druet, E., Potdevin, F. & Sapin, C. (1978) Immune type glomerulonephritis induced by $HgCl_2$ in the Brown-Norway rat. *Ann. Immunol.*, **129C**: 777-792

Duxbury, A.J., Ead, R.D., McMurrough, S. & Watts, D.C. (1982) Allergy to mercury in dental amalgam. *Br. dent. J.*, **152**: 47-48

Eggleston, D.W. & Nylander, M. (1987) Correlation of dental amalgam with mercury in brain tissue. *J. prosthet. Dent;*, **58**: 704-707

Elinder, C.-G., Gerhardsson, L. & Oberdoerster, G. (1988) Biological monitoring of metals. In: Clarkson, T.W., Friberg, L., Nordberg, G.F. & Sager, P., eds, *Biological Monitoring of Metals*, New York, Plenum Press, pp. 1-71

Fan, P.L. (1987) Safety of amalgam. *Can. dental Assoc. J.*, **September**: 34-36

Fillastre, J.-P., Druet, P. & Merg, J.-P. (1984) Proteinuric nephropathies associated with drugs and substances of abuse. In: Cameron, J.S. & Glasok, M.S.G., eds, *The Nephrotic Syndrome*, New York, Marcel Dekker, pp. 697-742

Finne, K., Göransson, K. & Winckler, L. (1982) Oral lichen planus and contact allergy to mercury. *Int. J. oral Surg.*, **11**: 236-239

Friberg, L. (1956) Studies on the accumulation, metabolism and excretion of inorganic mercury (Hg^{203}) after prolonged subcutaneous administration to rats. *Acta pharmacol. toxicol.*, **12**: 411-427

Friberg, L. & Mottet, N.K. (1989) Accumulation of methylmercury and inorganic mercury in the brain. *Biol. Trace. Elem. Res.* (in press)

Friberg, L., Hammarström, S. & Nyström, Å. (1953) Kidney injury after chronic exposure to inorganic mercury. *Arch. ind. Hyg. occup. Med.*, **8**: 149-152

Frykholm, K.O. (1957) Mercury from dental amalgam. Its toxic and allergic effects and some comments on occupational hygiene. *Acta odont. scand.*, **22**: 1-108

Hansson, M. (1986) [Changes in health after removal of toxic dental filling materials.] (in Swedish) *TF-Bladet*, **1**: 3-30

Henry, G.A., Jarnot, B.M., Steinhoff, M.M. & Bigazzi, P.E. (1988) Mercury-induced autoimmunity in the MAXX rat. *Clin. Immunol. Immunopathol.*, **49**: 187-203

Hirsch, F., Couderc, J., Sapin, C., Fournie, G. & Druet, P. (1982) Polyclonal effect of $HgCl_2$ in the rat, its possible role in an experimental autoimmune disease. *Eur. J. Immunol.*, **12**: 620-625

Houssin, D., Druet, E., Hinglais, N., Verroust, P., Grossetete, J., Bariety, J. & Druet, P. (1983) Glomerular and vascular IgG deposits in $HgCl_2$ nephritis: role of circulation antibodies and of immune complexes. *Clin. Immunol. Immunopathol.*, **29**: 167-180

Hultman, P. & Eneström, S. (1988) Mercury induced antinuclear antibodies in mice: characterization and correlation with renal immune complex deposits. *Clin. exp. Immunol.*, **71**: 269-274

Hultman, P., Skoog, T. & Eneström, S. (1989) Circulating and tissue immune complexes in mercury treated mice. *J. clin. Lab. Immunol.* (in press)

Hultman, P., Eneström, S., Pollard, K.M. & Tan, E.M. (1990) Antifibrillarin antibodies in mercury-treated mice. *Clin. exp. Immunol.* (in press)

Hursh, J.B., Clarkson, T.W., Cherian, M.G., Vostal, J.V. & Mallie, R.V. (1976) Clearance of mercury (Hg-197, Hg-203) vapor inhaled by human subjects. *Arch. environ. Health*, **31**: 302-309

Hursh, J.B., Greenwood, M.R., Clarkson, T.W., Allen, J. & Demuth, S. (1980) The effects of ethanol on the fate of mercury vapor inhaled by man. *J. Pharmacol. exp. Ther.*, **214**: 520-527

Jordi, A. (1947) [Mercury poisoning in ammunition workers.] (in German) *Schweiz. med. Wochenschr.*, **77**: 621

Kazantzis, G. (1978) The role of hypersensitivity and the immune response in influencing susceptibility to metal toxicity. *Environ. Health Perspect.*, **25**: 111-118

Kazantzis, G., Schiller, F.R., Asscher, A.W. & Drew, R.G. (1962) Albuminuria and the nephrotic syndrome following exposure to mercury and its compounds. *Q J. Med.*, **31**: 403-418

Kibukamusoke, J.W., Davies, D.R. & Hutt, M.S.R. (1974) Membranous nephropathy due to skin-lightning cream. *Br. med. J.*, **ii**: 646-647

Kosta, L., Byrne, A.R. & Zelenko, V. (1975) Correlation between selenium and mercury in man following exposure to inorganic mercury. *Nature*, **254**: 238-239

Langworth, S. (1987) Renal function in workers exposed to inorganic mercury. In: *International Congress on Occupational Health: Work for Health, Sydney, Australia, 27 September - 2 October, 1987,* Abstract, p. 237

Langworth, S., Elinder, C.G. & Åkesson, A. (1988) Mercury exposure from dental fillings. *Swed. dent. J.*, **12**: 69-70

Lauwerys, R., Bernard, A., Roels, H., Buchet, J.P., Gennart, J.P., Mahieu, P. & Foidart, J.M. (1983) Anti-laminin antibodies in workers exposed to mercury vapour. *Toxicol. Lett.*, **17**: 113-116

Lavstedt, S. & Sundberg, H. (1989) [Medical diagnosis and disease signs related to amalgam fillings.] (in Swedish) *Tandläkartidningen*, **3**: 81-88

Ledergerber, E. (1949) [Mortality and causes of death in ammunition factories.] (in German) *Schweiz. med. Wochenschr.*, **30**: 263

Lindqvist, K.J., Makene, W.J., Shaba, J.K. & Nantulya, V. (1974) Immunoflurescence and electron microscopic studies of kidney biopsies from patients with nephrotic syndrome, possibly induced by skin lightening creams containing mercury. *East Afr. med. J.*, **51**: 168-169

Michaelson, J.H., McCoy, J.P., Hirszel, P. & Bigazzi, P.E. (1985) Mercury-induced autoimmune glomerulonephritis in inbred rats. *Surv. synth. Pathol. Res.*, **4**: 401-411

Miller, E.G., Perry, W.L. & Wagner, M.J. (1987) Prevalence of mercury hypersensitivity in dental students. *J. prosthet. Dent.*, **58**: 235-237

Nakaaki, K., Fukabori, S. & Tada, O. (1975) [An experimental study on inorganic mercury vapour exposure.] (in Japanese with English summary) *J. Sci. Labour*, **51**: 705-716

Nakaaki, K., Fukabori, S. & Tada, O. (1978) [Evaluation of mercury exposure.] (in Japanese) *J. Sci. Labour*, **54**: 1-8

Nakayama, H., Niki, F., Shono, M. & Hada, S. (1983) Mercury exanthem. *Contact Dermatitis*, **9**: 411-417

Neal, P.A. & Jones, R. (1938) Chronic mercurialism in the hatters' fur-cutting industry. *J. Am. med. Assoc*, **110**: 337

Newton, D. & Fry, F.A. (1978) The retention and distribution of radioactive mercuric oxide following accidental inhalation. *Ann. occup. Hyg.*, **21**: 21-32

Nylander, M., Friberg, L. & Lind, B. (1987) Mercury concentrations in the human brain and kidneys in relation to exposure from dental amalgam fillings. *Swed. dent. J.*, **11**: 179-187

Nylander, M., Friberg, L., Eggleston, D. & Björkman, L. (1989) Mercury accumulation in tissues from dental staff and controls in relation to exposure. *Swed. dent. J.* (in press)

Olstad, M.L., Holland, R.I., Wandel, N. & Hensten Pettersen, A. (1987) Correlation between amalgam restorations and mercury concentrations in urine. *J. dent. Res.*, **66**:1179-1182

Reuter, R., Tressars, G., Vohr, H.-W., Gleichmann, E. & Lührmann, R. (1989) Mercuric chloride induces autoantibodies to small nuclear ribonucleoprotein in susceptible mice. *Proc. natl Acad. Sci. USA* (in press)

Riva, G. (1945) [The question of chronic mercury nephrosis.] (in German) *Helv. med. Acta*, **12**: 539

Roels, H., Gennart, J.-P., Lauwerys, R., Buchet, J.-P., Malchaire, J. & Bernard, A. (1985) Surveillance of workers exposed to mercury vapour: validation of a previously pro-posed biological threshold limit value for mercury concentration in urine. *Am. J. ind. Med.*, **7**: 45-71

Roman-Franco, A.A., Turiello, M., Albini, B., Ossi, E., Milgrom, F. & Andres, G.A. (1978) Anti-basement membrane antibodies and antigen-antibody complexes in rabbits injected with mercuric chloride. *Clin. Immunol. Immunopathol.*, **9**: 464-481

Rosenman, K.D., Valciukas, J.A., Glickman, L., Meyers, B.R. & Cinotti, A. (1986) Sensitive indicators of inorganic mercury toxicity. *Arch. environ. Health*, **41**: 208-215

Rudzki, E. (1979) Occupational dermatitis among health service workers. *Derm. Berufsverb. Umwelt*, **27**: 112

Sapin, C., Druet, E. & Druet, P. (1977) Induction of anti-glomerular basement membrane antibodies in the Brown-Norway rat by mercuric chloride. *Clin. exp. Immunol.*, **28**: 173-179

Schiele, R. (1988) In: [*Amalgam - Pro and Contra. Statements. Discussion*] (in German), ?, ?, pp. 123-131

Siblerud, R.L. (1988) *The Relationship between Dental Amalgam and Health*, PhD Thesis, Colorado State University, Denver

Socialstyrelsen (1987) [Mercury amalgam - health risks.] (in Swedish with English summary). Report by the LEK-Committee, Stockholm, National Board of Health and Welfare.

Stonard, M.D., Chater, B.V., Duffield, D.P., Nevitt, A.L., O'Sullivan, J.J. & Steel, G.T. (1983) An evaluation of renal function in workers occupationally exposed to mercury vapour. *Int. Arch. occup. environ. Health*, **52**: 177-189

Thomson, J. & Russell, J.A. (1970) Dermatitis due to mercury following amalgam dental restorations. *Br. J. Dermatol.*, **82**: 292-297

Vimy, M.J. & Lorscheider, F.L. (1985a) Intra-oral air mercury released from dental amalgam. *J. dent. Res.*, **64**: 1069-1071

Vimy, M.J. & Lorscheider, F.L. (1985b) Serial measurements of intra-oral air mercury: estimation of daily dose from dental amalgam. *J. dent. Res.*, **64**: 1073-1085

White, R.R. & Brandt, R.L. (1976) Development of mercury hypersensitivity among dental students. *J. Am. dent. Assoc.*, **92**: 1204-1207

World Health Organization (1976) *Environmental Health Criteria I - Mercury*, Geneva

World Health Organization (1980) *Recommended Health-based Limits in Occupational Exposure to Heavy Metals* (WHO Tech. Rep. Ser. No. 647), Geneva

World Health Organization (1990) *Environmental Health Criteria - Inorganic Mercury*, Geneva (in press)

Ziff, S. (1984) *Silver Dental Fillings - The Toxic Time Bomb. Can the Mercury in Your Dental Fillings Poison You?* New York, Aurora Press

IMMUNOTOXICOLOGY OF COBALT AND SELENIUM

F. Kayama, Y. Kodama, U. Yamashita & K. Tsuchiya

University of Occupational and Environmental Health
Iseigaoka, Kitakyushu 807, Japan

ABSTRACT

Immunological studies on cobalt are very few and mainly restricted to metal allergy; however, several papers suggest that cobalt can modulate the immune function, and most studies have shown suppression of the immune system in many modalities. At the same time, cobalt can cause allergic reactions. The mechanisms of nonspecific activation of lymphoid cells induced by cobalt should also be elucidated.

Selenium has been studied more extensively than cobalt. Selenium deficiency impairs both humoral and cellular immunity as well as nonspecific immune responses. In contrast, selenium supplementation at low concentrations enhances many immune responses, such as natural killer activity, delayed-type hypersensitivity response and antibody production. It also affects the secretion of some cytokines. These findings show that modulation of the immune system by selenium may be related to the intricate network of immunocompetent cell groups.

INTRODUCTION

Immunotoxicological effects of heavy metals were reviewed by Koller (1981). Although much research has been done on heavy metal immunotoxicity, reports on immunological alterations by cobalt are very limited and are mainly restricted to metal allergy. In contrast, the carcinogenesis and anticancerous effects of selenium have been studied for several decades, and the effects of selenium on immune responses were reviewed extensively by Kiremidjian-Schumacher and Stotzky (1987). The purpose of our review is to summerize the knowledge accumulated so far and to present recent evidence on cellular immunology and cytokines.

COBALT

Cobalt is a constituent of vitamin B_{12}, an essential nutrient for humans and many other animals; Other biological roles of this element are still unknown. Cobalt chloride functions as a nonspecific bone-marrow stimulating agent and is used in the treatment of certain refractory anaemias. It induces reticulocytosis and a rise in erythrocyte counts.

Currently, there is little knowledge about the influence of cobalt exposure on the immune system. Since the description of Derkach and Burmakina (1970) of suppression of the Arthus phenomenon by cobalt, several reports have described altered immune responses. It is now generally accepted that cobalt induces some functional changes in host resistance. These are summerized in Table 1.

Ward *et al.* (1975) showed that cobalt suppressed chemotaxis of rabbit polymorpho-nuclear leukocytes *in vitro*. Direct plaque-forming cells against sheep erythrocytes decreased from 35 to 49% during a five-day exposure *in vitro* to 10 µM or 100 µM cobalt chloride (Lawrence, 1981). To assess host resistance, CD-1 mice were exposed to 0.01 M cobalt

Immunotoxicity of Metals and Immunotoxicology, Edited by
A. D. Dayan *et al.*, Plenum Press, New York, 1990

Table 1. Immunological reactions to cobalt

Species	Response	Condition of exposure	Effect	Reference
Mouse	Arthus phenomenon		Decrease	Derkach & Burmakina (1970)
Mouse	T-Dependent antibody response	0.1, 1 μM *in vitro* for 5 days 10 μM *in vitro* for 5 days 100 μM *in vitro* for 5 days	35% decrease 49% decrease	Lawrence (1981)
Rabbit	Chemotaxis of polymorphonuclear leukocytes	1 mM *in vitro* for 1 h	Decrease	Ward *et al.* (1975)
Mouse	Experimental infection with encephalomyocarditis virus	47 ppm orally for 2.5 months	50% decrease	Gainer (1972)
Mouse	Rauscher leukaemia virus	0.01 M cobalt sulfate for 3-6 weeks	Decrease	Gainer (1973)
Guinea-pig	Optimization test	0.5% cobalt dichloride intradermally		Maurer *et al.* (1979)
Guinea-pig	Maximization test	0.1% cobalt dichloride epicutaneously 0.5% cobalt dichloride epicutaneously 1% cobalt dichloride epicutaneously	13% positive 83% positive 100% positive	Wahlberg & Boman (1978)
Guinea-pig	Nonspecific lympho-proliferation	0.01-1 μM cobalt dichloride	Increase	Nordlind (1982)

sulfate orally for three to six weeks and showed significant activation of Rauscher leukaemia virus (Gainer, 1973). Experimental challenges with encephalomyocarditis virus resulted in increased mortality of mice (up to 50%) after exposure to cobalt at 47 ppm for 2.5 months (Gainer, 1972).

Hypersensitivity reactions

Cobalt dichloride often sensitizes skin and induces allergic reactions among people working with metal. Allergic reactions to cobalt alloys, such as artificial joint implants and screws, have also been reported in clinical settings, especially in the field of orthopaedics (Merritt & Brown, 1981; Lewin *et al.*, 1982; Wigren, 1982).

In experimental animals, an epicutaneous application of 0.1, 0.5 or 1% solution of cobalt dichloride to guinea-pigs induced 13, 83 and 100% positive allergic responses, respectively (Wahlberg & Boman, 1978). Cobalt chloride has been reported to cause specific blast transformation of sensitized human lymphocytes. The possibility of diagnosing contact allergy by an in-vitro test has been suggested (Veien & Svejgaad *et al.*, 1978).

Humans exposed to cobalt showed altered immune and biochemical reactions, as observed with nickel: immunoglobulin analysis of workers exposed to cobalt revealed a significant increase in IgA level (Bencko *et al.*, 1984). Immunoglobulin values may be one of the parameters for monitoring degree of alteration of the immune system; extensive collaborative research should be undertaken in workers exposed to cobalt to investigate this area.

Nonspecific lymphocyte proliferation

There is increasing evidence that cobalt also induces nonspecific blastogenesis in unsensitized lymphoid cells. DNA synthesis in lymphoid cells from unsensitized guinea-pigs was tested by adding cobalt chloride, mercuric chloride, nickel sulfate and potassium dichromate at 10^{-8} to 10^{-6} M. All compounds stimulated DNA synthesis in both thymocytes and peripheral lymphocytes after 48 h of culture (Nordlind, 1982). Similar nonspecific stimulation of lymphocyte proliferation has been observed with lead, nickel and zinc, and a possible mechanism has been proposed by Warner and Lawrence (1988). All of these metals can elicit contact sensitivity reactions, implying that each may interact with self, thereby eliciting a positive immune response directed toward the metal-modified self.

Our experimental data indicate that the mechanism of nonspecific stimulation by cobalt is probably different from that of nickel and zinc. Although their activation mechanisms are still speculative, the development of cell surface marker analysis by flow fluorocytometry has made it possible to classify functionally diverse subsets of lymphoid cells and other immunocompetent cells. Cell-cell contact is probably important in generating this response (Warner & Lawrence, 1986a,b). While there is no evidence in the case of cobalt, lead, nickel and zinc induce proliferation of T cells *via* major histocompatibility complex class II, which requires activation of L3T4+ T cells and recognition of self Ia (Warner & Lawrence, 1988).

SELENIUM

Selenium is not categorized as a metal and occurs in the VI A subgroup of the periodic table with chemical properties similar to those of sulfur. There are many kinds of naturally occurring selenium compounds, and selenium can be substituted for the sulfur of the sulfur-containing amino acids, cysteine and methionine. Over the last few decades, the image of selenium has shifted drastically from that of a strong carcinogen to that of an essential trace element with the functions of an antioxidant and anticancerous agent. The toxicity of selenium has been recognized since the 1930s. Nelson *et al.* (1943) reported that oral administration of selenium could induce liver adenoma and hepatic carcinoma; however, Schwartz and Foltz (1957) demonstrated that it prevented liver necrosis in vitamin E-deficient rats, leading to the recognition of the biological essentiality of selenium as a trace element. Selenium deficiency syndrome in man was first seen in China, known as Keshan disease, a juvenile cardiomyopathy (Keshan Disease Research Group of the Chinese Academy of Medical Sciences, 1979). Rotruck *et al.* (1972) showed that serum glutathione peroxidase activity in erythrocytes was lowered in selenium-deficient rats but that the effect could be reversed by administration of the element.

Nonspecific immune responses: phagocytosis

The first encounter of the host with a foreign configuration leads to a stereotyped response that consists of mobilization of phagocytic cells into areas where the foreign configuration has been introduced. Neutrophils and macrophages engulf and kill the organisms by oxygen radicals in the phagosomes. Selenium deficiency not only impairs the ability of neutrophils to phagocytize but also impairs the capacity to kill the pathogenic organisms (Serfass & Ganther, 1975; Boyne & Arthur, 1981). These functional defects of the neutrophils are associated with changes in enzymatic activities and structural conformations of the cell surface and interior. Impaired scavenging of hydroxyl radicals by decreased glutathione peroxidase activity in cytoplasm is thought to inhibit their glucose catabolism *via* the glucose monophosphate shunt. The inhibition of glucose oxidation limits the supply of energy for the continuing production of hydroxyl radicals necessary for the microbicidal process (Arthur *et al.*, 1981).

Although selenium deficiency impairs the normal response of neutrophil functions, the outcome of microbial challenge to experimental animals is an increase or decrease in host resistance. Selenium deficiency increases the survival of rats infected with *Salmonella typhimurium* and of mice infected with *Plasmodium bergeii, Listeria monocytogenes* or *Pseudorabies* virus. In contrast, selenium deficiency increases susceptibility to *Diplococcus pneumoniae* Type 1 and *Staphylococcus aureus* infection. These differences in susceptibility to pathogens may partly explain the unavailability of selenium necessary for the growth of microorganisms (Boyne *et al.*, 1984).

Humoral immunity

There is considerable evidence that selenium supplementation enhances humoral immunity in animals, including rodents, against pathogenic microbes (Serfass *et al.*, 1974;

Spallholz, 1981). Selenium-supplemented (1-3 ppm) mice produced increased titres of IgM and IgG antibodies against sheep red blood cells (Spallholz *et al.*, 1973; Shackelford & Martin, 1980), and both primary and secondary immune responses to these cells are enhanced by selenium supplementation (Spallholz *et al.*, 1974; Koller *et al.*, 1979), which has been attributed to an increase in antibody-forming cells (Koller *et al.*, 1979). However, supplementation with higher doses of selenium (5 ppm) caused inhibition of antibody production in rats (Koller *et al.*, 1986). In contrast, selenium deficiency induced suppression of antibody synthesis and lower antibody titres in chicks (Marsh *et al.*, 1981a,b) and dogs (Sheffy & Schultz, 1978). In general, selenium supplementation enhances antibody production, and selenium deficiency results in a decrease in antibody titres.

Cellular immunity

Both T and B lymphocytes from selenium-deficient dogs (Sheffy & Schultz, 1979), mice (Parnham *et al.*, 1983) and rats (Eskew *et al.*, 1985) had significantly suppressed responsiveness to several mitogens. Lymphocytes from selenium-supplemented pigs (Larsen & Tollersrund, 1981) and lambs (1 ppm; Turner *et al.*, 1985), however, showed an increased ability to proliferate in response to stimulation by phytohaemagglutinin or pokeweed mitogen. This evidence shows that selenium can modulate cellular immune responsiveness.

Koller *et al.* (1986) studied the effect of selenium supplementation on cellular immunity. Selenium administered orally to female Sprague-Dawley rats for ten weeks at 0.5-2.0 ppm significantly enhanced natural killer activity. Delayed-type hypersensitivity response was suppressed at all doses, while antibody synthesis and prostaglandin E_2 synthesis were reduced only at the highest dose. T Cell-dependent antibody synthesis and interleukin-1 activity were not affected by selenium administration.

Recently, developments in cellular immunology enabled us to elucidate the intricate network of immunocompetent cell groups. This network is modulated by a variety of cytokines as well as by surface marker interactions. Selenium also affects secretion of cytokines from immunocompetent cells. For instance, lymphocytes from selenium-deficient goats showed reduced production of leukocyte migration inhibitory factor but no change in their ability to produce interleukin-2 (Aziz & Klesius, 1986). In contrast, selenium at 10 ng/ml enhanced interleukin-2 production in a primate lymphoid cell line (Brown *et al.*, 1985). Peripheral human lymphocytes incubated in the presence of 10^{-6} to 10^{-9} M selenium had enhanced ability to produce interferon (Watson *et al.*, 1986). Interleukin-1 production by peritoneal macrophages from selenium-supplemented rats was not affected (Koller *et al.*, 1986).

Epidemiological investigations have associated high dietary intakes of selenium with a decreased incidence of several types of cancer. A great deal of experimental evidence has accumulated on this interesting phenomenon (Schrauzer *et al.*, 1978): selenium prevents chemically induced tumours in animals (Medina *et al.*, 1983; Clark, 1985). Selenium at 2 ppm in drinking-water did not enhance peritoneal macrophage tumoricidal capacity, although it did result in a 60% reduction in mouse tumour burden (Watson *et al.*, 1987).

Mechanism of action

Hydrogen peroxide metabolism. Several selenoenzymes have been identified, although glutathione peroxidase is the only such enzyme known in mammals. It represents the major distribution compartment of selenium in the body and contains selenocysteine at its catalytic site. Behne and Walters (1983) and Hawkes *et al.* (1985) reported that 33-40% of the total body selenium is in the form of glutathione peroxidase. It acts to reduce both hydrogen peroxide and organic peroxides by using reduced glutathione as a hydrogen donor to produce oxidized glutathione and water.

In several cell types, such as neutrophils and macrophages, hydrogen peroxide is produced by an oxidation process and acts as a microbicidal agent but may also become toxic to phagocytes. There are several detoxication systems against autooxidation, including catalase and glutathione peroxidase, presumably metallothionein. Selenium deficiency induces enhanced formation of extracellular hydroxy radicals and increased lipid peroxidation in hepatic mitochondria and microsomes of chicks (Combs *et al.*, 1975) and rats (Hill & Burk, 1984) deficient in vitamin E and selenium.

Cell surface and intracellular modifications. Alterations in peroxide metabolism induced by selenium deficiency change the integrity of the cellular membranes and affect the function of immunocompent cells, because the cellular surface is involved in the recognition of antigens and major histocompatibility complexes and several cytokines, the transmission of signals to the interior, the release of soluble mediators, and subsequent lysis of foreign cells. Inhibition of the microtubule assembly inhibits not only cellular migration and phagocytosis, but also the topographical redistribution of appropriate surface receptors during stimulation of lymphocytes by antigen or mitogen (Nicolson, 1974).

Supplementation with selenium can prevent structural damage and disruption of cellular integrity caused by peroxidation of membranes and other cell components by enhancing the action of glutathione peroxidase on hydroperoxides of unsaturated fatty acids (Tappel, 1973; Ramstoeck *et al.*, 1980). Gabor *et al.* (1985) demonstrated that exposure of quartz-treated guinea-pig macrophages to nontoxic levels of selenium *in vitro* reduced the high rate of lipid peroxidation caused by the quartz treatment and enhanced cell viability and migration (Gabor *et al.*, 1985). This phenomenon can be potentiated by the addition of vitamin E.

Prostaglandin metabolism. In the first step of host resistance, macrophages phagocytize foreign organisms. If the cells fail to cope with this nonspecific reaction, macrophages act like antigen-presenting cells and transmit the antigens to T-cell lineages. The physiological role of prostaglandins on immunocompetent cells, investigated *in vitro* is to modulate the function of immunocompetent cells such as monocytes, neutrophils, macrophages and mast cells. These cells release arachidonic acid by the action of phospholipase A2, and the arachidonic acids are converted to prostaglandins by the arachidonate cascade, namely, the cyclooxygenase and lipoxygenase pathways. The first products of these two pathways are hydroxyperoxides, which may be affected by glutathione peroxidase. The first product of arachidonic acid released by platelet 12-lipoxygenase, 12-hydroperoxyarachidonic acid, is reduced by glutathione peroxidase and converted to 12-hydroxyarachidonic acid. Bryant and Bailey (1982) studied arachidonic acid metabolism in platelets of selenium-deficient rats and showed a decrease in 12-hydroxyarachidonic acid and an increase in THETE (a mixture of 8,9,12-trihydroxy-5,8,10,14-eicosatrienoic acid and 8,11,12-trihydroxy-5,9,14-eicosatrienoic acid) in the lipoxygenase pathway. 12-Hydroxy-arachidonic acid may therefore not be reduced due to insufficient glutathione peroxidase activity but is converted nonenzymatically to THETE.

Another example of the modulation of arachidonate metabolism in selenium-deficient rats is that exposure to cigarette smoke almost completely inhibits (>80 %) the zymosan-stimulated release of arachidonate metabolites LTB4 by pulmonary alveolar macrophages. In selenium-fed animals, release of the cyclooxygenase products, prostaglandin E_2 and thromboxin, remained unaffected by cigarette smoke, while an inhibition of approximately 50% in the release of the lipoxygenase product, LTB4, was observed in pulmonary alveolar macrophages (Gairola & Tai, 1986).

This evidence is contradictory to some extent, probably due to insufficient knowledge about the functions of prostaglandins in immunocompetent cells. Although the physiological role of glutathione peroxidase in prostaglandin metabolism is unknown, study of the functions of prostaglandins in immunocompetent cells will reveal the effects of selenium on immune function.

Unknown, physiologically active selenium compounds in serum. Evaluation of these results is complicated by the fact that addition of serum to culture media in the assessment of lymphoid cell activation is usually indispensable. Even after inactivation of fetal calf serum, it contains hundreds of biologically active proteins, some of which have inhibitory and others of which have stimulatory effects on immune responses. If it becomes possible to perform assays in serum-free media (Brown *et al*, 1985), we will be able to investigate the functions of various selenopeptides in serum. Various biological systems may be involved in the effects of selenium.

CONCLUSION

This is certainly a far from complete review of the literature on the immunotoxicity of cobalt and selenium. The experimental evidence cited here is contradictory and indicates the complexity of the responses. This is presumably because the immune system fulfills its complex functions by delicately regulated cooperation between not only several subsets of lymphoid cells but also other cell types. Therefore, it is necessary to investigate the role of the subsets and different cell types in selenium deficiency and selenium supplementation experiments.

Many metals appear to be chemically hyperactive in living organisms, in comparison with organic compounds. When the metals are incorporated into macromolecules, such as enzymes, they are usually located within or in the vicinity of the catalytic site. Since their potent chemical properties are often detrimental to the normal function of the systems, even low-level exposure may induce harmful effects in the immune system, because immuno-competent cells are vulnerable to chemical exposure. However, cobalt and selenium may also may be involved in activation of the immune system. Investigation of their mechanisms of activation will provide clues to understanding the delicate regulation of the immune system.

REFERENCES

Arthur, J.R., Boyne, R., Hill, H.A.O. & Okolow-Zubkowska, M.J. (1981) The production of oxygen-derived radicals by neutrophils from selenium-deficient cattle. *FEBS Lett.*, **135**: 187-190

Aziz, E.S. & Klesius, P.H. (1986) The effect of selenium deficiency in goats on lymphocyte production of leukocyte migration inhibitory factor. *Vet. Immunol. Immunopathol.*, **10**: 381-390

Behne, D. & Walters, W. (1983) Distribution of selenium and glutathione peroxidase in the rat. *J. Nutr.*, **113**: 456-461

Bencko, V., Wagner, V., Wagnerova, M. & Zavazal, V. (1984) Human exposure to nickel and cobalt: biological monitoring and immunobiochemical response. *Environ. Res.*, **40**: 399-410

Boyne, R. & Arthur, J.R. (1981) Effects of selenium and copper deficiency on neutrophil function in cattle. *J. comp. Pathol.*, **92**: 271-276

Boyne, R., Mann, S.O. & Arthur, J.R. (1984) Effect of *Salmonella typhimurium* infection on selenium deficient rats. *Microbios Lett.*, **27**: 83-87

Brown, R.L. Griffith, R.L., Ruscetti, F.W. & Rabin, H. (1985) Modulation of interleukin 2 release from a primate lymphoid cell line in serum-free and serum-containing media. *Cell. Immunol.*, **92**: 14-21

Bryant, R.W. & Bailey, J.M. (1982) Altered lipoxygenase metabolism and decreased glutathione peroxidase activity in platelets from selenium-deficient rats. *Biochem. biophys. Res. Commun.*, **92**: 268-272

Clark, L.D. (1985) The epidemiology of Se and cancer. *Fed. Proc.*, **44**: 2584-2589

Combs, G.F., Jr, Noguchi, T. & Scott, M.L. (1975) Mechanism of action of selenium and vitamin E in protection of biological membranes. *Fed. Proc.*, **34**: 2090-2095

Derkach, V.V. & Burmakina, L.I. (1970) The influence of cobalt on precipitin formation and development of Arthus phenomenon. Zn. *Mikrobiol. Epidemiol. Immunobiol.*, **47**: 59-62

Eskew, M.L., Scholz, R.W., Reddy, C.C., Todhunter, D.A. & Zarkower, A. (1985) Effects of vitamin E and selenium deficiencies on rat immune function. *Immunology*, **54**: 173-180

Gabor, S., Ciugudeann, M. & Surcel, K. (1985) Effects of selenium on quartz-induced cytotoxicity in macrophages. *Environ. Res.*, **37**: 293-299

Gainer, J.H. (1972) Increased mortality in encephalomyocarditis virus-infected mice consuming cobalt sulfate: tissue concentrations of cobalt. *Am. J. vet. Res.*, **33**: 2067-2073

Gainer, J.H. (1973) Activation of the Rauscher leukemia virus by metals. *J. natl Cancer Inst.*, **51**: 609-614

Gairola, C.G. & Tai, H.H. (1986) Cigarette smoke-induced alterations in the release of arachidonate metabolites by pulmonary alveolar macrophage from selenium-fed and selenium-deficient rats. *Biochem. Pharmacol.*, **35**: 2423-2428

Hawkes, W.C., Wilhemsen, E.C. & Tappel, A.L. (1985) Abundance and tissue distribution of selenocysteine-containing proteins in the rat. *J. inorg. Biochem.*, **23**: 77-92

Hill, K. & Burk, R.F. (1984) Influence of vitamin E and selenium on glutathione-dependent protection against microsomal lipid peroxidation. *Biochem. Pharmacol.*, **33**: 1065-1072

Keshan Disease Research Group of the Chinese Academy of Medical Sciences (1979) Observations on effect of sodium selenite in prevention of Keshan disease. *Chin. med. J.*, **92**: 471-476

Kiremidjian-Schumacher, L. & Stotzky, G. (1987) Review/ Selenium and immune responses. *Environ. Res.*, **42**: 277-303

Koller, L.D. (1981) Review/Commentary: immunotoxicology of heavy metals. *Int. J. Immunopharmacol.*, **2**: 269-279

Koller, L.D., Isaacson-Kerkvliet, N., Exon, J.H., Brauner, J.A. & Patton, N.M. (1979) Synergism of methylmercury and selenium producing enhanced antibody formation in mice. *Arch. environ. Health*, **34**: 248-252

Koller, L.D., Exon, J.H., Talcott, P.A., Osvorne, C.A. & Henningsen, G.M. (1986) Immune responses in rats supplemented with selenium. *Clin. exp. Immunol.*, **63**: 570-576

Larsen, H.J. & Tollersrund, S. (1981) Effect of dietary vitamin E and selenium on phytohaemagglutinin response of pig lymphocytes. *Res. vet. Sci.*, **31**: 301-305

Lawrence, D.A. (1981) *In vitro* effects of heavy metals on primary humoral immune responses. *Toxicol. appl. Pharmacol.*, **47**: 439-451

Lewin, J., Lindgren, U. & Wahlberg, J.E. (1982) Screw fixation in bone of guinea pigs sensitized to nickel and cobalt. *Acta orthop. scand.*, **53**: 675-680

Marsh, J.A., Combs, G.F. & Dietert, R.F. (1981a) Effects of selenium and vitamin E on development of humoral immunity of the chick. In: Spallholz, J.E., Martin, L.L. & Ganther, H.E., eds, *Selenium in Biology and Medicine*, Westport, CT, AVI Publications, pp. 358-365

Marsh, J.A., Dietert, R.R. & Combs, G.F., Jr (1981b) Influence of dietary selenium and vitamin E on the humoral immune response of the chick. *Proc. Soc. exp. Biol. Med.*, **166**: 228-236

Maurer, T., Thomann, N., Weinrich, E.G. & Hess, R. (1979) Predictive evaluation in animals of the contact allergenic potential of medically important substances. II. Comparisons of different methods of cutaneous sensitization with 'weak' allergens. *Contact Dermatitis*, **5**, 1-6

Medina, D., Lane, H.W. & Shepherd, F. (1983) Effect of dietary selenium levels on 7,12-dimethylbenzanthracene-induced mouse mammary tumorigenesis. *Carcinogenesis*, **4**: 1159-1163

Merritt, K. & Brown, S.A. (1981) Metal sensitivity reactions to orthopedic implants. *Int. J. Dermatol.*, **20**: 89-94

Nelson, A.A., Fitzhugh, O.G. & Calvery, H.O. (1943) Liver tumors following cirrhosis caused by selenium in rats. *Cancer Res.*, **3**: 230-236

Nicolson, G.L. (1974) The interactions of lectins with animal cell surfaces. *Int. Rev. Cytol.*, **39**: 89-90

Nordlind, K. (1982). Effect of metal allergens on the DNA synthesis of unsensitized guinea pig lymphoid cells cultured *in vitro*. *Int. Arch. Allergy appl. Immunol.*, **69**:12-17

Parnham, M.J., Winkelmann, J. & Leyck, S. (1983) Macrophage, lymphocyte, and chronic inflammatory responses in selenium deficient rodents: association with decreased glutathione peroxidase activity. *Int. J. Immunopharmacol.*, **5**: 455-461

Ramstoeck, F.R., Hoekstra, W.G. & Ganther, H.E. (1980) Trialkyllead metabolism and lipid peroxidation *in vitro* in vitamin E and selenium deficient rats, as measured by ethane production. *Toxicol. appl. Pharmacol.*, **54**: 251-257

Rotruck, J.T., Pope, A.L., Ganther, H.E. & Hoekstra, W.G. (1972) Prevention of oxidative damage to rat erythrocytes by dietary selenium. *J. Nutr.*, **102**: 689-696

Schrauzer, G.N., White, D.A. & Schneider, C.J. (1978) Selenium and cancer: effects of selenium and of the diet on the genesis of spontaneous mammary tumors in virgin inbred female C3H/ST mice. *Bioinorg. Chem.*, **8**: 387-396

Schwartz, G.N. & Foltz, C,M. (1957) Selenium as an integral part of factor 3 against dietary necrotic liver degeneration. *J. Am. chem. Soc.*, **79**: 3292-3296

Serfass, R.E. & Ganther, H.E. (1975) Defective microbicidal activity in glutathione peroxidase deficient neutrophils of Se deficient rats. *Nature*, **225**: 640-641

Serfass, R., Hinsdill, R.D. & Ganther, H.E. (1974) Protective effect of dietary selenium on *Salmonella* infection: relation to glutathione peroxidase and superoxide dismutase activity of phagocytes. *Fed. Proc.*, **33**: 094-702

Shackelford, J. & Martin, J. (1980) Antibody response of mature male mice after drinking water supplemented with selenium. *Fed. Proc.*, **39**: 339-342

Sheffy, B.E. & Schultz, R.D. (1978) Nutrition and the immune reponse. *Cornell Vet.*, **68** (Suppl. 7): 48-61

Sheffy, B.E. & Schultz, R.D. (1979) Influence of vitamin E and selenium on immune response mechanism. *Fed. Proc.*, **38**: 2139-2143

Spallholz, J.E. (1981) Selenium: What role in immunity and immune cytotoxicity? In: Spallholz, J.E., Martin, L.L. & Ganther, H.E., eds, *Selenium Biology and Medicine*, Westport, CT, AVI Publications, pp. 103-117

Spallholz, J.E., Martin, J.L., Gerlach, M.L. & Heinzerling, R.H. (1973) Immunologic responses of mice fed diets supplemented with selenium. *Proc. Soc. exp. Biol. Med.*, **143**: 685-689

Spallholz, J.E., Heinzerling, R.H., Gerlach, M.L. & Martin, J.L. (1974) The effect of selenite, tocopherol acetate and selenite, and tocopherol acetate on the primary and secondary immune responses of mice administered tetanus toxoid of sheep red blood cell antigen. *Fed. Proc.*, **33**: 694-704

Tappell, A.L. (1973) Lipid peroxidation damage to cell components. *Fed. Proc.*, **32**: 1870-1874

Turner, R.J., Wheatley, L.B. & Beck, N.F.G. (1985) Stimulatory effects of selenium on mitogen responses in lambs. *Vet. Immunol. Immunopathol.*, **8**: 119-124

Veien, N.K. & Svejgaad, E. (1978) Lymphocyte transformation in patients with cobalt dermatitis. *Br. J. Dermatol.*, **99**: 191-196

Wahlberg, J.E. & Boman, A. (1978). Sensitization and testing of guinea-pig with cobalt chloride. *Contact Dermatitis*, **4**: 123-128

Ward, P.A., Goldschmidt, P. & Greene, N.D. (1975) Suppressive effects of metal salts on leukocyte and fibroblastic functions. *J. Reticuloendoth. Soc.*, **18**: 313-318

Warner, G.L. & Lawrence, D.A. (1986a) Stimulation of lymphocytes by cations. *Cell. Immunol.*, **101**: 425-439

Warner, G.L. & Lawrence, D.A. (1986b) Cell surface and cell cycle analysis of metal induced murine T cell proliferation. *Eur. J. Immunol.*, **16**: 1337- 1342

Warner, G.L. & Lawrence, D.A. (1988) The effect on metals on IL-2 related lymphocyte proliferation. *Int. J. Immunopharmacol.*, **10**: 629-637

Watson, R.R., Moriguchi, S., McRae, B.K., Tobin, L., Mayverry, J.C. & Lucus, D. (1986) Effects of selenium in vitro on human T-lymphocyte functions and K-562 tumor cell growth. *J. Leuk. Biol.*, **39**: 447-457

Watson, R.R., Moriguchi, S. & Gensler, H.L. (1987) Effects on dietary retinyl palmitate and selenium on tumoricidal capacity of macrophages in mice undergoing tumor promotion. *Cancer Lett.*, **36**: 181-187

Wigren, A. (1982) Cobalt allergy reaction after knee arthroplasty with a walldius prosthesis. *Z. Orthop.*, **120**: 17-18

IMMUNOLOGICAL DIAGNOSIS OF CHRONIC BERYLLIUM DISEASE IN HUMANS AND ANIMALS

A.L. Reeves[1] & O.P. Preuss[2]

[1]Wayne State University, Detroit, MI 48202; and
[2]1393 Coyote Road, Prescott, Arizona 86303, USA

ABSTRACT

Chronic beryllium disease is an occupational disorder with immunological pathogenesis. Diagnostic tests based on detection of beryllium hypersensitivity include cutaneous reactivity, macrophage migration inhibition and lymphocyte blast transformation. The latter test can be done both on peripheral blood and on bronchoalveolar lavage fluid. Skin testing is unsuitable in clinical medicine because it involves exposure of the host to antigen; the macrophage migration inhibition test was found to be of limited clinical usefulness because it showed great sensitivity to immunosuppressive (steroid) therapy. The lymphocyte blast transformation test presently appears to be the diagnostic procedure of choice for the detection of beryllium hypersensitivity, especially if performed on bronchoalveolar lavage fluid. Experience with the last test, as compared with the results of lymphocyte blast transformation in peripheral blood, leads to a hypothesis of compartmentalized immune response involving only the lungs as the essential event in the development of chronic beryllium disease.

INTRODUCTION

Chronic beryllium disease (CBD) is a granulomatous inflammation of the lungs seen in person with occupational and/or environmental contact with certain beryllium compounds. The condition was first described by Hardy and Tabershaw (1946); the first satisfactory animal model was established by Policard (1950). Recent reviews are available on the clinical details of this syndrome as well as on its etiology, including specification of the molecular species capable of provoking it (Reeves & Preuss, 1985; Preuss, 1986).

CBD presented a considerable diagnostic problem to clinicians of past decades. A history of significant exposure and/or presence of beryllium in the lungs or elsewhere in the organism, and subtle clinical signs with concurrent nonspecific X-ray manifestations, were stressed by the early investigators (Hardy, 1961; Dattoli et al., 1964; Vorwald, 1966). Histopathological examination of tissue obtained at biopsy or autopsy was helpful in differentiating CBD from nongranulomatous diseases such as idiopathic pulmonary fibrosis or tuberculosis, but a purely histological distinction between the granuloma of CBD and of sarcoidosis or of certain cases of hypersensitivity pneumonitis caused by fungal microspores turned out to be difficult or impossible (Jones Williams 1958; Dudley, 1959). Even the concurrent chemical detection of beryllium in pulmonary tissue could not be regarded as absolute proof, because measurable quantities of this metal were found in the lungs of beryllium workers and of other persons without the disease (Lieben et al., 1963). The definitive differential diagnosis of CBD from histologically similar conditions had to wait until a better understanding of the pathogenesis of this condition was achieved.

Immunotoxicity of Metals and Immunotoxicology, Edited by
A. D. Dayan *et al.,* Plenum Press, New York, 1990

183

PATCH TEST IN HUMANS

An immunological pathogenesis for CBD was first proposed by Sterner and Eisenbud (1951). This then unconventional hypothesis was justified by the epidemiological distribution of CBD cases; the typical lack of a linear dose-response relationship; and the demonstrated ability of beryllium to cause cutaneous hypersensitivity in humans (De Nardi *et al.*, 1949; McCord, 1951). The patch test of Curtis (1951) was the first practical procedure with potential implications for an immunological diagnosis of CBD. It was found that application of unbuffered ionic beryllium (fluoride, chloride or sulfate) to the skin at concentrations of 1-2% produced a local allergic eczematous reaction in all of 13 workers with a history of dermatitis in a beryllium plant. Subsequent application of this technique in 32 CBD patients also led to a positive response in each case, whereas all but one of 19 patients with non-beryllium interstitial lung disease showed negative results (Curtis, 1959). Although a positive result appeared to indicate cutaneous hypersensitivity rather than pulmonary disease, it was nevertheless considered that a negative result and exposure history provided dependable criteria for ruling out CBD. One of the greatest drawbacks of the patch test was that it could produce contact sensitization in previously unexposed individuals, a feature reported in both of Curtis' papers. Further clinical experience with the test (Van Ordstrand, 1959; Niemöller, 1962; Groetenbriel *et al.* 1970) suggested that this was a serious problem, and might also exacerbate CBD in patients in a state of remission (Waksman, 1959; Zschunke & Folesky, 1969; Sarkar *et al.*, 1971). False-positive results due to a state of beryllium hypersensitivity without CBD and false-negative results due to a generalized cutaneous anergy were also encountered (Hardy, 1963). In one case, epitheloid-cell granuloma at the test site with severe generalized anaphylactoid reaction was reported (Sneddon, 1955). In view of these difficulties, patch testing with beryllium could never gain a foothold in clinical medicine and could not be recommended as a standard diagnostic measure.

CUTANEOUS HYPERSENSITIVITY IN ANIMALS

In spite of its unsuitability for clinical diagnosis, the Curtis patch test did prove that beryllium was antigenic and served to stimulate further research in this direction. In the USSR, Alekseeva (1965) found the guinea-pig to be a suitable animal model for the production of cutaneous hypersensitivity with intradermal injections of beryllium chloride. The reaction was of the delayed type and could be transferred passively with lymphoid cells of sensitized animals but not with serum; it did not involve, even together with homologous protein, humoral antibody formation (Alekseeva *et al.*, 1966). These studies established that beryllium hypersensitivity was cell-mediated. Treatment of guinea-pigs with a pulmonary nucleoprotein preparation in addition to beryllium, or with a bovine serum albumin complex of beryllium, produced more intense skin reactions than those due to beryllium alone, suggesting a possible autoimmune component of CBD (Alekseeva, 1967; Krivanek & Reeves, 1972). Formation of a pulmonary beryllium-protein complex or of a pulmonary nucleo-protein influenced by the presence of beryllium was also observed in rats (Vasilieva, 1969, 1972), but this species did not show a cutaneous reaction to beryllium comparable to that seen with the Curtis test.

Chiappino *et al.* (1968, 1969) in Italy were able to produce negative reactions to skin tests in guinea-pigs in which a state of beryllium hypersensitivity had been induced previously by intratracheal beryllium oxide treatments. All cutaneous reactivity could be abolished by treating the guinea-pigs with an anti-guinea-pig lymphocyte serum obtained from rabbits; the reaction of cytoplasmic and/or nuclear membrane components of sensitized guinea-pig lymphocytes with rabbit serum antibodies could be demonstrated by immunofluorescence.

In the USA, experimental work on the immunological tissue response to beryllium was pursued by Reeves *et al.* (1970, 1972), Marx and Burrell (1973), Reeves and Krivanek (1974) and Palazzolo and Reeves (1975) and was summarized by Reeves (1976, 1983). More recent work was reported by Barna *et al.* (1984a). The animal of choice in these experiments was the Hartley guinea-pig, which is commercially available as an immunologically 'responding' (to poly-L-lysine) substrain. The parameters and histological criteria for a positive skin reaction were defined and differentiated from those of a mere cutaneous irritation. It was found that hypersensitivity to beryllium, at least in this guniea-pig strain, did not parallel the responsiveness to poly-L-lysine conjugates. The ability to respond was transmitted to progeny as a simple Mendelian dominant, non-sex-linked characteristic (Polak *et al.*, 1968).

MACROPHAGE MIGRATION INHIBITION TEST IN HUMANS

Clinical difficulties with immunological tests that involved the patient as host stimulated interest in in-vitro procedures that do not require contact of the subject with the presumed antigen. Bloom and Bennett (1966) demonstrated a soluble factor elaborated by sensitized lymphocytes which could inhibit the free migration of macrophages *in vitro*. The 'migration inhibitor factor' (MIF) appeared to be highly antigen-specific but not cell- or species-specific. It appeared possible to culture populations of lymphocytes from human blood in the presence of antigen and then test the supernatant of such a culture on guinea-pig peritoneal exudate cells. Inhibition of migration of the latter cells was observed if, and only if, the source of the lymphocytes was a sensitized patient.

The MIF test was first applied to CBD patients by Henderson *et al.* (1972), who showed that beryllium oxide-stimulated lymphocytes from these patients, but not from healthy controls, produced the inhibitory factor. Marx and Burrell (1973) studied seven patients with CBD and found positive results in all, while the results for six healthy workers and for two non-CBD pulmonary patients were negative. It was also found, however, that corticosteroid therapy could substantially suppress results in the MIF test (Jones Williams *et al.*, 1972): among seven CBD patients receiving such therapy, a positive result was obtained in only one. Price *et al.* (1976) studied five CBD patients along with 50 healthy beryllium workers and 20 healthy controls. One of the five patients who was not on corticosteroid therapy showed a pronounced MIF titre, which reverted to normal when the therapy was instituted; the reverse effect was seen in another patient whose corticosteriod therapy was suspended. It was clear that the value of MIF as a diagnostic test for CBD was severely limited by its extraordinary sensitivity to corticosteroid suppression.

THE MIF TEST IN ANIMALS

The guinea-pig turned out to be a suitable experimental model for assessment of the MIF test as a measure of beryllium hypersensitivity. Marx and Burrell (1973) tested 13 beryllium-sensitized guinea-pigs (compared with 19 'naive' negative controls and 11 tuberculin-sensitized positive controls) with beryllium antigens and a commercial purified protein derivative. Migration of peritoneal macrophages harvested from sensitized animals was clearly inhibited and clearly antigen-specific. The results of the MIF test and of skin tests in sensitized animals showed a 75% positive correlation. Palazzolo and Reeves (1975) established that a size threshold of 3.5-mm diameter in a positive skin test corresponded to a migration inhibition threshold of about 18%. The correlation coefficient for degree of migration and skin reaction diameter at 48 h was calculated to be moderately strong at - 0.45 but improved with better definition of optimal conditions for the performance of the MIF test. On the one hand, skin reactivity and macrophage migration inhibition may be interrelated facets of the same phenomenon; on the other hand, it is clear that both of these tests provide a measure of the state of beryllium hypersensitivity rather than the condition of CBD. On the basis of available evidence, Reeves (1980) concluded that:
  (1) Immunological tests involving beryllium antigen were diagnostic for the state of beryllium hypersensitivity, not CBD.
  (2) The state of beryllium hypersensitivity can exist without clinically manifest CBD.
  (3) Clinically manifest CBD involves hypersensitivity to beryllium, unless modified by immunosuppression.

LYMPHOCYTE TRANSFORMATION IN HUMANS

The role of lymphoid cells in beryllium hypersensitivity has been noted (Alekseeva, 1965, 1967; Chiappino *et al.*, 1968, 1969), and lymphocytes also play a known role in the formation of gramulomata (Epstein, 1967). This relationship is demonstrated by the phenomenon of transformation *in vitro* of small lymphocytes to large lymphoblasts in response to granuloma-producing antigens (Robbins, 1964; Oppenheim, 1968). This lymphocyte transformation test (LTT) was first applied to CBD cases by Hanifin *et al.* (1970), who showed that beryllium compounds caused striking transformation *in vitro* of lymphocytes obtained from the peripheral blood of beryllium-sensitive subjects, but that lymphocytes from normal, nonsensitive subjects were not transformed.

The reaction proved to be reasonably antigen-specific. Deodhar *et al.* (1973) reported that 25 of 35 CBD patients (71%) had positive results in the LTT, even though they were being treated with immunosuppressive corticosteroids. There was also a correlation between the severity of the clinical disease and the degree of lymphocyte transformation. The incidence of positive results in control groups was low: two of 30 healthy beryllium workers, three of 19 healthy subjects with no known exposure and one of 11 patients with other lung diseases with no known exposure. The results of sequential tests in 16 CBD patients showed considerable individual variability in eight of them (Preuss *et al.*, 1980).

Increasing experience with the procedure was associated with improved accuracy of the results, suggesting that the early false-positive and false-negative results may have been due to imperfect technique. As a quantitative response indicator, pulsing with tritiated thymidine of cells challenged with beryllium salts and of unstimulated controls became a generally accepted procedure. Differences in scintillation counts between the two cell groups are expressed by a stimulation index representing the ratio of counts for stimulated cells to control cells. Williams and Jones Williams (1982a) developed an improved form of the test, utilizing purified lymphocytes suspended in 20% serum, with beryllium added in the nanomole (10^{-8} g) range. When the beryllium concentration was significantly higher, transformation was inhibited, apparently due to suppressed DNA biosynthesis (Van Ganse *et al.*, 1972; Jones & Amos, 1974, 1975).

An important further development occurred when Epstein *et al.* (1982) first reported use of the LTT on pulmonary lymphocytes obtained by bronchoalveolar lavage (BAL) fluid from a CBD patient. Significantly more uniform and more specific responses could be obtained from BAL lymphocytes than from circulating blood lymphocytes; these initial observations were confirmed by Chibara *et al.* (1983) and Rossman *et al.* (1988). The following parameter charges were observed in CBD patients in comparison with normal persons:

(1) The absolute number of all cells in BAL fluid was $33.6\pm9.4 \times 10^4$/ml (*vs.* $6.4\pm1.7 \times 10^4$/ml), an increase of three to nine fold.

(2) Of all cells, $58.8\pm6.7\%$ (*vs.* $10.9\pm2.0\%$) were lymphocytes, an increase of 4.0-7.4 times.

(3) Of all lymphocytes, $80.3\pm5.8\%$ (*vs.* $58.2\pm4.1\%$) were T lymphocytes (as tested with the monoclonal antibody OKT 3), an increase of 1.2-1.6 times.

(4) Of all T lymphocytes, $67.8\pm4.9\%$ (*vs.* $35.5\pm6.9\%$) were helper cells (as tested with OKT 4) and $19.1\pm3.8\%$ (*vs.* $28.0\pm5.8\%$) were suppressor cells (as tested with OKT 8), an increase of 1.5-3.2 times and a decrease of 0-2.2 times, respectively.

(5) The above percentages yielded a helper:suppressor ratio of 4.7 ± 0.1 (*vs.* 1.6 ± 0.5), an increase of 2.2-4.4 times.

(6) When BAL lymphocytes from all CBD patients were challenged with beryllium floride or sulfate, they had a significantly higher stimulation index than peripheral blood lymphocytes from the same patients.

(7) BAL lymphocytes from control cases, including sarcoidosis patients, patients with non-beryllium pulmonary disease and healthy unexposed individuals, had normal stimulation indices.

These observations clearly establish the BAL-LTT as a significant advancement in the clinical diagnosis of CBD. In the series of Rossman *et al.*, 1988), one beryllium worker who had a history of accidental high exposure showed lung granulomata on transbronchial biopsy, but no clinically manifest disease according to physiological and radiological evaluation. Results of the BAL-LTT were positive. This case may represent a subclinical state of CBD leading eventually to manifest disease, or perhaps to an immune state similar to the course of events that take place in most individuals following infection with tuberculosis. The possibility of 'immunization' to CBD was observed earlier in animal experiments (Reeves *et al.*, 1972; Reeves, 1976).

A relative disadvantage of the BAL-LTT is the requirement for BAL, which may not be feasible in individual cases for clinical or logistic reasons. However, material for this highly specialized evaluation can often be obtained by local chest physicians trained in bronchoscopy, and shipped to a laboratory experienced with this test (BAL cells can survive *in vitro* for nearly 20 h). Although it is an invasive procedure, BAL, if performed skilfully, is well tolerated by most patients, and it provides the opportunity for transbronchial biopsy of lung tissue for an affirming histopathological analysis with less inconvenience than an open lung biopsy.

THE LTT IN ANIMALS

The first attempt at application of the LTT to experimental animals treated with beryllium was reported by Kang *et al.* (1977). New Zealand rabbits were sensitized by the intradermal route (Reeves, 1972), and lymphocytes were obtained from the popliteal lymph nodes. The results of the tests were negative, even though the animals appeared to be hypersensitive to beryllium, as assessed by skin testing and macrophage migration inhibition. Barna *et al.* (1981, 1984b), however, observed a significantly elevated percentage of T lymphocytes in the BAL fluid of beryllium-sensitive guinea-pigs.

Harmsen *et al.* (1986) and Haley *et al.* (1989) reported on use of the BAL-LTT in beagle dogs exposed to beryllium oxide calcined at 500 and 1000°C. Serial necropsies for the purpose of evaluating lung burden and histopathological response were performed at 8, 32, 64, 180 and 365 days; additional dogs were studied by BAL at 3, 6, 7, 11, 15, 18 and 22 months and necropsied at 24 months. Lymphocyte numbers and percentages were increased in BAL samples from all dogs exposed to the 500°C compound at three months but returned to normal thereafter; the response of the dogs exposed to the 1000°C compound was variable and insignificant at all times. Only the 500°C compound caused manifest CBD, and only in those animals that attained a high initial lung burden of beryllium (> 40 mg/kg), which showed a positive result in the BAL-LTT at six and seven months. Application of the LTT to peripheral blood gave less consistent responses; the stimulation index tended to be highest at 18 months. When blood and BAL samples from the same animal both gave positive results, the stimulation indices with BAL were always higher. The authors concluded that a compartmentalized immune response in the lungs, as opposed to a systemic response consistently involving the blood lymphocytes as well, is the key event in the pathogenesis of CBD. This suggests that BAL lymphocytes may provide a better index of an individual's reactivity to beryllium, and his propensity for developing CBD, than peripheral blood lymphocytes. Similar findings were made in relation to other hypersensitivity diseases of the lung (Bice *et al.*, 1980; Bice & Shopp, 1988) and in pulmonary sarcoidosis (Hunninghake & Crystal,1981).

CONCLUSION

As an immunological test for the diagnosis of CBD, the skin test of Curtis (1951, 1959) had to be rejected, because it required contact of the subject with the allergen, resulting in de-novo sensitizations and/or exacerbations.

In-vitro tests that have been developed include the LTT (Hanifin *et al.*, 1970) and the MIF test (Henderson *et al.*, 1972), both of which require only blood samples from the host. Williams and Jones Williams (1982b) made a clinical comparison of these two tests and concluded that the LTT had clear advantages because it is easier to perform, has better reproducibility and undergoes less suppression by steroid therapy. However, in peripheral blood, the LTT also produces false-negative results. Furthermore, although proliferation ratios of beryllium-stimulated *vs.* non-stimulated lymphocytes greater than 2.0 or 2.5 have been generally accepted as clinically positive, those under 3.0 were frequently found to be nonspecific. A suggestion has been made that the LTT be used on peripheral blood in the routine surveillance of beryllium workers (Williams & Jones Williams, 1982b), but experience with a large factory population (O.P. Preuss, personal observation) casts doubt on the usefulness of this approach. Several individuals with interstitial lung disease, later independently confirmed as CBD by the BAL-LTT, had persistently negative scores in blood-LTT. A large-scale study of this question is currently in progress at the National Jewish Center for Immunology and Respiratory Medicine in Denver, CO, USA. Its protocol includes long-term follow-up of workers with suspected granulomatous tissue reaction and the degree to which this can be correlated with the results of the blood-LTT and BAL-LTT.

Pending the outcome of this study, which could provide important additional information on the natural history of CBD, present evidence favours the BAL-LTT as the procedure of choice for the clinical diagnosis of CBD. BAL from CBD patients appears to give higher stimulation indices and more specific test results than peripheral blood lymphocytes, with a good dose-response relationship. These observations support the concept of a 'compartmentalized' immune response and the view that CBD may be a special case of hypersensitivity pneumonitis. In that case, positive results in the BAL-LTT signify not simply a state of systemic beryllium hypersensitivity, as do skin tests, the MIF test and possibly the blood-LTT, but a specific response in the lungs, i.e., CBD itself, or perhaps an immune state resulting from a successfully arrested case of CBD. The latter possibility in particular requires further clarification.

REFERENCES

Alekseeva, O.G. (1965) [Inquiry into the ability of beryllium compounds to produce allergy of the delayed type.] (in Russian) *Gig. Tr. prof. Zabol.*, **xi**: 20-25

Alekseeva, O.G. (1967) [Experimental study of the influence exerted by pulmonary nucleoprotein sensitization on the intensity of the Curtis patch test in berylliosis.] (in Russian) *Gig. Tr. prof. Zabol.*, **ix**: 29-34

Alekseeva, O.G., Volkova, A.O. & Svinkina, N.V. (1966) [Mechanism underlying the action of beryllium in the body.] (in Russian) *Farmakol. Toksikol.*, **iii**: 353-355

Barna, B.P., Chiang, T., Pillarisetti, S.G. & Deodhar, S.D. (1981) Immunologic studies of experimental beryllium lung disease in the guinea pig. *Clin. Immunol. Immunopathol.*, **20**: 402-411

Barna, B.P., Deodhar, S.D., Chiang, T., Gautam, S. & Edinger, M. (1984a) Experimental beryllium-induced lung disease. I: Differences in immunologic responses to beryllium compounds in strains 2 and 13 guinea pigs. *Int. Arch. Allergy appl. Immunol.*, **73**: 42-48

Barna, B.P., Deodhar, S.D., Gautam, S., Edinger, H., Chiang, T. & McMahon, J.T. (1984b) Experimental beryllium-induced lung disease. II: Analyses of bronchial lavage cells in strains 2 and 13 guinea pigs. *Int. Arch. Allergy appl. Immunol.*, **73**: 49-55

Bice, D.E. & Shopp, G.M. (1988) Antibody responses after lung immunization. *Exp. Lung Res.*, **14**:133-155

Bice, D.E., Harris, D.L., Bill, J.O., Muggenburg, B.A. & Wolff, R.K. (1980) Immune responses after localized lung immunizations in dogs. *Am. Rev. respir. Dis.*, **122**: 755-760

Bloom, B.R. & Bennett, B. (1966) Mechanism of a reaction in vitro associated with delayed-type hypersensitivity. *Science*, **153**: 80-82

Chiappino, G., Barbiano di Belgiojoso, G. & Cirla, A.M. (1968) [Hypersensitivity to beryllium compounds: inhibition mediated by anti-lymphocyte serum of the intradermal reaction in the guinea-pig.] (in Italian) *Boll. Ist. Sieroter. Milan.*, **47**: 669-677

Chiappino, G., Cirla, A.M. & Vigliani, E.C. (1969) Delayed-type hypersensitivity reactions to beryllium compounds. *Arch. Pathol.*, **87**: 131-140

Chihara, J., Nagai, S., Fujimura, N., Hirata, T. & Izumi, T. (1983) Bronchoalveolar lavage lymphocyte findings in chronic beryllium disease. *Am. Rev. respir. Dis.*, **127** (Suppl):64

Curtis, G.H. (1951) Cutaneous hypersensitivity to beryllium. *Arch. Dermatol. Syphilol.*, **640**: 470-482

Curtis, G.H. (1959) Diagnosis of beryllium disease, with special reference to the patch test. *Arch. ind. Health*, **19**: 150-153

Dattoli, J.A., Lieben, J. & Bisbing, J.(1964) Chronic beryllium disease. *J. occup. Med.*, **6**: 189-194

De Nardi, J.M., Van Ordstrand, H.S. & Carmody, M.G. (1949) Acute dermatitis and pneumonitis in beryllium workers. *Ohio State med. J.*, **45**: 567-575

Deodhar, S.D., Barna, B. & Van Ordstrand, H.S. (1973) Study of the immunologic aspects of chronic berylliosis. *Chest*, **63**: 309-313

Dudley, R.H. (1959) Pathologic changes of chronic beryllium disease. *Arch. ind. Health*, **19**: 184-189

Epstein, P.E., Dauber, J.H., Rossman, M.D. & Daniele, R.P. (1982) Bronchoalveolar lavage in a patient with chronic berylliosis: evidence for hypersensitivity pneumonitis. *Ann. intern. Med.*, **97**: 213-216

Epstein, W.L. (1967) Granulomatous hypersensitivity. *Prog. Allergy*, **ii**: 36-88

Groetenbriel, C., Van Ganse, W. & Oleffe, J. (1970) [A case of chronic beryllium poisoning: pathogenic considerations and the validity of the 'patch-test' for diagnosis.] (in French) *Acta tuberc. pneumol. belg.*, **61**: 363-376

Haley, P.J., Finch, G.L., Mewhinney, J.A., Harmsen, A.G., Hahn, F.F., Hoover, M.D. & Bice, D.E. (1989) Granulomatous lung disease in dogs from inhaled beryllium oxide. *Am. Rev. respir. Dis.* (in press)

Hanifin, J.M., Epstein, W.L. & Cline, M.J. (1970) In vitro studies of granulomatous hypersensitivity to beryllium. *J. invest. Dermatol.,* **55**: 284-288

Hardy, H.L. (1961) Beryllium disease: a continuing diagnostic problem. *Am. J. med. Sci.,* **242**: 150-156

Hardy, H.L. (1963) Beryllium disease. *Ann. N.Y. Acad. Sci.,* **107**: 525-538

Hardy, H.L. & Tabershaw, I.R. (1946) Delayed chemical pneumonitis occurring in workers exposed to beryllium compounds. *J. Ind. Hyg.,* **28**: 197-211

Harmsen, A.G., Finch, G.L., Mewhinney, J.A., Muggenburg, B.A. & Bice, D.E. (1986) Lung cellular response and lymphocyte blastogenesis in beagle dogs exposed to beryllium oxide. In: Muggenburg, B.A. & Bice, D.E., eds, *Annual Report, Inhalation Toxicology Research Institute,* Albuquerque, NM, Lovelace Biomedical & Environmantal Research Institute, pp. 291-295

Henderson, W.R., Fukuyama, K., Epstein, W.L. & Spitler, L.E. (1972) In vitro demonstration of delayed hypersensitivity in patients with berylliosis. *J. invest. Dermatol.,* **58**: 5-8

Hunninghake, S.W. & Crystal, R.G. (1981) Pulmonary sarcoidosis: disorder mediated by excess helper T-lymphocytic activity at sites of disease activity. *New Engl. J. Med.,* **305**: 429-434

Jones, J.M. & Amos, H.E. (1974) Contact sensitivity in vitro. I: Activation of actively allergized lymphocytes by a beryllium complex. *Int. Arch. Allergy,* **46**:161-171

Jones, J.M. & Amos, H.E. (1975) Contact sensitivity in vitro. II: Effect of beryllium preparations on the proliferative response of specifically allergized lymphocytes and normal lymphocytes stimulated with PHA. *Int. Arch. Allergy,* **48**: 22-29

Jones Williams, W. (1958) Histological study of the lungs in 52 cases of chronic beryllium disease. *Br. J. ind. Med.,* **15**: 84-91

Jones Williams, W., Grey, J. & Pioli, E. (1972) Diagnosis of beryllium disease. *Br. med. J.,* **iv**: 175

Kang, K.Y., Bice, D.E., Hoffmann, E., D'Amato, R., & Salvaggio, J. (1977) Experimental studies of sensitization to beryllium, zirconium, and aluminum compounds in the rabbit. *J. Allergy clin. Immunol.,* **59**: 425-436

Krivanek, N.D. & Reeves, A.L. (1972) Effect of chemical forms of beryllium on the production of the immunological response. *Am. ind. Hyg. Assoc. J.,* **33**: 45-52

Lieben, J., Dattoli, J.A. & Vought, V.M. (1963) Quantitative beryllium studies in postmortem lungs. *Arch. environ. Health,* **7**:183-187

Marx, J.J. & Burrell, R. (1973) Delayed hypersensitivity to beryllium compounds. *J. Immunol.,* **11**: 590-598

McCord, C.P. (1951) Beryllium as sensitizing agent. *Ind. Med. Surg.,* **20**: 336

Niemöller, H.R. (1962) [On the beryllium skin test of Curtis and its modifications.] (in German) *Int. Arch. Gewerbepathol. Gewerbehyg.,* **19**: 27-34

Oppenheim, J.J. (1968) Relationship of in vitro lymphocyte transformation to delayed hypersensitivity in guinea pigs and man. *Fed. Proc.,* **27**: 21-28

Palazzolo, M.J. & Reeves, A.L. (1975) Hypersensitivity to beryllium in guinea pigs. *Toxicologist,* **14**: 13

Polak, L., Barnes, J.M. & Turk, J.L. (1968) Genetic control of contact sensitivity to inorganic metal compounds in guinea pigs. *Immunology,* **14**: 707-711

Policard, A. (1950) Histological studies of the effects of beryllium oxide (glucine) on animal tissues. *Br. J. ind. Med.,* **7**: 117-121

Preuss, O.P. (1975) Beryllium and its compounds. In: Zenz, C., ed., *Occupational Medicine,* 2nd ed., Chicago, Year Book Medical Publishers, pp. 619-636

Preuss, O.P., Deodhar, S.D. & Van Ordstrand, H.S. (1980) Lymphoblast transformation in beryllium workers. In: Jones Williams, W. & Davies, B.H., eds, *Sarcoidosis and Other Granulomatous Disorders,* Cardiff, Alpha Omega, pp. 711-714

Price, C.D., Pugh, A., Pioli, E. & Jones Williams, W. (1976) Beryllium macrophage migration inhibition test. *Ann. N.Y. Acad. Sci.,* **278**: 204-211

Reeves, A.L. (1976) Berylliosis as an autoimmune disorder. *Ann. clin. Lab. Sci.,* **6**: 256-262

Reeves, A.L. (1980) Delayed hypersensitivity in experimental pulmonary berylliosis. In: Jones Williams, W. & Davies, B.H., eds, *Sarcoidosis and Other Granulomatous Disorders,* Cardiff, Alpha Omega, pp. 715-721

Reeves, A.L. (1983) Immunotoxicology of beryllium. In: Gibson, G.G., Hubbard, R. & Parke, D.V., eds, *Immunotoxicology,* London, Academic Press, pp. 261-282

Reeves, A.L. & Krivanek, N.D. (1974) Influence of cutaneous hypersensitivity to beryllium on the development of experimental pulmonary berylliosis. *Trans. N.Y. Acad. Sci.,* **36**: 78-93

Reeves A.L. & Preuss, O.P. (1985) Immunotoxicity of beryllium. In: Dean, J.H., Luster, M.I., Munson A.E. & Amos, H., eds, *Immunotoxicology and Immunopharmacology,* New York, Raven Press, pp. 441-455

Reeves, A.L., Swanborg, R.H., Busby, E.K. & Krivanek, N.D. (1970) Role of immunologic reactions in pulmonary berylliosis. In: Walton, W.H., ed., *Inhaled Particles III,* Old Woking, Unwin Bros, pp. 599-608

Reeves, A.L., Krivanek, N.D., Busby, E.R. & Swanborg, R.H. (1972) Immunity to pulmonary berylliosis in guinea pigs. *Int. Arch. occup. Health*, **29**: 209-220

Robbins, J.H. (1964) Tissue culture studies of the human lymohocyte. *Science*, **146**:1648-1654

Rossman, M.D., Kern, J.A., Elias, J.A., Cullen, M.R., Epstein, P.E., Preuss, O.P., Markham, T.N. & Daniele, R.P. (1988) Proliferative response of bronchoalveolar lymphocytes to beryllium. *Ann. intern. Med.*, **108**: 687-693

Sarkar, T.K., Jones, E.R. & Lutwyche, V.U. (1971) Diagnosis of beryllium lung disease. *Br. J. Dis. Chest*, **65**:182-195

Snetton, I.B. (1955) Berylliosis: a case report. *Br. med. J.*, **1**:1448-1450

Sterner, J.H. & Eisenbud, M. (1951) Epidemiology of beryllium intoxication. *Arch. ind. Hyg.*, **4**:123-151

Van Ganse, W.F., Oleffe, J., Van Howe, W. & Groetenbriel, C. (1972) Lymphocyte transformation in chronic pulmonary berylliosis. *Lancet*, **1**: 1023

Van Ordstrand, H.H. (1959) Diagnosis of beryllium disease. *Arch. ind. Health*, **19**: 157-159

Vasilieva, E.V. (1969) [Immunological assessment of a model for experimental berylliosis.] (in Russian) *Byull. eksp. Biol. Med.*, **iii**: 74-77

Vasilieva, E.V. (1972) [Changes in the antigen composition of the lungs in experimental berylliosis]. (in Russian) *Byull. eksp. Biol. Med.*, **ii**: 76-80

Vorwald, A.J. (1966) Medical aspects of beryllium disease. In: Stokinger, H.E., ed., *Beryllium: Its Industrial Hygiene Aspects*, New York, Academic Press, pp. 167-200

Waksman, B.H. (1959) Diagnosis of beryllium disease, with special reference to the patch test. *Arch. ind. Health*, **19**: 154-156

Williams, W.R. & Jones Williams, W. (1982a) Development of beryllium lymphocyte transformation tests in chronic beryllium disease. *Int. Arch. Allergy*, **67**: 175-180

Williams, W.R. & Jones Williams, W. (1982b) Comparison of lymphocyte transformation and macrophage migration inhibition tests in the detection of beryllium hypersensitivity. *J. clin. Pathol.*, **35**: 684-687

Zschunke, E. & Folesky, H. (1969) [Experimental study on beryllium sensitization.] (in German) *Hautarzt*, **20**: 403-404

EFFECT OF ORGANOTIN COMPOUNDS ON LYMPHOID ORGANS AND LYMPHOID FUNCTIONS: AN OVERVIEW

A.H. Penninks, N.J. Snoeij[1], R.H.H. Pieters & W. Seinen

Research Institute of Toxicology (RITOX), University of Utrecht
NL-3508 TD Utrecht, The Netherlands

ABSTRACT

The structure-activity relationships of various di- and trisubstituted organotin compounds on lymphoid organs and the subsequent disturbances of immune function are presented and discussed, and the lymphocytotoxicity of di- and trisubstituted organotins *in vitro* is summarized. Special attention is paid to selective thymic effects. On the basis of the similarity in thymic effects of various di- and triorganotin compounds, a fast metabolism of trisubstituted compounds to the corresponding disubstituted homologues is proposed. The disubstituted compounds are held to be responsible for the observed thymic effects. Mechanistic studies performed in relation to the selective thymic effects are reviewed and supplemented with current ideas on cellular interactions of organotins in the thymus.

INTRODUCTION

Organotin compounds are chemicals that contain at least one bond between tin and carbon. The subgroups, which are used in a variety of technical applications (Lewis & Hedges, 1957; Ross, 1965; Luijten, 1971; Van der Kerk, 1978; Wilkinson, 1984), are referred to as di- and trisubstituted organotins, R_2SnX_2 and R_3SnX, respectively. Usually, R stands for an alkyl or aryl group and X for chloride, fluoride, oxide, hydroxide, acetate, carboxylate or thiolate. The dialkyltin compounds, and in particular di-*n*-butyltin-, di-*n*-octyltin- and, to a lesser extent, diethyltin derivatives, are used primarily as stabilizers for polyvinylchloride plastics. For polyvinylchloride plastics that come into contact with food, the US Food and Drug Administration permits the use of di-*n*-octyltin maleate, di-*n*-octyltin-*S,S'*-bis(iso-octyl-mercaptoacetate) and octyltin-*S, S'', S''*-tris(iso-octylmercaptoacetate), as well as bis(β-carbo-butoxyethyl)tin bis(iso-octylmercaptoacetate and β-carbobutoxyethyltin tris(iso-octyl-mercapto acetate).

The toxicity of organotins has been reviewed extensively by Barnes and Stoner (1959), Luijten (1971), Piver (1973), Snoeij *et al.* (1987), Nicklin and Robson (1988) and Boyer (1989) and in a report of the World Health Organization (1980). Until the first report by Seinen and Willems (1976) of the immunotoxic potential of di-*n*-octyltin dichloride, hepatotoxicity and bile-duct proliferation were the most obvious mammalian effects of dimethyl- to dihexyl-substituted compounds. Di-*n*-octyltin compounds were considered not to be toxic by the oral route (Barnes & Magos, 1968). Further studies have revealed that not only di-*n*-octyltin compounds but also other disubstituted organotins primarily affect lymphoid organs, the thymus being the most sensitive (Seinen *et al.*, 1977a; Seinen & Penninks, 1979).

The trisubstituted organotins are widely used as biocides. Tributyltin oxide (TBTO; bis(tri-*n*-butyltin)oxide or hexa-*n*-butyldistannoxane) is used for the preservation of paper and wood, for disinfection of surfaces and cooling water, and as an active ingredient in antifouling paints. Controlled-release formulations of TBTO and tri-*n*-butyltin fluoride (TBTF) have been proposed as molluscicides for the control of the snails that are

---

[1]Present address: Duphar BV, PO Box 900, NL-1380 DA Weesp, The Netherlands

Immunotoxicity of Metals and Immunotoxicology, Edited by
A. D. Dayan *et al.,* Plenum Press, New York, 1990

intermediate hosts for the trematode parasite that causes schistosomiasis in man (Cardarelli, 1976; Duncan, 1980). Triphenyltin compounds have become important agricultural fungicides due to their specific activity against two important major plant diseases, late blight on potatoes and leaf spot in sugar beets. The lower homologues within the series of trioganotin compounds, trimethyl- and triethyltin compounds, are neurotoxic. Trimethyltin compounds induce neuronal necrosis in the central nervous system, whereas triethyltin compounds induce interstitial oedema of the white matter of the brain and spinal cord without obvious neuronal damage (for references see Snoeij et al., 1987).

Despite the large amount of toxicological data, the effects of trialkyltins on the immune system have been reported only recently, although the first indications of the potential immunotoxicity of certain organotin compounds came from toxicity studies of Verschuuren et al. (1966) with triphenyltin acetate and triphenyltin hydroxide. Effects on the lymphoid tissue of TBTO were first described by Ishaaya et al. (1976); more extensive studies were reported by Vos et al. (1984a), Krajnc et al. (1984) and, for tri-n-butyltin chloride (TBTC), Seinen and Penninks (1979) and Snoeij et al. (1985, 1988a). This paper presents a survey of the immunotoxic properties of di- and triorganotin compounds, with special emphasis on dibutyl-, dioctyl- and tributyltin compounds.

GENERAL EFFECTS OF DIALKYLTIN COMPOUNDS ON LYMPHOID TISSUE

Effects of di-n-octyltin on lymphoid tissue after oral administration to rats

A selective action of dialkyltin compounds on the immune system was first described by Seinen and Willems (1976) in relation to di-n-octyltin dichloride (DOTC). A remarkable, dose-related decrease in thymic weight was observed in male and female weanling rats fed 50 or 150 ppm DOTC in the diet for six weeks. In this time-response study, thymic weights of rats given 150 ppm were already significantly lower after a four-day feeding period, and decreased progressively over 14 days to approximately 50 and 20% of the control value in the groups receiving 50 and 150 ppm, respectively. This reduction remained almost constant during the additional four-week feeding period. The reduced thymic weight was accompanied by a less pronounced, dose-related decrease in the weight of spleen and lymph nodes, without obvious effects on other organs. The number of cells in thymus and spleen was also decreased by feeding DOTC, whereas no effect was observed on cell counts in bone-marrow cells (Seinen & Willems, 1976). Histologically, lymphocyte depletion was seen in the thymus and in thymus-dependent areas of the spleen (periarteriolar lymphocyte sheaths) and lymph nodes (paracortical areas). In the thymus gland in particular, the cortical area was depleted of thymocytes, resulting in loss of corticomedullary boundaries. Since lymphocytotoxicity was observed in DOTC-treated rats at concentrations that did not induce generalized toxicity or myelotoxicity, it was concluded that DOTC exerted a selective effect on lymphocytes in the thymus and thymus-dependent areas of peripheral lymphoid organs.

Seinen et al. (1977a) subsequently showed that the diminished thymic weight induced by four-week feeding with 150 ppm DOTC was followed by a fast recovery. Within two weeks' feeding of the stock diet, thymic weights of rats previously treated with DOTC returned to control values, suggesting that DOTC has a short half-life.

This marked effect of DOTC on the thymus was confirmed by other groups in different strains of rats (Miller et al., 1982, 1984; Miller & Scott, 1985; Smialowicz et al., 1988). After feeding diets containing 75 ppm DOTC for up to 12 weeks, similar reductions in thymic weight and cellularity were observed in six- to eight-week-old PVG rats (Miller & Scott, 1985; Nicklin et al., 1985). After two weeks' exposure, overt thymic atrophy was observed, as demonstrated by a thymic weight loss of 75%. Thymic atrophy was found to be almost complete after four weeks' exposure and remained constant for the rest of the 12-week period. The thymic atrophy observed was accompanied by some loss of circulating leukocytes, due to a decreased number of lymphocytes, which was first apparent four weeks after commencement of treatment but showed little further decrease over time. After eight and 12 weeks of treatment, the number of peripheral blood lymphocytes was decreased by approximately 25% (Miller & Scott, 1985; Nicklin et al., 1985). Additional analysis of T-cell subpopulations in the circulating blood lymphocytes indicated a preferential loss of cells expressing the T helper phenotype (detected with Mab W3/25). The absolute number of

W3/25-positive lymphocytes was decreased by 30% in DOTC-fed animals after 12 weeks' feeding, whereas no difference between treated and control rats was found in cells expressing the T non-helper phenotype (detected with Mab MRC Ox8). In studies of Smialowicz et al. (1988), acute oral dosing of fully developed adult female rats (Fischer 344, 80 days of age) with DOTC at 20, 40, 60 or 80 mg/kg body weight daily by gavage in 0.5 ml of peanut oil for ten consecutive days resulted in severe thymic weight reduction at all doses. Spleen weight was reduced significantly only at the highest dose level; however, the dramatic, significant effects on body weights at doses above 20 mg/kg bw per day (almost equivalent to the amount ingested by rats on a 150-ppm DOTC diet) indicate that additional effects, like stress, cannot be excluded at higher dose levels. In an additional study with young adult (eight-week-old) male rats dosed with DOTC at 10 or 20 mg/kg bw per day three times a week for a total of ten doses, severe thymic atrophy (reduced to 50%) was observed three days after the last dose. Within four weeks, this effect had disappeared and thymic weight returned to normal. This finding is consistent with those of Seinen et al. (1977a) but not with the observations of Miller et al. (1982, 1984), who observed that return to a normal diet after feeding of diets containing 150 ppm DOTC for four weeks to young adult rats resulted in increased cellularity in the thymus but thymic weight was still significantly reduced after a four-week recovery period. Although different rat strains were used in these studies, as well as different regimes and durations of dosing, age at commencement of treatment may be the most important factor governing the absence of complete recovery in thymic weight in the studies of Miller et al. Seinen et al. (1977a) started with weanling rats, but Miller et al. used young adult rats; therefore, the recovery period in the study of Miller et al. may have coincided with physiological age-dependent thymic involution. The experiments of Smialowicz et al. (1988) may support this explanation: they also started with young adult rats, but their treatment period was shorter (ten days), and complete recovery of thymic weight occurred.

In order to study whether the developing immune system suffers greater adverse effects than the mature system, Seinen et al. (1979) exposed rats from day 2 of pregnancy to diets containing DOTC at 0, 50 or 150 ppm/kg up to six weeks after the birth of offspring, so that pups were exposed prenatally by transplacental passage and postnatally via the milk of the dams and directly via food from the moment they started to eat the DOTC-containing diet. In groups on the 150-ppm DOTC diet, growth was stunted and 80% of pups died sometime after starting to eat the diet, with no major pathology except for severe atrophy of the lymphoid organs (Seinen et al., 1979). Some animals receiving 150 ppm DOTC weighed 20 g at one month of age, whereas controls and those receiving 50 ppm DOTC weighed an average of 100 g. No mortality occurred in the group receiving 50 ppm; they had a slight weight gain and reduced lymphoid organ weight.

Prenatal (days 10-20 of gestation), pre- and postnatal (days 11-20 of gestation and days 2-11 of age) or postnatal (days 2-13 of age) administration of DOTC at 20-50 mg/kg bw per day did not affect thymic and spleen weights in offspring (Smialowicz et al., 1988); however, lymphoid organ weights and immune function were recorded in offspring aged 4-12 weeks. In view of the fast reversibility of effects on lymphoid organs, the time between the last dose and necropsy would have been long enough for a complete recovery. Since in neither the study of Seinen et al. (1979) nor that of Smialowicz et al. (1988) were lymphoid organ weights measured or pathological examination performed on the day of birth of the pups or just before they started to eat the diet, it is questionable whether DOTC was transported via the placenta or milk and whether the amount was sufficient to affect the developing lymphoid tissues (see results with di-n-dibutyltin dichloride (DBTC) below). When two-day-old pups were dosed orally with DOTC at 5 or 15 mg/kg bw thrice weekly by gavage until day 25, very severe thymic effects were observed (Seinen et al., 1979), and the number of lymphocytes that could be isolated from the thymus was diminished to 9 and 3% of that in the control animals, respectively, in a dose-related fashion. Smialowicz et al. (1988) also demonstrated that direct dosing of rat pups with DOTC at 5, 10 or 15 mg/kg bw, beginning at day 3 of age and then thrice a week up to 24 days of age, resulted in a severe reduction in thymic weight of three-week-old pups at all dose levels. A slight but significant reduction in spleen weight was observed at the highest dose level only. No difference in lymphoid organ weight was seen four weeks after the last dose, corroborating the finding that the effects of DOTC on lymphoid tissue weight are completely reversible.

Structure-activity relationships of the effects of disubstituted organotin compounds after oral administration to rats

Comparative short-term feeding studies in rats at dose levels of 50 and 150 ppm showed that DOTC and other dialkyltin compounds caused lymphoid atrophy in thymus and thymus-dependent areas of spleen and lymph nodes (Seinen et al., 1977a). The extent of dialkyltin-induced thymic atrophy, which was found to be the most sensitive parameter, is strongly related to the length of the alkyl chain and probably dependent on the water-lipid distribution of the homologues. The more water-soluble lower homologues, dimethyltin (DMTC) and diethyltin (DETC) dichlorides, induce no and slight thymic atrophy, respectively, whereas DBTC and di-n-octyltin dichloride, both almost insoluble in water, induced almost equally severe thymic atrophy. With the extremely lipophilic homologues didodecyltin and dioctadecyltin dichloride, no thymic atrophy was observed. With DBTC and DOTC, reduction in thymic weight was observed at dietary concentrations as low as 5 mg/kg feed (Seinen, 1981). A single oral administration by gastric intubation of DBTC at 5-35 mg/kg bw also reduced thymic weight in a dose-related fashion and was maximal four days after intubation (Snoeij et al., 1988a). Thymic weight reverted to normal within nine days.

The higher potency of DETC compared to DMTC in producing atrophy of the thymus was also demonstrated in five-week-old female Sprague-Dawley rats administered the compounds via the drinking-water during a treatment period of five weeks (Miller, 1978). At 62.5 ppm and 125 ppm DMTC, there was no observable effect on growth or lymphoid tissue weight; at the highest dose level (250 ppm), a significant relative reduction in thymic weight was observed, but this effect was associated with significantly lower body weight and increased adrenal weight, indicating that additional stress cannot be excluded at the highest dose level tested. In a similar study with 125 and 250 ppm DETC in the drinking-water of male and female rats, the highest dose was overtly toxic, resulting in severe growth retardation and death of all animals after approximately four weeks of exposure. At 125 ppm, growth retardation was less severe; after ten days of treatment, when body weights were not yet affected, a significant reduction in thymic weight was apparent in animals of each sex, whereas spleen weight was significantly lower only in males. In comparative studies in which DMTC, DBTC and DOTC were administered to rats by gastric intubation, the minimal effective dose that induced thymic atrophy was found to increase in the order DBTC<DOTC<DMTC (Renhof et al., 1980).

The effects of DBTC on the developing immune system were also studied by pre- and postnatal exposure of rats to 50, 150 and 450 ppm in the diet (A. Penninks & W. Seinen, unpublished results). Exposure from day 2 of pregnancy did not affect body weight gain of the mothers or the weight (day 1) or number of offspring up to levels of 150 ppm DBTC; however, 450 ppm DBTC induced overt maternal toxicity, as demonstrated by severe weight loss and the absence of any offspring. Histopathology on one-day-old pups revealed no change in the thymus or spleen, indicating that if transplacental passage of DBTC occurs it is not sufficient to affect the morphology of the developing lymphoid organs. Autopsy of young rats at weaning (four weeks) showed a selective, dose-related reduction in relative thymic weight. Although the tin content (measured by tin activation) of one-day-old fetuses and of milk isolated from the stomach of two-day-old fetuses increased with dose (A. Penninks, unpublished results), the observed effects on thymic weight at weaning may have been due to the diet.

The diester tin compounds bis(ß-carbobutoxyethyltin) dichloride (CBETC) and bis(ß-carbomethoxyethyltin) dichloride did not induce lymphoid atrophy in two-week feeding studies at levels up to 1350 ppm (Penninks & Seinen, 1982). Since CBETC showed lymphocytotoxicity comparable to that of DBTC in vitro, a rapid metabolic conversion (hydrolysis of the ester bond) in vivo is suggested to yield the water-soluble bis(ß-carboxyethyl)tin dichloride. This hypothesis is supported by the fact that this compound is not lymphocytotoxic in vivo or in vitro (Penninks & Seinen, 1982) and that the only detectable metabolite after oral or intravenous administration of CBETC was bis(ß-carboxyethyl)tin dichloride (Penninks & Seinen, 1985).

Only limited information is available on the aryl-substituted diphenyltin dichlorides. After two-week feeding of 150 ppm diphenyltin dichlorides, moderate thymic atrophy was observed, similar to that observed with a dietary concentration of 150 ppm DETC (Seinen & Penninks, 1979).

Species differences and parenteral application of dialkyltin compounds

In contrast to rats, no selective lymphoid atrophy occurred in DOTC- or DBTC-fed mice, Japanese quail or guinea-pigs. Four-week feeding of mice with diets containing DBTC at up to 150 ppm did not affect body weight or the weight of thymus, spleen or liver (Seinen et al., 1977a); however, comparable thymic effects were readily produced in rats and mice after intravenous administration of DBTC or DOTC, suggesting that interspecies differences in susceptibility after oral administration of these compounds may be due to differences in gastrointestinal absorption, distribution, metabolism or elimination. The reduction in thymic weight in mice after intravenous administration was confirmed by Hennighausen et al. (1980) with di-n-alkyltin compounds of different chain lengths (C4-C8). Hennighausen and Lange (1980) showed that the thymic weight reduced four days after a single intravenous administration of DOTC at 8 mg/kg returned to the control level within 14 days. Although Lange et al. (1980) observed a 50% reduction in thymic weight after oral application of DOTC to mice at 500 mg/kg bw, the dose would have been too high to exclude additional effects.

No selective organotin-induced lymphoid atrophy could be established in guinea-pigs, although weaning animals fed 150 ppm DOTC died within three weeks. These animals were emaciated and showed abdominal oedema and enlarged caecums filled with fluid (Seinen et al., 1977a). At 100 and 150 ppm, thymic weight was decreased after four weeks' feeding but was associated with a greatly reduced body weight and increased adrenal weights. Histologically, marked depletion of cortical thymocytes was associated with a starry sky appearance, indicating that in this instance thymic atrophy was indirectly caused by stress, probably as a result of gastrointestinal disturbances. Because of the antibacterial activity of dialkyltins (Kaars Sijpesteijn et al., 1969), in particular against gram-positive bacteria which are the predominant flora in the gastrointestinal tract of guinea-pigs, caecal fermentation was disturbed. Almost complete inhibition of free fatty acid production in the caecum was also demonstrated (H. Winkels & W. Seinen, unpublished results), and atrophy of the villi was observed in the gastrointestinal tract of these guinea-pigs.

Japanese quail appeared to be very insensitive to the toxic effects of dialkyltin compounds, since feeding of levels up to 600 ppm for four weeks neither affected the weight of the thymus and bursa of Fabricius nor induced any other sign of toxicity (Seinen et al., 1977a). In contrast, Renhof et al. (1980) reported a slight decrease in thymic weight in chickens administered DOTC by gavage for 14 days at levels of 100 and 500 mg/kg bw. This effect was apparent only when DOTC was emulsified in methylcellulose and not if administered as a solution in peanut oil.

In rats, single or repeated intravenous doses of as little as 1 mg/kg of DBTC or DOTC readily induced thymic atrophy (Seinen et al., 1977a). At doses up to 24 mg/kg bw, DMTC was not active, whereas DETC slightly depressed thymic weights at 6 and 12 mg/kg bw. Di-n-dodecyltin dichloride was inactive after repeated intravenous administration, as after oral administration. Therefore, the absence of effects on lymphoid tissues of oral doses of lower (DMTC) and higher homologues (di-n-dodecyltin dichloride) cannot be explained by differences in uptake only. Neither the estertin compound CBETC nor its proposed hydrolysis product bis(ß-carboxyethyl)tin dichloride affected thymic weight after single intravenous or intraperitoneal doses of up to 10 mg/kg bw, indicating that CBETC might be easily hydrolysed to its inactive metabolite dicarboxylic acid tin dichloride in the periphery (Penninks & Seinen, 1982).

Interference of dialkyltins with immune function

Since the thymus and thymus-dependent lymphocytes play a central role in the immune system, a decrease in cell number in thymus and thymus-dependent areas of peripheral lymphoid organs induced by organotin may result in an impairment of T cell-dependent immunity in particular, and consequently in decreased resistance to bacterial infections. Susceptibility of rats to infection with Listeria monocytogenes, a T cell-dependent phenomenon, was markedly increased by DBTC and DOTC. Within ten days after an intravenous injection with 0.5 x 10⁶ *Listeria*, four of six rats fed 150 ppm DOTC and all animals fed DBTC for four weeks from weaning age had died; all controls and animals fed 50 ppm DBTC or DOTC remained alive (Seinen, 1981).

In order to investigate various immune reactions in which T lymphocytes participate, Seinen *et al.* (1979) exposed weanling Wistar rats to DBTC or DOTC at levels of 50 and 150 mg/kg of diet. The delayed-type hypersensitivity reaction to tuberculin was decreased in a dose-related fashion in rats fed DOTC for six weeks. Allograft rejection, another cell-mediated immune response, was significantly delayed in animals receiving DBTC or DOTC at the 150-ppm level. The developing immune system of rats appeared to be particularly vulnerable, as the effect of DBTC on allograft rejection was most pronounced when exposure to DBTC started immediately after birth. Rejection times were significantly increased in animals given oral doses of DBTC at 1 or 3 mg/kg bw three times a week over nine weeks. Thymus-dependent humoral immunity was inhibited, as shown by a reduction in plaque-forming cells in the spleen and by suppressed haemagglutinin and haemolysis titres against sheep red blood cells (SRBC) in the serum of DBTC- and DOTC-exposed rats. However, the antibody response to *Escherichia coli* lipopolysacharide, a thymus-independent antigen, was unaffected. In a subsequent study, graft-*versus*-host activity was found to be significantly decreased in the spleens of rats exposed to DBTC or DOTC at 50 or 150 mg/kg diet (Seinen *et al.*, 1979). The results of Seinen *et al.* (1977b) in respect to the antibody response to SRBC following exposure to DOTC are not consistent with those of Miller and Scott (1985) or Smialowicz *et al.* (1988). The former saw no effect of DOTC on haemagglutinin titres to SRBC in rats fed 75 mg/kg diet for eight or 12 weeks, and graft-*versus*-host activity of lymph node cells was not depressed. Smialowicz *et al.* (1988) reported that acute oral dosing of adult rats with DOTC at 20, 40, 60 or 80 mg/kg per day for ten consecutive days did not affect the primary antibody response to SRBC, as measured in the IgM/plaque-forming cell assay; however, a reduction in the number of plaque-forming cells per 10⁶ spleen cells was seen with the lowest dose of DOTC, which was even more pronounced when calculated on a total spleen basis. At 40 mg/kg, the IgM/plaque-forming response was not affected; it was not determined at the two highest dose levels. These inconsistent findings may be due to differences in the conduct of the various studies, such as dose, length of exposure, rat strain and age of rats at commencement of the studies (weanling *versus* young adult).

The mitogen responsiveness of cell suspensions from lymphoid organs and blood isolated from dialkyltin-exposed rats were studied by various investigators. To assess the lymphoproliferative response of thymocytes and spleen cells, Seinen *et al.* (1979) gavaged rat pups with DOTC at 5 or 15 mg/kg from the second day after birth three times a week for four weeks. The response of lymphocytes from thymus and spleen to the T-cell mitogens phytohaemagglutinin (PHA) and concanavalin A (Con A) was severely depressed in a dose-related fashion and approached the zero level. The response of spleen cells to the B-cell mitogen lipopolysaccharide was not impaired. Smialowicz *et al.* (1988) showed that direct oral dosing of rat pups with DOTC at 5-15 mg/kg, beginning at three days of age and then three times per week up to 24 days of age for a total of ten doses resulted in severe suppression of the lymphoproliferative response of splenocytes to the T-cell mitogens PHA and Con A and also to the T- and B-cell pokeweed mitogen (PWM) and the B-cell mitogen *Salmonella typhimurium*, when measured at three weeks of age (just after the last dose). Four weeks after the last dose of DOTC, Con A and PHA stimulation in splenocytes was still significantly decreased at all dose levels. PWM and *S. typhimurium* stimulation were significantly depressed only at the highest dose levels. The mitogenic responsiveness of splenocytes to PHA was still significantly suppressed seven weeks after the last dose and returned to control levels only two weeks later. In a comparative study of young adult rats (eight weeks old) given DOTC at 10 or 20 mg/kg bw under identical conditions, suppression of the proliferative response to Con A, PHA and PWM, but not to the B-cell mitogen *S. typhimurium*, was observed three days after the last dose; however, four and eight weeks after the last dose, the lymphoproliferative response of splenocytes to these mitogens was no longer affected. These studies indicate that suppression of the lymphoproliferative response after exposure to DOTC was more persistent during development of the immune system than during adulthood. Prenatal, pre- and postnatal or postnatal oral dosing of dams with DOTC at 20-50 mg/kg did not consistently alter lymphocyte stimulation in the offspring

(Smialowicz et al., 1988), owing to the limited exposure of the offspring and the fact that lymphocyte proliferation was determined only three weeks after the last dose.

The proliferative response of peripheral blood lymphocytes to PHA was also significantly suppressed in PVG rats fed DOTC at 75 ppm for eight weeks (Miller & Scott, 1985; Nicklin et al., 1985). In the same studies, marked reduction in alloantigenic stimulation was observed, as measured by the mixed leukocyte reaction (MLR) in vitro, and was explained by a DOTC-induced decrease in the number of circulating lymphocytes of the helper/inducer type.

Natural killer (NK) cell activity of splenocytes to YAC-1 mouse lymphoma cells and W/F4 rat lymphoma cells was not affected by DOTC given by any of the dosing regimens employed by Smialowicz et al. (1988). Moreover, in the limited number of studies available, macrophages do not appear to be compromised by dialkyltin compounds, since the number of blood monocytes and phagocytizing capacity, as measured by the clearance of carbon particles, were not affected by DOTC in rats (Seinen et al., 1977b, 1979).

Probably because lymphoid atrophy does not occur in other animal species (mice, guinea-pigs and chickens) after oral administration of dialkyltins, only a few studies of immune function have been carried out in these species. In male mice fed DBTC at up to 150 ppm in the diet for four weeks, no difference in antibody response to SRBC was found (Seinen et al., 1977b), and in guinea-pigs the delayed hypersensivity reaction to tuberculin was not affected by feeding of DBTC at 50 ppm for five or seven weeks. Miller et al. (1986) intubated mice with DOTC at 0, 20, 100 or 500 mg/kg bw at weekly intervals for eight weeks. Humoral responsiveness, measured by antibody response to self erythrocytes and rat erythrocytes, was affected only at the highest dose level. Since thymic atrophy was also seen at this dose, although it had not previously been observed in mice treated orally, stress cannot be excluded as a cause. The delayed-type hypersensitivity reaction to oxazolone, a measure of cell-mediated immunity, was not affected.

Studies of effects on immune function have not been reported for other dialkyl-substituted organotins, nor for diaryl-substituted diphenyltin compounds.

GENERAL EFFECTS OF TRIALKYLTIN COMPOUNDS ON LYMPHOID TISSUE

Effects of tri-n-butyltin on lymphoid tissue after oral administration to rats

Explorative studies by Seinen and Penninks (1979) showed that TBTC, like some dialkyltins, induced thymic atrophy in weanling rats after two weeks feeding of 50 or 150 ppm. Funahashi et al. (1980) reported that TBTO given by gavage in olive oil at levels of 6 or 12 mg/kg bw per day on five days a week for 13 or 26 weeks resulted in a marked, significant, dose-related reduction in absolute and relative thymic weight; the effect was not seen with 3 mg/kg bw per day for 13 weeks. Spleen weight was also diminished at 6 and 12 mg/kg bw per day for 13 or 26 weeks, although only significantly so at 6 mg/kg for 13 weeks and at 12 mg/kg for 26 weeks. However, at doses of 6 mg/kg bw per day (26 weeks only) and higher, growth of rats was markedly inhibited, whereas relative adrenal weights were significantly increased. The additional hypertrophy and hyperactivity of the adrenal cortex, together with an increased serum cortisol level at the higher doses, indicate that at these doses the effects on lymphoid organs are exerted not only directly but also indirectly. After a single oral dose of TBTO at 100 mg/kg bw to five-week-old male Sprague-Dawley rats, Funahashi et al. (1980) observed a reduction in relative thymic weight after three days; the effect was most pronounced at day 6. A slow recovery became apparent on day 8, but which was incomplete by day 21. At this dose level, rats lost weight and showed an increase in relative adrenal weight. These effects, together with the histological observations of pyknosis, karyorrhexis and increased macrophage activity in the thymic cortex are more consistent with an additional indirect stress effect that with a direct effect of TBTO on the thymus only.

In a recent study by Snoeij et al. (1988a), the effects of a single oral dose of TBTC on thymus were studied in more detail in weaned rats over a dose range of 5-60 mg/kg bw. At doses of 10 mg/kg bw and above, a statistically significant reduction in thymic weight was seen, which was maximal four days after intubation. A single dose of 29 mg/kg bw was calculated to cause an approximately 50% reduction in relative thymic weight; recovery from the thymic involution occurred with seven days. Krajnc *et al.* (1984) reported the effects of feeding diets containing TBTO at 0, 5, 20, 80 or 320 mg/kg diet to young SPF-Wistar rats for four weeks: absolute and relative thymic weights were significantly reduced in both male and female rats at 80 and 320 mg/kg diet and in females at 20 mg/kg diet; absolute spleen weight was reduced at the two higher dose levels in males and at the highest level in females. Probably because of decreased body weight, the relative spleen weight was significantly increased in males receiving 320 mg/kg diet. At 80 and 320 mg/kg diet, absolute mesenteric lymph node weights were also reduced.

In a subsequent study, Vos *et al.* (1984a) showed that the reduced lymphoid organ weight seen after feeding TBTO at 80 and 320 mg/kg diet was associated with a time-dependent (three, eight and 20 days' exposure) reduction in cell count and cell viability in thymus and spleen and in cell count in bone marrow, particularly after prolonged exposure (20 days) to 320 ppm. After nine weeks' exposure to TBTO at 20 or 80 mg/kg diet, lymphocyte subpopulations were analysed in spleen by immunostaining; the diminished number of spleen lymphocytes was seen to result from a reduction in the number of T lymphocytes (Vos *et al.*, 1984a). No effect was observed on the ratio between T helper and T non-helper subsets. Microscopically, lymphocyte depletion of the thymic cortex was noted with TBTC at 80 and 320 mg/kg diet, resulting in indistinct corticomedullary junctions. In addition, an increased density of ceroid/lipofuscin-loaded macrophages was found. In spleen, a diffuse atrophy of the white pulp, in particular in the T cell-dependent perarteriolar lymphocyte sheets, was noted in the highest dose group. As determined by pan T immunostaining, predominantly T lymphocytes were depleted. Atrophy of the mesenteric lymph nodes increased with dose and was evident in all animals treated with TBTO at 320 mg/kg diet. Both the size and cellularity of the paracortex and medulla of lymph nodes were reduced as well as the size and number of follicles. B Lymphocyte areas also showed low-level activity, as indicated by the presence of fewer follicles and inconspicuous germinal centres. A remarkable finding in the mesenteric lymph nodes was that the sinusoidal content of erythrocytes increased with dose, and red blood cells were frequently associated with mononuclear cells, forming rosettes. The total number of blood leukocytes was decreased in rats fed TBTO at 80 mg/kg (males) or 320 mg/kg (males and females), due to a marked decrease in the number of lymphocytes.

In a two-week feeding study in rats with TBTC at 0, 15, 50, 100 and 150 ppm/kg (Snoeij *et al.*, 1985), a severe, dose-related reduction in thymic and spleen weights was also observed from 50 mg/kg diet. Erythrocyte rosettes were found in the sinuses of some mesenteric lymph nodes, evident macroscopically by reddening of some nodes in each dosage group. After a single oral dose of TBTC at 10 mg/kg or more, erythrocyte rosettes were frequently observed around mononuclear cells in the sinuses of mesenteric lymph nodes. The severe thymic atrophy induced by TBTC was shown to be completely reversible, like that observed with DOTC. When diets were changed to normal after four weeks of treatment with TBTC at 100 mg/kg, thymic weights returned to the control level within one week. The early effects on spleen weight, observed at 50 mg/kg in the two-week study, were considered to be transient since spleen weight was not affected after feeding 100 mg/kg for four weeks (Snoeij *et al.*, 1985). This result is consistent with the observations of Krajnc *et al.* (1984), who found no effect on spleen weight after a four-week feeding period with TBTO at 80 mg/kg diet. In long-term studies with weaned male rats exposed to diets containing TBTO at 0, 0.5, 5 or 50 mg/kg for up to two years (Krajnc *et al.*, 1987; Wester *et al.*, 1987; Vos *et al.*, 1990; Wester *et al.*, 1990), a slight but significant reduction in thymic weight was observed at the highest dose level after 4.5 months' exposure. Body and spleen weights were not significantly depressed. After one year of exposure, thymic atrophy was no longer observed; this effect was suggested to be due to a masking of physiological thymic involution at older ages (Wester *et al.*, 1987, 1990). Erythrocyte rosettes occurred in the sinuses of mesenteric lymph nodes (which were a sensitive parameter in the short-term studies) only incidentally in the long-term study and were considered a transient effect. Exposure to TBTO at 5 or 50 mg/kg diet for six or 18 months reduced the relative count of T lymphocytes and consequently increased the percentage of B lymphocytes in mesenteric lymph nodes, as quantified by flow cytometric analysis. When calculated per whole node, the numbers of T cells were diminished by approximately 50%, whereas the total number of B lymphocytes appeared to be unaltered (Vos *et al.*, 1990). The number of blood leucokytes tended to decrease in animals of each sex at the dietary level of 50 mg/kg. Differential counts showed that this effect was due to a decrease in the number of lymphocytes, which was significant in females after 12 (5 and 50 mg/kg) and 24 months (50 mg/kg) and in males after 24 months (50 mg/kg) (Wester *et al.*, 1990). General effects on lymphoid tissues were not seen later during the two-year study, although several specific tests of immune function were performed.

In order to study the effects of TBTO on aged rats, one-year-old males were fed TBTO for five months at levels of 0, 0.5 and 5 and 50 mg/kg. As in young animals, a reduction in thymic weight was observed at the highest dose after five months' exposure, whereas body and spleen weights were not affected (Vos *et al.*, 1990). Data on administration of TBTO during early postnatal life are lacking. Some information on its toxicity in rats exposed pre- and postnatally was described recently by Crofton *et al.* (1989), although their study was not designed to investigate immunotoxic effects.

Structure-activity relationships of trisubstituted organotin compounds after oral administration to rats

Comparative two-week feeding studies with 0, 15, 50 or 150 mg/kg diet of a series of trialkyltin compounds and triphenyltin chloride (TPhTC) on the lymphoid organs of weaned male rats were reported by Snoeij *et al.* (1985). As for dialkyltin compounds, the extent of the effects of trialkyltins on lymphoid organs was strongly related to the length of the alkyl chain. The lower homologues trimethyltin chloride and triethyltin chloride were extremely neurotoxic and were therefore not considered. Although atrophy of the thymus and spleen was observed in rats dosed with either compound at 15 mg/kg diet, the effect was suggested to be caused by stress and emaciation; the increase in adrenal weight supported this assumption. The most striking effects on the lymphoid system were observed with tripropyltin chloride (TPTC) and TBTC. Feeding of these compounds for two weeks resulted in a dose-related reduction in thymic weight from 15 mg/kg diet for TPTC and 50 mg/kg diet for TBTC, whereas spleen weights were significantly diminished with both compounds from 15 mg/kg diet. The higher trialkyltin homologues tri-*n*-hexyltin and tri-*n*-octyltin chloride had no or a slight effect on the weight of the thymus at 150 mg/kg diet, respectively (Snoeij *et al.*, 1985). As with TBTC, the early effects of TPTC on spleen weight after two weeks' feeding was transient, since after four weeks' feeding of TPTC at 100 mg/kg diet, the relative spleen weight was not affected. Also, after four weeks' feeding of tri-*n*-octyltin chloride at 100 mg/kg diet, lymphoid organ weights were not affected. As with TBTC, the severe reduction in thymic weight induced by TPTC at 100 mg/kg diet was followed by recovery within one week of feeding stock diet.

The effects of aromatic TPhT compounds on the immune system were first described by Verschuuren *et al.* (1966). In short-term toxicity studies in rats fed diets containing triphenyltin acetate (TPhTA) or triphenyltin hydroxide (TPhTH) at levels ranging from 0- 50 mg/kg diet for 90 days, they found a dose-related decrease in the number of peripheral blood lymphocytes at the end of week 12. Some animals were reported to show atrophy of the splenic white pulp. In the comparative two-week feeding studies of Snoeij *et al.* (1985), the effects of TPhTC resembled those of TPTC and TBTC but were less severe. Reductions in thymic and spleen weight were noted with doses from 15 and 50 mg/kg diet, respectively. Erythrocyte rosettes were not observed with TPhTC in these studies. The findings on lymphoid organ weights confirm the observations of Seinen and Penninks (1979) with TPhTC and of Vos *et al.* (1983, 1984b) with TPhTH. Gaines and Kimbrough (1968) also reported reduced spleen weights in rats after oral exposure to TPhTH.

Species differences and parenteral application of trisubstituted organotin compounds

Only limited information is available in the open literature concerning the effects of trisubstituted organotin compounds on lymphoid tissue in different animal species. In contrast to rats, thymic and spleen weights of mice were decreased only at a relatively high dietary level of TBTC (150 mg/kg diet), which was associated with a significantly decreased body weight (Snoeij, 1987). Ishaaya *et al.* (1976) described a decrease in spleen weights of mice fed TBTO at approximately 150 mg/kg diet for seven days, but they did not determine thymic weights. Whether this reduction in spleen weight is transient, as was found for rats, is not known, although the histology of the affected spleens was similar in the two animal species. TPhTA was also active on the lymphoid system of mice, as demonstrated by the induction of lymphopenia and reduced spleen weight after administration of dietary levels of approximately 30, 100 and 300 mg/kg (Ishaaya et al., 1976).

Japanese quail appeared to be very resistant to TBTC (Snoeij, 1987). Feeding of this compound at concentrations up to 450 mg/kg diet for two weeks did not affect growth, feed consumption, organ weights, blood cell count or haemoglobin concentration. Hens also tolerated oral administration of the homologues tri-n-ethyltin hydroxide (Barnes & Stoner, 1958) and TPhTA (Stoner, 1966) but were killed by relatively low parenteral dosages. The resistance of fowl to oral administration of triorganotin compounds was suggested to result from limited intestinal absorption or from detoxification in the intestinal tract.

In short-term studies with guinea-pigs fed diets containing TPhT compounds, Verschuuren et al. (1966) observed a significant lymphopenia in males and females fed TPhTH at levels of 10 and 2.5 mg/kg diet, respectively. In guinea-pigs fed TPhTA, decreased numbers of peripheral blood lymphocytes were observed from a level of 10 ppm in males and 5 ppm in females.

In contrast to oral exposure, intravenous administration of TBTC did not reduce thymic weight in rats (Snoeij, 1987). When given via this route, TBTC was rapidly lethal at a dose of 6 mg/kg bw; even at a dose of 4 mg/kg bw, three out of five rats rapidly died, but they tolerated intravenous doses of 2.5, 1 or 0.5 mg/kg bw. They grew normally, and four days after injection all organ weights, including that of the thymus, were at the control level. This observation is at variance with the results for DBTC. Although after oral administration both DBTC and TBTC induce thymic atrophy, intravenous injection caused thymic atrophy only in the case of DBTC. Intravenous administration of tri-n-octyltin chloride at doses up to 10 mg/kg did not affect lymphoid organ weight nor any of the other parameters studied (Snoeij, 1987).

Interference of triorganotins with immune function

Assessment of immune function in trialkyltin-exposed animals has been limited to TBTO. Vos et al. (1984a) investigated the functional aspects of the effects of TBTO on lymphoid tissues in weaned rats both in vivo and ex vivo after at least six weeks' feeding with 20 or 80 mg/kg diet. In peripheral blood, a dose-related (80 and 320 mg/kg diet) increase in serum IgM and a decreased IgG level were observed from day 14 onwards, which became more pronounced after longer exposure. This finding was interpreted to indicate that TBTO alters the humoral responses of rats to natural stimulation as a result of suppressed T helper cell function. As demonstrated in various functional studies, thymus-dependent immunity was markedly suppressed. At both 20 and 80 mg/kg diet, TBTO induced significant suppression of delayed-type hypersensitivity reactions to ovalbumin and tuberculin. The thymus-dependent antibody response of rats exposed to TBTO at 20 or 80 mg/kg diet for at least six weeks was assessed in relation to SRBC, tetanus toxoid, ovalbumin and Trichinella spiralis. Exposure to 80 mg/kg had a strong effect on the secondary mercaptoethanol-resistant (presumably IgG) haemagglutination titre to SRBC, whereas the primary response was unaffected. The mean IgM and IgG titres to ovalbumin were the same in treated and control animals. A marginal but statistically nonsignificant effect was seen in response to tetanus toxoid. Although the IgM and IgG antibody titres to T. spiralis were not affected, a significant, dose-related reduction in the IgE response was measured. Resistance to infection by T. spiralis was diminished at both doses of TBTO, and the numbers of worm larvae in muscle and of adult worms in the small intestine were significantly increased in a dose-dependent manner. Histologically, the inflammatory reaction around larvae-containing muscle cells in sections of the tongue was reduced after TBTO treatment.

The nonspecific resistance of rats exposed to TBTO was studied in vivo and in vitro. In vivo, host resistance was monitored in rats fed TBTO at 20 or 80 mg/kg diet by clearance of Listeria monocytogenes from the spleen at days 1 and 2 after intravenous infection. On the second day after infection, statistically significant increases in the number of viable bacteria were noted in rats treated at 80 mg/kg diet for six or seven weeks. *In vitro*, the phagocytosis and killing of *L. monocytogenes* by spleen (after six weeks' exposure) from male rats was reduced after exposure to 20 and 80 mg/kg diet; the effect was not seen in peritoneal cells after ten weeks' exposure. The total number of adherent peritoneal and spleen cells was found to decrease, in particular at the higher dose level, indicating that the impaired splenic bacterial clearance seen *in vivo* might be due to a reduction in the number of adherent spleen cells and of bacterial digestion on a cell-for-cell basis (Vos *et al.*, 1984a). Extracellular killing of macrophages and NK cells was studied by determining the capacity to kill YAC-lymphoma cells *in vitro*. The spontaneous killing activity of spleen cells was reduced in animals fed 80 mg/kg and was significantly depressed when calculated for the whole spleen. The cytotoxic activity of the total population of peritoneal cells and of the nonadherent fraction (NK cells) was not affected, whereas the activity of adherent cells was significantly suppressed in treated animals. In a subsequent study (Van Loveren *et al.*, 1990) of rats at dietary levels of 20 and 80 mg/kg for six weeks, suppressed NK activity was observed in the lung. The susceptibility of rats to endotoxin was not affected, as mortality from endotoxic shock occurred with the same concentrations of lipopolysaccharide in the control and treated groups (Vos *et al.*, 1984a).

Mitogenic stimulation of thymocytes and splenocytes was also affected by dietary exposure of rats to TBTO at 80 mg/kg for six weeks. Incorporation of ^{3}H-thymidine into DNA of thymus cells was strongly suppressed after stimulation with the T-cell mitogens PHA and ConA and the T- and B-cell mitogen PWM. The response of spleen cells to T-cell mitogens was also reduced on a cell-for-cell basis, while the responses to PWM and the B-cell mitogen lipopolysaccharide were increased; when calculated on the basis of the whole spleen, the responses to PHA and ConA were suppressed and those to PWM and lipopolysaccharide unaltered. These results are in line with the observed relative increase in B cells as a result of a reduction in the number of T cells.

The effect of TBTO on specific and nonspecific immunity was also determined in a long-term study (Krajnc *et al.*, 1987; Vos *et al.*, 1990). Weaned male rats were fed diets containing TBTO at 0, 0.5, 5 or 50 mg/kg for two years, and immune function studies were performed after four to six and 15-17 months of exposure. As assessed by resistance to *T. spiralis* infection, a dose-related suppression of thymus-dependent immunity occurred. At five and 16 months, the yield of muscle larvae was increased and specific IgE responses were significantly reduced at 5 and 50 mg/kg diet. As seen in the short-term study, there was no consistent effect on specific IgM and IgG responses to *T. spiralis* and ovalbumin. Total circulating IgM and IgG concentrations were altered in the same way as in the short-term study: increased IgM and decreased IgG, particularly at the 50 mg/kg diet level in females. The IgG response to SRBC, tested after 16 months' exposure, was not affected, whereas in the short-term studies it was decreased at 80 mg/kg diet. The T-cell mitogen response of thymocytes (measured after four to six months' exposure) and of splenocytes (measured after four to six and 15-17 months) was no longer affected. In contrast to the results of the short-term study, delayed-type hypersensitivity reactions to tuberculin and ovalbumin were unaltered.

Nonspecific resistance, measured by splenic clearance of *L. monocytogenes*, was reduced at five and 17 months only with the highest dose. The natural cell-mediated cytotoxicity of adherent peritoneal cells was not affected after four to six months, whereas splenic NK cell activity was reduced after 16 months at all dose levels tested.

In the same study, TBTO-containing diets were fed to aged (one-year-old) rats for five months at the same dose levels. Only limited immune function tests were performed at the end of the treatment period. Reductions in host resistance to *T. spiralis* (decreased expulsion of adult worms, increased yield of muscle larvae and decreased inflammatory reaction around muscle larvae) and to *L. monocytogenes* (reduced splenic clearance) were seen in the group fed 50 mg/kg diet. Splenic NK cell activity was not affected. Although the difference in dose per body weight should be considered (young rats ingest twice the dose of adult rats), it was concluded that the immune system of rats becomes less sensitive to immunotoxic insult by TBTO with age, so that starting exposure at an advanced age results in less pronounced effects.

The effects of TPhT compounds on immune function were evaluated in studies by Verschuuren *et al.* (1970) in guinea-pigs and Vos *et al.* (1983, 1984b). After 49, 77 or 104 days of exposure of three-week-old guinea-pigs to TPhTA at 15 mg/kg diet, serum Ig levels to tetanus toxoid and the number of Ig-producing plasma cells in the popliteal lymph node were reduced (Verschuuren *et al.*, 1970). In weanling rats fed TPhTH at dietary levels of 0 or 25 ppm for three or four weeks, and in rats exposed pre- and postnatally up to the age of five weeks (Vos *et al.*, 1983, 1984b), no distinct immunosuppressive activity was seen. Delayed-type hypersensitivity reactions to ovalbumin and tuberculin were significantly depressed in rats fed 25 ppm TPhTH, but other cell-mediated immune reactions, such as allograft rejection, resistance to *L. monocytogenes* infection and splenic clearance of *L. monocytogenes*, were not affected. Lymphocyte transformation tests carried out on spleen and thymus cells showed that the capacity of these cells to respond to various T- and B-cell mitogens was not affected by TPhTH treatment; only the PHA response of spleen cells was slightly depressed. The humoral immune response was not affected, and IgM and IgG levels were the same in treated and control groups; after immunization with tetanus toxoid or *E. coli* lipopolysaccharide, the IgM and IgG antibody titres were the same in treated groups and controls.

MECHANISM OF ORGANOTIN-INDUCED THYMIC ATROPHY

Of the organotin compounds, DBTC, DOTC and TBTC have been studied most extensively to elucidate the mechanism of their thymolytic activity. In general, it is agreed that the anion(s) attached to the Sn are of less relevance to the cellular interactions, because, when absorbed, the organotins will be present as cations (DBT[++], TBT[+]), a salt (chloride or carbonate) or attached to proteins. The ultimate reactive organotin species is probably the cation. Therefore, mechanistic studies with, e.g., TBTC are considered to be of relevance for TBTO. A striking resemblance is evident in the effects of various dialkyltins and trialkyltins on the thymus. The histology of the involuted thymus, studied under the light (Seinen & Willems, 1976; Snoeij *et al.*, 1985) and electron microscope (Penninks *et al.*, 1985; N.J. Snoeij, unpublished observations), showed indistinct corticomedullary junctions due to loss of cortical thymocytes, with no overt sign of cellular destruction, after exposure to dialkyl- (DBTC, DOTC) and trialkyl- (TBTC, TBTO) tin compounds. Various indirect mechanisms could explain organotin-induced thymic atrophy. Serum corticosteroid levels have not been measured in rats exposed to dialkyltin, but they were not elevated in TBTO-treated rats. There are other indications that stress is not involved: (1) Neither adrenal weight nor the histology of the adrenal cortex was affected after exposure to DBTC (Seinen & Willems, 1976), TBTC (Snoeij *et al.*, 1985) or TBTO (Krajnc *et al.*, 1984). (2) Thymic weight was reduced equally in adrenalectomized and sham-operated rats fed DBTC (Seinen & Willems, 1976), DOTC (Miller *et al.*, 1984) or TBTC (Snoeij *et al.*, 1985). Diminished growth hormone production is also not likely to be involved. Treatment of rats with growth hormone in amounts that reversed hypophysectomy-induced thymic atrophy did not restore the DOTC-induced involution of the thymus (Penninks *et al.*, 1985). Furthermore thymic atrophy in dialkyltin-treated rats was much more pronounced than that observed in hypophysectomized rats and was not associated with severe growth retardation.

Whether a disturbance of the humoral function of the thymus is involved is still doubtful. On the basis of morphological criteria, conflicting conclusions have been drawn with regard to interference with the production and/or secretion of thymic hormones. In thymus glands from DOTC-fed rats, Miller *et al.* (1984) observed vacuolization of reticular epithelial cells, together with normal epithelial cells containing an increased amount of secretory droplets. Vacuolization of epithelial cells was also observed by Penninks *et al.* (1985), but only when the thymus was already involuted; after repopulation of the thymic cortex, the vacuolization rapidly disappeared. The increased amount of secretory granules noted by Miller *et al.* (1984) was not observed. Since the latter studies were performed on rats fed DOTC for at least two weeks, the observed vacuolization may be a consequence, rather than a cause, of thymocyte depletion. This conclusion is supported by the fact that extensive vacuolization of reticular epithelial cells is a common finding in the acutely involuted thymus when the reticular network is collapsed by depletion of cortical thymocytes (Van Haelst, 1967). Evans *et al.* (1986) discredited the hypothesis of dysfunction of the thymic epithelial cells as a primary event in DOTC-induced thymic injury.

Studies of the distribution of alkyltin compounds, either by measuring tissue tin content (Hennighausen *et al.*, 1981) or by using radiolabelled compounds (Penninks & Seinen, 1983a; Nicklin *et al.*, 1985; Penninks *et al.*, 1987; Snoeij, 1987), revealed that the selectivity is not due simply to an accumulation of these compounds in the thymus.

Interference of dialkyltins with bone-marrow stem cells was also considered; however, neither the number and viability nor the mitotic activity of bone-marrow cells was affected after exposure to dialkyltin compounds *in vivo* (Penninks & Seinen, 1983a; Penninks *et al.*, 1985). Furthermore, colony formation was similar in DBTC-treated and control bone-marrow cells (Seinen & Penninks, 1979; Penninks *et al.*, 1985). The current theory that prothymocytes mature within the thymus for approximately 12 days before starting to proliferate and the fact that thymic atrophy occurs more rapidly (maximal within three to four days) may definitely exclude any interference with the influx of prothymocytes, either by affecting their production in bone marrow or their traffic and influx into the thymus (Scollay & Shortman, 1983).

In a recent study (Snoeij *et al.*, 1988a), the striking resemblance of various aspects of the effects of DBTC and TBTC on the thymus was studied in more detail. When DBTC and TBTC were given at 5-60 mg/kg bw as a single oral dose to rats, the log dose-effect relationships were found to be linear and parallel. Although TBTC appeared to be approximately 40% less effective than DBTC in reducing thymic weights, these observations suggest a similar mode of action. The two compounds induce the same histological appearance of the involuted thymus, the same species dependence, the same absence of stress involvement, and the same kinetics in effects on thymocyte subsets and thymocyte proliferation after exposure *in vivo*. Snoeij *et al.* (1988a) suggested that these observations indicate that TBTC-induced thymic atrophy in the rat is caused by its metabolite DBTC. In the few studies on the metabolism of tributyltin compounds (Kimmel *et al.*, 1977; Iwai *et al.*, 1981), it is clear that tributyltin is dealkylated to dibutyltin and monobutyltin in rodents; however, the amount of dialkylation and the site of conversion are not unequivocally established. In a preliminary study (Snoeij, 1987), tributyltin, dibutyltin and monobutyltin were detected in the blood of rats 3 h after a single oral dose of ^{14}C-TBTC. In addition, monobutyltin trichloride (Snoeij *et al.*, 1988a) and monooctyltin trichloride (Seinen *et al.*, 1977a) had no effect on the thymus.

On the basis of these studies, an indirect effect of organotin compounds cannot be ruled out; however, a direct interaction with thymocytes is more likely. Both dialkyltin and trialkyltin compounds exert cytotoxic and cytostatic effects on several cell types, including thymocytes (Penninks & Seinen, 1980, 1983a,b; Penninks *et al.*, 1986; Snoeij *et al.*, 1986a,b,c; Penninks & Seinen, 1987). *In vitro*, TBTC was more cytotoxic than DBTC, probably because of different intrinsic properties, as evidenced by their dissimilar effects on energy metabolism. At lower doses, both DBTC and TBTC exerted antiproliferative effects. With DBTC, this effect is assumed to result from an interference with protein synthesis, which was found to be most sensitive, whereas in the case of TBTC the effect was suggested to result from interference with energy production (Snoeij *et al.*, 1986b).

Exposure of rats *in vivo* to DBTC (Penninks & Seinen, 1987; Vos & Penninks, 1987), DOTC (Volsen *et al.*, 1989) or TBTC (Snoeij *et al.*, 1988a) also resulted in early, rapid reduction of the proliferative activity of thymocytes. A single oral dose of DBTC or TBTC (Snoeij *et al.*, 1988a) or a single intravenous dose of DBTC (Vos & Penninks, 1987) induced a marked reduction in the proliferating activity of thymocytes and in the number of large proliferating thymoblasts within 24 h, well before thymic atrophy was evident. From day 2 on, the large population of small, non-dividing cells that populate the thymic cortex gradually decreased and was maximally affected at day 4, when the number of thymoblasts had returned almost to normal. Within seven to nine days, thymic weight and thymocyte cell counts were also back to the control level. It was concluded that thymic atrophy caused by DBTC or TBTC is due to a selective effect on the population of large, rapidly proliferating cells. This selective effect on thymoblasts would generate fewer small cortical thymocytes and, together with the continual physiological dying off of most of these cells, would result in a marked depletion of cortical thymocytes and, consequently, in a reduction in thymic weight (Penninks *et al.*, 1985; Vos & Penninks, 1987; Snoeij *et al.*, 1988a). In subsequent immunohistochemical studies, this hypothesis was supported by an observed increase from day 2-5 of immature cortical thymocytes, phenotypically characterized as CD4- and CD8-negative Ox44+ cells (Pieters et al., 1989 a,b). A disturbance during differentiation of this early thymocyte subpopulation might result in a decreased number of proliferating thymocytes, which probably originate from this double-negative Ox44+ subpopulation (Kampinga & Aspinall, 1989).

At the cellular level, it is doubtful whether the antiproliferative effects of di- and tributyltins observed in vitro (see above) would account for this selective interaction in vivo. Firstly, the mechanisms by which DBTC and TBTC affect proliferative activity in vitro cannot explain the selectivity for thymocytes. Secondly, observed differential effects of DBTC (A. Penninks and others, unpublished results) and TBTC (Snoeij et al., 1988b) on the proliferation of various subpopulations of thymocytes in vitro are not compatible with the effects observed in vivo. Therefore, more subtle interactions probably underlie the selective action of dialkyltins on thymic lymphoblasts in vivo. A possible explanation for the anti-differentiating effect of DBTC on thymocytes at an early stage of the maturation process could be a disturbance of the interaction between thymocytes and thymic epithelial cells. It has been suggested that the SRBC-receptor or CD2 antigen, present on thymocytes, and its ligand, the lymphocyte function-associated antigen-3, present on thymic epithelial cells, may be an activating signal in this maturation process in the human thymus (Meuer et al., 1984; Reinherz, 1985). Monoclonal antibodies directed against CD2 and the lymphocyte function-associated antigen were shown to inhibit thymocyte binding to human thymic epithelial cells (Vollger et al., 1987) and human thymic epithelium-dependent thymocyte activation (Denning et al., 1987, 1988). Since Seinen et al. (1979) observed that DBTC inhibits SRBC-rosette formation in human thymocytes, DBTC might disturb the interaction of early thymocytes and thymic epithelial cells by interfering with CD2, resulting in disturbed maturation and proliferation. In a recent study, Volsen et al. (1989) suggested that the reduction in the proliferative signal might be a rapid down-regulation of intrathymic interleukin-2, either by a general reduction in the level of interleukin-2 gene expression on medullary thymocytes or a specific depletion of high interleukin-2 producing cells. Further research will be necessary to study the various hypotheses in relation to inhibition of early thymocyte proliferation by dialkyltins. Ultimately, this may result in finding the cellular and molecular target of dialkyltins in the thymus.

REFERENCES

Barnes, J.M. & Magos, L. (1968) The toxicology of organometallic compounds. *Organometal. chem. Rev.*, **3**: 137-150

Barnes, J.M. & Stoner, H.B. (1958) Toxic properties of some dialkyl and trialkyltins salts. *Br. J. ind. Med.*, **15**: 267-279

Barnes, J.M. & Stoner, H.B. (1959) The toxicology of tin compounds. *Pharmacol. Rev.*, **11**: 211-232

Boyer, I.J. (1989) Toxicity of dibutyltin, tributyltin and other organotin compounds to humans and to experimental animals. *Toxicology*, **55**: 253-298

Cardarelli, N.F. (1976) *Controlled-release Pesticide Formulations*, Cleveland, OH, CRC Press

Crofton, K.M., Dean, K.F., Boncek, V.M., Rosen, M.B., Sheets, L.P., Chernoff, N. & Reiter, L.W. (1989) Prenatal or postnatal exposure to bis(tri-n-butyltin)oxide in the rat: postnatal evaluation of teratology and behavior. *Toxicol. appl. Pharmacol.*, **97**: 113-123

Denning, S.M., Tuck, D.T., Vollger, L.W., Springer, T.A., Singer, K.H. & Haynes, B.F. (1987) Monoclonal antibodies to CD2 and lymphocyte function-associated antigen 3 inhibit human thymic epithelial cell-dependent mature thymocyte activation. *J. Immunol.*, **139**: 2573-2578

Denning, S.M., Dustin, M.L., Springer, T.A., Singer, K.H. & Haynes, B.F. (1988) Purified lymphocyte function-associated antigen-3 (LFA-3) activates human thymocytes via CD2 pathway. *J. Immunol.*, **144**: 2980-2985

Duncan, J. (1980) The toxicology of molluscicides. The organotins. *Pharmacol. Ther.*, **10**: 407-429

Evans, J.G., Scott, M.P. & Miller, K. (1986) The effect of pregnancy on dioctyltin dichloride-induced thymic. *Thymus*, **8**: 319-320

Funahashi, N., Iwasaki, I. & Ide, G. (1980) Effects of bis(tri-n-butyltin)oxide on endocrine and lymphoid tissues of male rats. *Acta pathol. jpn.*, **30**: 955-966

Gaines, T.B. & Kimbrough, R.D. (1968) Toxicity of fentin hydroxide to rats. *Toxicol. appl. Pharmacol.*, **12**: 397-403

Henninghausen, G. & Lange, P. (1980) Immunotoxic effects of dialkyltins used for stabilization of plastics. *Pol. J. Pharmacol. Pharm.*, **32**: 119-124

Henninghausen, G., Lange, P. & Merkord, J. (1980) The relationship between the length of the alkyl chain of dialkyltin compounds and their effects on thymus and bile ducts in mice. *Arch. Toxicol.*, **Suppl. 4**: 175-178

Henninghausen, G., Karnstedt, U. & Lange, P. (1981) Organotin concentrations in liver, spleen and thymus of rats after a single administration of di-n-octyltin dichloride. *Pharmazie*, **36**: 710-711

Ishaaya, I., Engel, J.L. & Casida, J.E. (1976) Dietary triorganotins affect lymphatic tissues and blood composition of mice. *Pestic. Biochem. Physiol.*, **6**: 270-279

Iwai, H., Wada, O. & Arakawa, Y. (1981) Determination of tri-, di- and monobutyltin and inorganic tin in biological materials and some aspects of their metabolism in rats. *J. anal. Toxicol.*, **5**: 300-306

Kaars Sijpesteijn, A., Luijten, J.G.A. & Van der Kerk, G.J.M. (1969) Organometallic fungicides. In: Torgeson, D.C., ed., *Fungicides*, New York, Academic Press, pp. 331-366

Kampinga, J. & Aspinall, R. (1989) A concept of T cell differentiation. *Thymus Update*, **2**: 2

Kimmel, E.C., Fish, R.H. & Casida, J.E. (1977) Bioorganotin chemistry. Metabolism of organotin compounds in microsomal monooxygenase systems and in mammals. *J. Agric. Food Chem.*, **25**: 1-9

Krajnc, E.I., Wester, P.W., Loeber, J.G., Van Leeuwen, F.X.R., Vos, J.G., Vaessen, H.A.M.G. & Van der Heijden, C.A. (1984) Toxicity of bis(tri-n-butyltin)oxide in the rat. I. Short-term effects on general parameters and on the endocrine and lymphoid systems. *Toxicol. appl. Pharmacol.*, **75**: 363-386

Krajnc, E.I., Vos, J.G., Wester, P.W., Loeber, J.F. & Van der Heijden, C.A. (1987) Toxicity of bis(tri-n-butyltin)oxide (TBTO) in rats. In: *Toxicology and Analytics of the Tributyltins - The Present Status*, Berlin(West), ORTEP Association, pp. 35-53

Lange, P., Henninghausen, G. & Karnstedt, U. (1980) Pharmacokinetics and immunotoxicity. *Arch. Toxicol.*, **Suppl. 4**: 132-137

Lewis, W.R. & Hedges, E.S. (1957) Applications of organotin compounds. *Adv. Chem. Ser.*, **23**: 190-203

Luijten, J.G.A. (1971) Applications and biological effects or organotin compounds. In: Sawyer, A.K., ed., *Organotin Compounds*, New York, Marcel Dekker, pp. 931-974

Meuer, S.C., Hussey, R.E., Fabbi, M., Fox, D., Acuto, O., Fitzgerald, K.A., Hodgon, J.C., Protentis, J.P., Schlossman, S.F. & Reinherz, E.L. (1984) An alternative pathway of T-cell activation: a functional role for the 50 kd T11 sheep erythrocyte receptor protein. *Cell*, **36**: 897-906

Miller, K. & Scott, M.P. (1985) Immunological consequences of dioctyltin dichloride (DOTC)-induced thymic injury. *Toxicol. appl. Pharmacol.*, **78**, 395-403

Miller, K., Scott, M.P. & Foster, J.R. (1982) Sequential effects of dioctyltin dichloride on the rat thymus: new toxicology for old. *Arch. Toxicol.*, **Suppl. 5**, 328-330

Miller, K., Scott, M.P. & Foster, J.R. (1984) Thymic involution in rats given diets containing dioctyltin dichloride. *Clin. Immunol. Immunopathol.*, **30**: 62-70

Miller, K., Maisey, J. & Nicklin, S. (1986) Effect of orally administered dioctyltin dichloride on murine immunocompetence. *Environ. Res.*, **39**, 434-441

Miller, R.R. (1978) *Effects of Dialkyltins on the Thymus and Thymocytes of Rats.* PhD thesis, University of Michigan, Dearborn, MI

Nicklin, S. & Robson, M.W. (1988) Organotins: toxicology and biological effects. *Appl. Organomet. Chem.*, **2**: 487-508

Nicklin, S., Scott, M.P., Evans, J. & Miller, K. (1985) The effect of dioctyltin dichloride on the thymus and T-cell differentiation of the rat. In: Klans, G., ed., *Proceedings 8th Germinal Centre Conference*, London, Plenum Press, pp. 357-365

Penninks, A.H. & Seinen, W. (1980) Toxicity of organotin compounds. IV. Impairment of energy metabolism of rat thymocytes by various dialkyltin compounds. *Toxicol. appl. Pharmacol.*, **56**: 221-231

Penninks, A.H. & Seinen, W. (1982) Comparative toxicity of alkyltin and estertin stabilizers. *Food Chem. Toxicol.*, **20**: 909-916

Penninks A.H. & Seinen, W. (1983a) The lymphocyte as target of toxicity: a biochemical approach to dialkyltin induced immunosuppression. In: Hadden, J.W., Chedid, L., Dukor, P., Spreafico, F. & Willoughby, D., eds, *Advances in Immunopharmacology*, Oxford, Pergamon Press

Penninks, A.H. & Seinen. W. (1983b) Immunotoxicity of organotin compounds. In: Gibson, G.G., Hubbard, R., & Parke, D.V., eds, *Immunotoxicity*, London, Academic Press

Penninks, A.H. & Seinen, W. (1985) Detoxification of the estertin stabilizer bis-(b-carbobutoxyethyl)tin dichloride in rats by hydrolysis of the ester bond. *Toxicology*, **37**: 285-295

Penninks, A.H. & Seinen, W. (1987) Immunotoxicity of organotin compounds. A cell biological approach to dialkyltin-induced thymic atrophy. In: Berlin, A., Dean, J., Draper, M.H., Smith, E.M.B. & Spreafico, F., eds, *Immunotoxicology. Proceedings of the International Seminar on the Immunological System as a Target for Toxic Damage*, Dordrecht, Martinus Nijhoff

Penninks, A.H., Kuper, F., Spit, B.J. & Seinen, W. (1985) On the mechanism of dialkyltin-induced thymus involution. *Immunopharmacology*, **10**: 1-10

Penninks, A.H., Snoeij, N.J. & Seinen, W. (1986) Thymocytes as target of dialkyltin toxicity. In: Chedid, L., Hadden, J.W., Spreafico, F., Dukor, P. & Willoughby, D., eds, *Advances in Immunopharmacology*, Oxford, Pergamon Press

Penninks, A.H., Hilgers, L. & Seinen, W. (1987) The absorption, tissue distribution and excretion of di-n-octyltin dichloride in rats. *Toxicology*, **44**: 107-120

Pieters, R.H.H., Kampinga, J., Snoeij, N.J., Bol-Schoenmakers, M., Lam, A.W., Penninks, A.H. & Seinen, W. (1989a) An immunohistochemical study of dibutyltin-induced thymic atrophy. *Arch. Toxicol.*, **Suppl. 13**: 175-178

Pieters, R.H.H., Kampinga, J., Bol-Schoenmakers, M., Lam, A.W., Penninks, A.H. & Seinen, W. (1989b) Organotin-induced thymic atrophy concerns the OX44⁺ immature thymocytes: relation to the interaction between early thymocytes and thymic epithelial cells? *Thymus*, **14**: 79-88

Piver, W.T. (1973) Organotin compounds: industrial applications and biological investigation. *Environ. Health Perspect.*, **4**: 61

Reinherz, E.L. (1985) A molecular basis for thymic selection: regulation of T11 induced thymocyte expansion by T3-Ti antigen/MHC receptor pathway. *Immunol. Today*, **6**: 75-79

Renhof, M., Kretzer, U., Schurmeyer, T., Skopnik, H. & Kemper, F.H. (1980) Toxicity of organotin compounds in chicken and rats. *Arch. Toxicol.*, **Suppl. 4**: 148-150

Ross, A. (1965) Industrial application of organotin compounds. *Ann. N.Y. Acad. Sci.*, **125**, 107-123

Scollay, R. & Shortman, K. (1983) Thymocyte subpopulations: an experimental review including flow cytometric cross-correlations between the major murine thymocyte markers. *Thymus*, **5**: 245-295

Seinen, W. (1981) Immunotoxicity of alkyltin compounds. In: Sharma, R.P., ed., *Immunological Considerations in Toxicology*, Boca Raton, FL, CRC Press, pp. 104-119

Seinen, W. & Penninks, A.H. (1979) Immune suppression as a consequence of a selective cytotoxic activity of certain organometallic compounds on thymus and thymus-dependent lymphocytes. *Ann. N.Y. Acad. Sci.*, **320**: 499-517

Seinen, W. & Willems, M.I. (1976) Toxicity of organotin compounds. I. Atrophy of thymus and thymus-dependent lymphoid tissue in rats fed di-n-octyltin dichloride. *Toxicol. appl. Pharmacol.*, **35**: 63-75

Seinen, W., Vos, J.G., Van Spanje, I., Snoek, M., Brands, R. & Hooykaas, H. (1977a) Toxicity of organotin compounds. II. Comparative in vivo and in vitro studies with various organotin and organolead compounds in different animal species with special emphasis on lymphocyte cytotoxicity. *Toxicol. appl. Pharmacol.*, **42**: 197-212

Seinen, W., Vos, J.G., van Krieken, R., Penninks, A.H., Brands, R. & Hooykaas, H. (1977b) Toxicity of organotin compounds. III. Suppression of thymus dependent immunity in rats by di-n-butyltindichloride and di-n-octyltin dichloride. *Toxicol. appl. Pharmacol.*, **44**: 213-224

Seinen, W., Vos, J.G., Brands, R. & Hooykaas, H. (1979) Lymphocytotoxicity and immunesuppression by organotin compouds. Suppression of GvH activity, blast transformation and E-rosette formation by di-n-butyltin dichloride and di-n-octyltin dichloride. *Immunopharmacology*, **1**: 343-355

Smialowicz, R.J., Riddle, M.M. & Rogers, R.R. (1988) Immunologic effects of perinatal exposure of rats to dioctyltin dichloride. *J. Toxicol. environ. Health*, **25**: 403-422

Snoeij, N.J. (1987) *Triorganotin Compounds in Immunotoxicology and Biochemistry*. PhD Thesis, University of Utrecht, The Netherlands

Snoeij, N.J., Van Iersel, A.A.J., Penninks, A.H. & Seinen, W. (1985) Toxicity of triorganotin compounds: comparative in vivo studies with a series of trialkyltin compounds and triphenyltin chloride in male rats. *Toxicol. appl. Pharmacol.*, **81**: 274-286

Snoeij, N.J., Van Iersel, A.A.J., Penninks, A.H. & Seinen, W. (1986a) Triorganotin-induced cytotoxicity to rat thymus, bone marrow and red blood cells as determined by several in vitro assays. *Toxicology*, **39**: 71-83

Snoeij, N.J., Punt, P.M., Penninks, A.H. & Seinen, W. (1986b) Effects of tri-n-butyltin chloride on energy metabolism, macromolecular synthesis, precursor uptake and cyclic AMP production in isolated rat thymocytes. *Biochim. biophys. Acta*, **852**: 234-243

Snoeij, N.J., Van Rooijen, H.J.M., Penninks, A.H. & Seinen, W. (1986c) Effects of various inhibitors of oxidative phosphorylation on energy metabolism, macromolecular synthesis and cyclic AMP production in isolated rat thymocytes. *Biochim. biophys Acta*, **852**: 244-253

Snoeij, N.J., Penninks, A.H. & Seinen, W. (1987) Biological activity of organotin compounds - an overview. *Environ. Res.*, **44**: 335-353

Snoeij, N.J., Penninks, A.H. & Seinen, W. (1988a) Dibutyltin and tributyltin compounds induce thymic atrophy in rats due to a selective action on thymic lymphoblasts. *Int. J. Immunopharmacol.*, **10**: 891-899

Snoeij, N.J., Bol-Schoenmakers, M., Penninks, A.H. & Seinen, W. (1988b) Differential effects of tri-n-butyltin chloride on macromolecular synthesis and ATP levels of rat thymocyte subpopulations obtained by centrifugal elutration. *Int. J. Immunopharmacol.*, **10**: 29-37

Stoner, H.B. (1966) Toxicity of triphenyltin. *Br. J. ind. Med.*, **23**: 222-229

Van der Kerk, G.J.M. (1978) The organic chemistry of tin. *Chem. Technol.*, **8**: 356-365

Van Haelst, U. (1967) Light and electron microscopic study of normal and pathological thymus of the rat. II. The acute thymic involution. *Z. Zellforsch.*, **80**: 153

Van Loveren, H., Krajnc, E., Rombout, P.J.A., Blommaert, F.A. & Vos, J.G. (1990) Effects of ozone, hexachlorobenzene and bis(tri-n-butyltin)oxide on natural killer activity in the rat lung. *Toxicol. appl. Pharmacol.*, **102**: 21-33

Verschuuren, H.G., Kroes, R, Vink, H.H. & Van Esch, G.J. (1966) Short-term toxicity with triphenyltin compounds in rats and guinea-pigs. *Food Cosmet. Toxicol.*, **4**: 35-45

Verschuuren, H.G., Ruitenberg, E.J., Peetoom, F., Helleman, P.W. & Van Esch, G.J. (1970) Influence of triphenyltin acetate on lymphatic tissue and immune responses in guinea-pigs. *Toxicol. appl. Pharmacol.*, **16**: 400-410

Vollger, L.W., Tuck, D.T., Springer, T.A., Haynes, B.F. & Singer, K.H. (1987) Thymocyte binding to human thymic epithelial cell inhibited by monoclonal antibodies to CD2 and LFA-3 antigens. *J. Immunol.*, **138**: 358-363

Volsen, S.G., Barrass, N., Scott, M.P. & Miller, K. (1989) Cellular and molecular effects of di-n-octyltin dichloride on the rat thymus. *Int. J. Immunopharmacol.*, **11**: 703-715

Vos, J.G. & Penninks, A.H. (1987) Dioxin and organotin compounds as model immunotox chemicals. In: De Matteis, F. & Lock, E.A., eds, *Selectivity and Molecular Mechanisms of Toxicity*, London, MacMillan, pp. 85-102

Vos, J.G., Krajnc, E., Beekhof, P. & Van Logten, M. (1983) Methods for testing immune effects of toxic chemicals. Evaluation of the immunotoxicity of various pesticides in the rat. *IUPAC Pestic. Chem.*, **1**: 479-504

Vos, J.G., de Klerk, A., Krajnc, E.I., Kruizinga, W., van Ommen, B. & Rozing, J. (1984a) Toxicity of bis(tri-n-butyltin)oxide in the rat. II. Suppression of thymus dependent immune responses and of parameters of non-specific resistance after short-term exposure. *Toxicol. appl. Pharmacol.*, **75**: 387-408

Vos, J.G., Van Logten, M.J., Kreeftenberg, J.G. & Kruizinga, W. (1984b) Effect of triphenyltin hydroxide on the immune system of the rat. *Toxicology*, **29**: 325-336

Vos, J.G., De Klerk, A., Krajnc, E.I., Van Loveren, H. & Rozing, J. (1990) Immunotoxicity of bis(tri-n-butyltin)oxide in the rat: effects on thymus-dependent immunity and on nonspecific resistance following long-term exposure in young versus aged rats (submitted for publication)

Wester, P.W., Krajnc, E.I. & Van der Heijden, C.A. (1987) Chronic toxicity and carcinogenicity study with bis(tri-n-butyltin)oxide (TBTO) in rats. In: *Toxicology and Analytics of the Tributyltins - The Present Status*, Berlin (West), ORTEP Association, pp. 54-65

Wester, P.W., Krajnc, E.I., Van Leeuwen, F.X.R., Loeber, J.G., Van der Heijden, C.A., Vaessen, H.A.M.G. & Helleman, P.W. (1990) Chronic toxicity and carcinogenicity of bis(tri-n-butyltin)oxide (TBTO) in the rat. *Food Chem. Toxicol.* (in press)

Wilkinson, R.R. (1984) Technoeconomic and environmental assessment of industrial organotin compounds. *Neurotoxicology*, **5**: 141-158

World Health Organization (1980) *Tin and Organotin Compounds. A Preliminary Review (Environmental Health Criteria 15)*, Geneva

IMMUNOTOXICITY OF LEAD, CADMIUM AND ARSENIC: EXPERIMENTAL DATA AND THEIR RELEVANCE TO MAN

J. Descotes, F. Verdier, J.P. Brouland & C. Pulce

Laboratoire d'Immunotoxicologie Fondamentale et Clinique
INSERM U80-CNRS URA1177-UCBL, Faculté de Médecine Alexis Carrel
69008 Lyon, France

ABSTRACT

The influence of lead, cadmium and arsenic on the immune system is still ill-established. Exposure to lead *in vitro* and *in vivo* has been found to impair humoral and cellular immune responses as well as phagocytosis in rodents; resistance towards infection proved to be markedly decreased. In contrast, low-level and/or short-term exposures were usually associated with marginally enhanced phagocytosis and/or resistance toward infection. As very few data have been reported in man, the relevance of these findings remains to be determined in terms of human correlates and possible clinical consequences. Immune alterations induced by cadmium have also been studied extensively; the findings suggest a more subtle influence on the immune system. Resistance towards infection usually proved to be impaired. The clinical relevance of these findings is also unknown, as are the mechanisms involved in the induction of lead- and cadmium-related immune alterations. T Lymphocytes, instead of B lymphocytes or macrophages, have been proposed as probable targets. Finally, the influence of arsenic compounds on the immune system has only seldom been studied, and conflicting results were reported.

Our current knowledge of the effects of lead, cadmium and arsenic on the immune system is very limited and mostly restricted to rodents, with few of the studies conducted in accordance with currently accepted toxicological standards. The need for relevant studies in man should be stressed.

INTRODUCTION

Heavy metals are known to exert toxic effects on a variety of target organs, and the toxicity of lead, cadmium and arsenic, among others, is of major concern. Recently, numerous authors have focused on the possible immunotoxic effects of these metals and other heavy metals (for review, see Descotes, 1988). Unfortunately, the majority of published investigations were performed *in vitro* or using short-term tests with high-level exposure, thus having little relevance to real human exposure conditions.

LEAD

Some experimental evidence suggests that lead may exert varied adverse effects on the immune system of rodents, even though discrepancies can be noted in published reports.

Immunotoxicity of lead in rodents

Humoral immune responses. Early studies of humoral immune responses demonstrated that lead is an immunodepressive compound in both mice (Koller & Kovacic, 1974) and rats (Luster *et al.*, 1978). By contrast, Lawrence (1981) could find no change in humoral immunity *in vivo* in various strains of mice exposed to 0.08-10 mM lead orally.

Interestingly, Koller and Roan (1980) failed to show any change in humoral response following a ten-week oral treatment with 13, 130 or 1300 ppm in the diet, in sharp contrast to the results of a previous 56-day study (Koller & Kovacic, 1974).

Lipopolysaccharide-induced B-lymphocyte proliferation was shown to be enhanced dose-dependently following short-term exposure of mice to lead *in vitro* or *in vivo* (Shenker *et al*, 1977; Lawrence, 1981), or marginally inhibited (Koller *et al.*, 1979).

Cell-mediated responses. Delayed-type hypersensitivity responses were found to be depressed by prior treatment with lead acetate (Muller *et al.*, 1977; Laschi-Loquerie *et al.*, 1984) or lead chloride, but an opposite effect was noted when lead oxide, lead nitrate or lead carbonate was used (Descotes *et al.*, 1984). *In vitro*, lead enhanced T-lymphocyte proliferation induced by concanavalin A or phytohaemagglutinin, as well as in mixed lymphocyte culture (Lawrence, 1981), in disagreement with an earlier report (Gaworski & Sharma, 1978).

Nonspecific host defences. Studies on the influence of lead on phagocytosis also provide conflicting results: single (Schlick & Friedberg, 1981) or repeated (Koller & Roan, 1977) low-level exposure increased phagocytosis, whereas repeated exposure to higher doses depressed phagocytosis (Tam & Hindschill, 1984).

Host resistance assays. Most studies showed significantly impaired resistance of lead-exposed animals towards a wide range of pathogens, including *Salmonella typhimurium, S. enteritides, Klebsiella pneumoniae* and encephalomyocarditis virus (Koller, 1980); however, short-term exposure immediately before the infectious challenge was associated with an enhanced resistance toward *K. pneumoniae* (Laschi-Loquerie *et al.*, 1987).

Tumour resistance assays have seldom been used for assessing the immunotoxicity of lead but usually evidenced a decrease in rodent resistance (Koller, 1980).

Mechanism of lead immunotoxicity. As reviewed briefly above, numerous discrepancies can be seen in animal studies of lead immunotoxicity. The biological significance of most findings is therefore at least doubtful, as opposite results have sometimes been obtained depending upon the level or duration of exposure, the route of administration and the strain used. The mechanism of lead-associated immune alterations is unexpectedly still unknown, even though T lymphocytes were suggested to be a more likely target than B lymphocytes or macrophages (Lawrence *et al.*, 1987).

Immunotoxicity of lead in humans

Unfortunately, published studies are of no help in determining whether lead can actually interfere negatively with the human immune system, and little is known about the immunotoxicity, if any, of the various lead salts in humans.

A significant but negative relation was noted between blood lead concentrations and serum levels of complement C3 and IgG in lead-exposed workers. In contrast, a significant and positive correlation was observed with salivary IgA levels (Ewers *et al.*, 1982). Interestingly, influenza infections and colds were slightly more frequent in workers exposed to lead than in a control population. The results of this study are, however, in sharp contrast with those of a previous study by Reigart and Graber (1976), who found no difference in complement and immunoglobulin levels and the anamnestic response to tetanus toxoid in 12 lead-exposed children. Similarly, Kimber *et al.* (1986) found no change in IgG, IgA or IgM serum levels or T-lymphocyte or natural killer cell functions in lead-exposed workers with blood lead concentrations similar to those associated with immune alterations in rodents.

Recently, exposure to lead *in vitro* was reported to depress human neutrophil functions, i.e., phagocytosis and chemotaxis (Governa *et al.*, 1987). Interestingly, a statistically significant depression of both spontaneous and directed chemotaxis (agarose technique) was noted in workers with mean blood lead levels seven times higher than those of matched controls, whereas phagocytosis (assayed by chemiluminescence generation) was slightly but not significantly impaired (Bergeret *et al.*, 1990). Guillard and Lauwerys (1989) also found no change in the chemiluminescence generation of neutrophils from lead-exposed workers.

CADMIUM

The immunotoxic effects of cadmium also remain controversial, even though available data suggest a more subtle influence of cadmium on the immune system than that of lead.

Immunotoxicity of cadmium in animals

Humoral immune responses. Mostly conflicting results are available in this respect, since cadmium has been shown to enhance (Malavé & De Ruffino, 1984), depress (Borgman *et al.*, 1986) and exert no influence (Thomas *et al.*, 1985) on the humoral immune responses of rodents exposed orally for long periods. Interestingly, differences related to the use of T-dependent and T-independent antigens (Blakley & Tomar, 1986), together with the duration and level of exposure or the route of entry, are likely to account for these conflicting results.

Cell-mediated responses. In contrast to humoral immune responses, cell-mediated responses have been shown more consistently to be depressed following short-term (Fujimaki *et al.*, 1983) as well as long-term (Thomas *et al.*, 1985) oral exposure. In-vitro T-lymphocyte proliferation assays, e.g., mitogenic responses and mixed lymphocyte culture, provided evidence for a depressive effect of cadmium (Thomas *et al.*, 1985).

Nonspecific host defences. Phagocytosis was markedly decreased (Greenspan & Morrow, 1984), except in the study of Thomas *et al.* (1985), who noted a 48-61% increase in the phagocytosis of *K. pneumoniae* by peritoneal macrophages of B6C3F1 mice exposed to 10, 50 or 250 ppm for 90 days. Administration of cadmium *in vivo* was also reported to inhibit natural killer cell functions in rats exposed to 4 mg/kg per day orally for two to six weeks (Stacey *et al*, 1988).

Host resistance assays. Resistance towards infection of cadmium-exposed mice was consistently found to be depressed (Koller, 1980). Resistance of B6C3F1 mice toward *Listeria monocytogenes*, influenza virus and herpes HSV-1 and HSV-2 viruses was depressed following 10, 50 or 250 ppm for 90 days (Thomas *et al.*, 1985).

Mechanism of cadmium immunotoxicity. The mechanism of cadmium immunotoxicity is not yet fully established. A differential sensitivity of T and B cells to cadmium exposure has recently been reported, with an inhibition of antigen-specific T-cell responses by the activation of a nonspecific suppressor system (Hurtenbach *et al.*, 1988), suggesting that cadmium exposure may induce subtle alterations in immunocompetence.

Immunotoxicity of cadmium in humans

Extremely few data are available regarding the influence of cadmium on the immune system in humans. Williams *et al.* (1983) were unable to provide evidence that chronic cadmium disease is associated with significant alterations in immunological parameters *in vitro* (i.e., phytohemagglutinin- and purified protein derivative-induced lymphocyte proliferation, nitroblue tetrazolium reduction and antibody-dependent cellular cytotoxicity). Significantly reduced generation of chemiluminescence by neutrophils was noted in cadmium-exposed workers (Guillard & Lauwerys, 1989), the clinical consequence of which remains to be fully assessed.

ARSENIC

Although arsenic is a human carcinogen, few studies are available regarding the influence of arsenic compounds on the immune system. Exposure of mice to 2.5, 25 or 100 ppm arsenic in drinking-water for 10-12 weeks was not associated with immuno-suppression (Isaacson Kerkvliet *et al.*, 1980), whereas inhalation of arsenic trioxide decreased pulmonary bactericidal activity (Aranyi *et al.*, 1985). In contrast to these results, other investigators suggest that arsenic might enhance the immune responsiveness of exposed hosts. Thus, low-level exposure to both sodium arsenate and arsenite *in vitro* was reported to increase phytohaemagglutinin-induced proliferation of bovine as well as human lymphocytes (McCabe *et al.*, 1983). Similarly, Yoshida *et al.* (1988) found increased plaque-forming cell responses to sheep erythrocytes *in vitro* following exposure to 50 ng/ml, with a decreased response at 100 ng/ml. Finally, high doses of arsenicals were associated with impaired resistance to several viral infections in mice (Gainer & Pry, 1972).

Recently, Rosenthal *et al.* (1988) reported that female B6C3F1 mice exposed to 0.5, 2.5 or 5.0 ppm arsine by inhalation for 14 days demonstrated a dose-dependent decrease in splenic T-lymphocyte numbers, natural killer cell activity, cytotoxic T-lymphocyte function and mitogen-induced T-lymphocyte proliferation. Interestingly, these functional alterations were correlated with a decrease in host resistance to challenge with *L. monocytogenes* and *Plasmodium yoelii.* In contrast, B-cell functions were not altered.

The relevance of these findings with respect to human exposure is unknown. Bencko *et al.* (1988) observed that lower serum IgM levels were their only significant finding in workers at a thermal power plant burning arsenic-rich coal.

CONCLUSION

Lead, cadmium and, to a lesser extent, arsenic are a matter of concern for immunotoxicologists. A number of studies suggest that the immune competence of exposed animals may be significantly altered; however, studies have seldom been conducted according to current ad-hoc standards, particularly in terms of exposure level, duration of exposure and route of administration, so that the extrapolation of these findings to man should be done extremely carefully or, preferably, avoided.

Further investigations are warranted to determine whether lead, cadmium and arsenic can induce in acutely or subchronically exposed humans functional immune alterations similar to those noted in rodents. Epidemiological studies would be helpful for confirming whether such immune alterations are associated with relevant clinical consequences, e.g., more frequent and/or more severe infectious diseases.

REFERENCES

Aranyi, C., Bradof, J.N., O'Shea, W.J., Graham, J.A. & Miller, F.J. (1985) Effects of arsenic trioxide inhalation exposure on pulmonary antibacterial defenses in mice. *J. Toxicol. environ. Health,* **15**:163-172

Bencko, V., Wagner, V., Wagnerova, M. & Batora, J. (1988) Immunological profiles in workers of a power plant burning coal rich in arsenic content. *J. Hyg. epidemiol. Microbiol. Immunol.,* **32**: 137-146

Bergeret, A., Poujet, E., Tedone, R., Meygret, T., Cadot, R. & Descotes, J. (1990) Neutrophil functions in lead-exposed lead workers. *Exp. human Toxicol.* (in press)

Blakely, B.R. & Tomar, R.S. (1986) The effect of cadmium on antibody responses to antigens with different cellular requirements. *Int. J. Immunopharmacol.,* **8**: 1009-1015

Borgman, R.F., Au, B. & Chandra, R.K. (1986) Immunopathology of chronic cadmium administration in mice. *Int. J. Immunopharmacol.,* **8**: 813-817

Descotes, J. (1988) *Immunotoxicology of Drugs and Chemicals,* 2nd ed., Amsterdam, Elsevier Science

Descotes, J., Evreux, J.C., Laschi-Loquerie, A. & Tachon, P. (1984) Comparative effects of various lead salts on delayed hypersensitivity in mice. *J. appl. Toxicol.,* **4**: 265-266

Ewers, U., Stiller-Winkler, R. & Idel, H. (1982) Serum immunoglobulin, complement C3 and salivary IgA levels in lead workers. *Environ. Res.,* **29**: 351-357

Fujimaki, H., Shimizu, F., Kawamura, R. & Kubota, K. (1983) Inhibition of delayed hypersensitivity reaction in mice by cadmium. *Toxicol. Lett.,* **19**: 241-245

Gainer, J.H. & Pry, T.W. (1972) Effects of arsenicals on viral infections in mice. *Am. J. vet. Res.,* **33**: 2579-2586

Gaworski, C.L. & Sharma, R.P. (1978) The effects of heavy metals on ³H-thymidine uptake in lymphocytes. *Toxicol. appl. Pharmacol.,* **46**: 305-313

Governa, M., Valentino, M. & Visona, I. (1987) In vitro impairment of human granulocyte functions by lead. *Arch. Toxicol.,* **59**: 421-425

Greenspan, B.J. & Morrow, P.E. (1984) The effects of in vitro and aerosol exposures to cadmium on phagocytosis by rat pulmonary macrophages. *Fundam. appl. Toxicol.,* **4**: 48-57

Guillard, O. & Lauwerys, R. (1989) In vitro and in vivo effect of mercury, lead and cadmium on the generation of chemiluminescence by human whole blood. *Biochem. Pharmacol.,* **38**: 2819-2823

Hürtenbach, U., Oberbarnscheidt, J. & Gleichmann, E. (1988) Modulation of murine T and B cell reactivity after short-term cadmium exposure in vivo. *Arch. Toxicol.*, **62**: 22-28

Isaacson Kerkvliet, N., Baecher Steppan, L., Koller, L.D. & Exon, J.H. (1980) Immunotoxicology studies of sodium arsenate - effects of exposure on tumor growth and cell-mediated tumor immunity. *J. environ. Pathol. Toxicol.*, **4**: 65-79

Kimber, I., Stonard, M.D., Giglow, D.A. & Niewola, Z. (1986) Influence of chronic low-level exposure to lead on plasma immunoglobulin concentration and cellular immune function in man. *Int. Arch. occup. environ. Health*, **57**: 117

Koller, L.D. (1980) Immunotoxicology of heavy metals. *Int. J. Immunopharmacol.*, **2**: 269-279

Koller, L.D. & Kovacic, S. (1974) Decreased antibody formation in mice exposed to lead. *Nature*, **250**: 148-150

Koller, L.D. & Roan, J.G. (1977) Effects of lead and cadmium on mouse peritoneal macrophages. *J. Reticuloendothel. Soc.*, **21**: 7-12

Koller, L.D. & Roan, J.G. (1980) Effects of lead, cadmium and methylmercury on immunological memory. *J. environ. Pathol. Toxicol.*, **4**: 47-52

Koller, L.D., Roan, J.G. & Isaacson Kerkvliet, N. (1979) Mitogen stimulation of lymphocytes in CBA mice exposed to lead and cadmium. *Environ. Res.*, **19**: 177-188

Laschi-Loquerie, A., Descotes, J., Tachon, P. & Evreux, J.C. (1984) Influence of lead acetate on hypersensitivity. Experimental study. *J. Immunopharmacol.*, **6**: 87-93

Laschi-Loquerie, A., Eyraud, A., Morisset, D., Sanou, A., Tachon, P., Veysseyre, C. & Descotes, J. (1987) Influence of heavy metals on the resistance of mice toward infection. *Immunopharmacol. Immunotoxicol.*, **9**: 235-242

Lawrence, D.H. (1981) In vivo and in vitro effects of lead on humoral and cell-mediated immunity. *Infect. Immun.*, **31**: 136-143

Lawrence, D.H., Mudzinski, S., Rudofsky, U. & Warner, E. (1987) Mechanisms of metal-induced immunotoxicity. In: Berlin, A., Dean, J., Draper, M.H., Smith, E.M.B. & Spreafico, F., eds, *Immunotoxicology*, Dordrecht, Martinus Nijhoff, pp. 293-307

Luster, M.I., Faith, R.E. & Moore, J.A. (1978) Depression of humoral immunity in rats following chronic developmental lead exposure. *J. environ. Pathol. Toxicol.*, **1**: 397-402

Malavé, I. & De Ruffino, D.T. (1984) Altered immune response during cadmium administration in mice. *Toxicol. appl. Pharmacol.*, **74**: 46-56

MacCabe, M., Maguire, D. & Nowak, M. (1983) The effects of arsenic compounds on human and bovine lymphocyte mitogenesis in vitro. *Environ. Res.*, **31**: 323-331

Müller, S., Gillert, K.E., Krause, C., Gross, U., L'Age-Stehr, J. & Diamantstein, T. (1977) Suppression of delayed-type hypersensitivity of mice by lead. *Experientia*, **33**: 667-668

Reigart, J.R. & Graber, C.D. (1976) Evaluation of the humoral immune response of children with low-level lead exposure. *Bull. environ. Contam. Toxicol.*, **16**: 112-117

Rosenthal, G.J., Fort, M.M., Germolec, D.R., Ackermann, M.F., Blair, P., Lamm, K.R. & Luster, M.I. (1988) Effects of subchronic exposure to arsine on immune function and host resistance. *Toxicologist*, **8**: 74

Schlick, E. & Friedberg, K.D. (1981) The influence of low lead doses on the reticuloendothelial system and leucocytes of mice. *Arch. Toxicol.*, **47**: 197-207

Shenker, B.J., Matarazzo, W.J., Hirsch, R.L. & Gray, I. (1977) Effect of trace metals in the cultures on in vitro transformation of B lymphocytes. *Cell Immunol.*, **34**: 19-24

Stacey, N.H., Craig, G. & Muller, L. (1988) Effects of cadmium on natural killer and killer cell functions in vivo. *Environ. Res.*, **45**: 71-77

Tam, P.A., Hindschill, R.D. (1984) Evaluation of immunomodulatory chemicals: alterations of macrophage function in vitro. *Toxicol. appl. Pharmacol.*, **76**: 183-194

Thomas, P.T., Ratajczak, H.V., Aranyi, C., Gibbons, R. & Fenters, J.D. (1985) Evaluation of host resistance and immune function in cadmium-exposed mice. *Toxicol. appl. Pharmacol.*, **80**: 446-456

Williams, W.R., Kagamimori, S., Watanabe, M., Shinmura, T. & Hagino, N. (1983) An immunological study on patients with chronic cadmium disease. *Clin. exp. Immunol.*, **53**: 651-658

Yoshida, T., Shimamura, T. & Shigeta, S. (1987) Enhancement of the response in vitro by arsenic. *Int. J. Immunopharmacol.*, **9**: 411-415

IMMUNOTOXICOLOGY OF LEAD

I. Kimber

ICI Central Toxicology Laboratory
Alderley Park, Macclesfield
Cheshire SK10 4TJ, UK

ABSTRACT

The capacity of lead to influence the resistance of rodents to infectious challenge or tumour growth has been reported by a number of investigators. A variety of experimental approaches has been adopted to examine whether such changes in host resistance are wholly or partly attributable to the effect of lead on components of the immune system. In this report, the evidence regarding the immunotoxic properties of lead in rodents and its influence of the human immune system is critically reviewed.

INTRODUCTION

Lead ores are widely distributed on earth, and man has been aware of this metal for many millennia. It is clear that the mobilization of lead into the environment has been significantly accelerated by human activity. The widespread distribution of lead and its application in a variety of industries has stimulated considerable interest in the toxicology of this metal and, in particular, its effect on the haem biosynthetic pathway (Moore *et al.*, 1980). Over the last two decades, the capacity of lead to influence the functional integrity of the immune system has attracted the attention of many investigators, and much of the information available has been reviewed elsewhere (Treagan, 1975; Koller, 1980; Dean *et al.*, 1982; Lawrence, 1985).

Immunotoxicology as a discipline is approaching, but has perhaps not yet reached, maturity. Analysis of the effects of any agent on immune function is plagued by many difficulties, not least of which is the complexity of the immune system itself. Superimposed upon this is the fact that the immunotoxicity exerted by a chemical or drug is inevitably influenced by the species, strain and maturity of the animal, the test concentration employed, the route and duration of exposure and the indices of immune activity chosen for study. Interpretation of the physiological significance of changes in one or more immune parameters is particularly difficult, as only in recent years have studies attempted to examine the functional reserve of the immune system and to address the question of the degree of perturbation that is likely to result in a sustained and important depression of immune capacity. It is, of course, the concern of modern immunotoxicology that such changes in immune status may potentially result in significant impairment of host defence mechanisms and an associated increase in susceptibility to infectious and/or malignant disease. Consequently, it is perhaps appropriate for the purpose of this paper to first identify whether there exists a question to answer - that is, the extent to which experimental exposure to lead has been found to result in an alteration of host resistance.

HOST RESISTANCE

In fact, several lines of evidence suggest that exposure to lead salts may adversely influence host resistance mechanisms. A number of independent reports have described a 'sensitization' to bacterial endotoxins in lead-exposed mice (Seyle *et al.*, 1966; Seyberth *et al.*,

1972), rats (Filkin, 1970; Trejo & Di Luzio, 1971; Trejo *et al.*, 1972; Cook & Di Luzio, 1973; Cook et al., 1974), chickens (Truscott, 1970) and baboons (Holper *et al.*, 1973). Moreover, lead also appears to increase the susceptibility of animals to bacterial infection. Thus, Hemphill *et al.* (1971) found that chronic administration of lead reduced the resistance of mice to *Salmonella typhimurium.* Cook *et al.* (1975) observed a similar phenomenon in rats and reported that the intravenous administration of lead as lead acetate resulted in an approximately 1000-fold increase in susceptibility to *Escherichia coli.* Selected references summarizing the evidence for an impairment of host resistance to pathogens associated with exposure to lead are listed in Table 1.

The influence of lead on viral infection has been ascribed to the capacity of the metal to inhibit interferon production (Gainer, 1974). With respect to bacterial infection, it was originally proposed that increased susceptibility was the result of changes in the reticuloendothelial system and the functional activity of mononuclear phagocytes (Seyle *et al.*, 1966). Although Tam and Hinsdill (1984) reported that culture of murine peritoneal macrophages with noncytotoxic concentrations of lead acetate reduced the proportion of cells capable of ingesting yeast, other studies *in vivo* suggest that lead acetate fails to influence or even potentiates macrophage phagocytosis (Koller & Roan, 1977; Schlick & Friedberg, 1981; Dean & Adams, 1985). It may therefore be difficult to resolve the issue of lead and bacterial resistance in terms of phagocyte function alone. The situation may in fact be complex and involve changes in other organ systems, including hepatic parenchymal cell function (Cook *et al.*, 1974).

Exposure to lead has also been shown to enhance the growth and/or incidence of tumours in rodents (Hinton *et al.*, 1979; Kerkvliet & Baecher-Steppan, 1982), a phenomenon which may or may not be wholly attributable to the putative immunosuppressive properties of the metal.

The difficulties associated with the analysis of lead-induced changes in host resistance have recently been further emphasized by the report of Laschi-Loquerie *et al.* (1987), in which it was observed that the susceptibility of mice to *Klebsiella* was either enhanced or depressed by lead acetate according to the time of administration relative to infectious challenge. The authors argue that the variable influence of lead on *Klebsiella* infection is compatible with the natural history of resistance to this bacterium. Thus, exposure to lead prior to infection enhanced protection through potentiation of phagocytosis. At later stages of the infectious cycle, antibodies are elaborated, and if lead was administered 5 h following bacterial challenge the resultant enhancement of phagocytosis was no longer decisive and the observed increase in susceptibility was secondary to an impairment of humoral immunity (Laschi-Loquerie *et al.*, 1987). It is therefore relevant to consider the influence of lead on components of the adaptive immune system.

HUMORAL IMMUNITY

Antibody responses can be measured in a variety of ways, the most popular of which in immunotoxicology studies is currently the Jerne plaque assay, in which the frequency of

Table 1. Impairment of host resistance to infectious microorganisms following exposure to lead

Species	Pathogen	Reference
Mouse	*Salmonella typhimurium*	Hemphill *et al.* (1971)
Mouse	Rauscher leukaemia virus	Gainer (1973)
Mouse	Encephalomyocarditis virus	Gainer (1974)
Mouse	*Staphylococcus aureus*	Salaki *et al.* (1975)
Mouse	Langat virus	Thind & Khan (1978)
Mouse	*Serratia marcescens*	Schlipkoter & Freiler (1979)
Mouse	*Listeria monocytogenes*	Lawrence (1981a)
Rat	*Escherichia coli*	Cook *et al.* (1975)

antibody-producing (plaque-forming) cells is measured (Bick *et al.*, 1985; Thomas *et al.*, 1985; Dean & Thurmond, 1987). Humoral immune responses can also be assessed as a function of circulating antibody titre to a test antigen, and this was the approach employed by Koller (1973) who first demonstrated that, compared with control animals, rabbits exposed to lead acetate exhibited a significant decrease in specific antibody levels following challenge with psuedo-rabies virus. Subsequent studies in mice revealed that chronic exposure to lead in fact caused a decrease in the frequency of nucleated splenocytes producing IgG and IgM antibodies to sheep red blood cells (Koller & Kovacic, 1974). The situation regarding the effect of lead on humoral immunity is, however, complex, for a number of reasons.

Thus, for instance, although the studies of Koller and Kovacic (1974) and a number of other reports (Luster *et al.*, 1978; Blakley *et al.*, 1980) record that chronic exposure to lead impairs specific antibody levels, a single administration of lead given either intraperitoneally or orally was found to augment IgM antibody responses; IgG antibody responses were, however, suppressed (Koller *et al.*, 1976). Moreover, in a recent study, the administration of 10 mM lead acetate in drinking-water for eight weeks failed to influence the frequency of plaque-forming cells or circulating antibody or the serum concentrations of IgM, IgG and IgA in any of several strains of mice examined (Mudzinski *et al.*, 1986). In those instances in which reduced antibody levels have followed lead exposure, the mechanism of suppression is unclear. The influence of lead appears to be greater on the response to those antigens that require T-lymphocyte activation to elicit an antibody response (T-dependent antigens) (Luster *et al.*, 1978; Blakley & Archer, 1981). Although Koller and Brauner (1977) reported a decrease in the frequency of complement receptor-bearing splenic lymphocytes following exposure of mice to lead acetate, these data do not provide compelling evidence for a reduction in B-lymphocyte numbers, and one may speculate that the primary lesion is at the level of T lymphocytes. Alternatively, it has been reported that the observed reduction in plaque-forming cells following administration of lead is secondary to an impairment of accessory cell function and can be corrected with the macrophage substitute 2-mercapto-ethanol (Blackley & Archer, 1981).

Rather than inhibiting humoral immunity, lead may actually potentiate B-lymphocyte activation and antibody production. In a series of in-vitro experiments in which the influence of a variety of heavy metals on murine primary immune responses was examined, it was observed that lead augmented the frequency of plaque-forming cells (Lawrence, 1981b). In the same study, lead was also observed to enhance the proliferative response induced by the selective B-lymphocyte mitogen lipopolysaccharide. A similar potentiation of mitogen-induced B lymphocyte proliferation was reported in other studies of exposure to lead *in vitro* (Shenker *et al.*, 1977; Gallagher *et al.*, 1979; Lawrence, 1981a,c) and *in vivo* (Lawrence, 1981a). Some caution is necessary, however, as at least one other report has described some impairment of lipolysaccharide-driven blastogenesis following exposure of mice to relatively high concentrations of lead (Koller *et al.*, 1979). Taken together, these data lead to the tentative conclusion that, although under some circumstances, and largely following chronic exposure, lead may impair antibody responses, it is, on balance, unlikely that this effect is mediated by a direct inhibition of B lymphocyte function. Lead may, however, have the capacity to cause changes in B lymphocytes resulting in enhanced mitotic activity. These and similar data prompted Lawrence (1985) to speculate that exposure to lead (and some other heavy metals) may be a predisposing factor in the development of autoimmune disease. Certainly, the reported capacity of lead to enhance B-lymphocyte activation would be compatible with this hypothesis. Of relevance in this context is the possibility that lead may influence suppressor T lymphocyte, which are considered to play a role of some importance in the prevention of autoimmunity. Hambach *et al.* (1983) found that mice fed a diet containing lead acetate, resulting in a blood lead concentration of approximately 50 µg/100 ml, exhibited a significant increase in IgG and IgM secreting spleen cells following challenge with sheep erythrocytes. Higher blood lead levels resulted in an inhibition of antibody responses. As lead exposure also abrogated antigenic competition, it was concluded that relatively low levels of lead selectively influence the activity of suppressor T lymphocytes (Hambach *et al.*, 1983). It is not unreasonable to suggest therefore that the primary cellular target of lead-induced changes in humoral immune status may be critically dependent upon the level of exposure, and that at relatively low doses lead may in fact augment humoral immunity through either a direct potentiation of B lymphocytes or a selective impairment of suppressor cell activity.

CELLULAR IMMUNE FUNCTION

The influence of lead on cellular immune function, in contrast to humoral immunity, has attracted attention only relatively recently. The integrity of T-lymphocyte activity may be conveniently measured *in vitro* as a function of mitogen-induced proliferative responses. The mitogens favoured in such studies, phytohaemagglutinin (PHA) and concanavalin A (Con A), are relatively, or wholly, selective for T lymphocytes. This strategy has been adopted by a number of investigators to examine the effect of lead on cell-mediated immunity. An inhibition of the responsiveness of splenic lymphocytes to PHA following chronic exposure of mice to high concentrations of lead (2000 ppm) was reported by Gaworski and Sharma (1978). Acute exposure to lead has also been shown to result in transient alteration of T-cell function. Burchiel *et al.* (1987) found that a single intraperitoneal administration of lead acetate to mice was associated with a significant depression of proliferative responses to Con A and PHA one and three days following treatment, but that normal responsiveness to both mitogens was fully restored within five days. Effects on T-lymphocyte proliferation have also been described in rats: animals exposed pre- and postnatally to lead exhibited reduced thymic weight and a significant impairment of both PHA- and Con A-driven spleen cell proliferation (Faith *et al.*, 1979). Here again, however, the available data are not unequivocal, as other studies have failed to demonstrate similar effects on mitogen responses. For instance, splenocytes prepared from mice that had received lead acetate (1300 ppm) in drinking-water for ten weeks displayed normal proliferative activity following culture with Con A (Koller *et al.*, 1979). Likewise, studies performed in this laboratory have revealed that rats treated with 1000 ppm lead as lead acetate in drinking-water, and which displayed elevated blood lead concentrations and reduced blood 5-aminolaevulinic acid dehydratase activity, possessed normal splenic T-cell function in terms of PHA responsiveness (Kimber *et al.*, 1986a).

Although the matter is clearly unresolved, it would appear that lead treatment results in some impairment of rodent splenic T-cell function under certain experimental conditions, when high concentrations and/or prolonged exposure periods are used. The effect is, however, rather inconsistent, and it is appropriate to consider whether other manifestations of T-lymphocyte function are altered following exposure to lead.

One approach that has been used is to examine changes in the ability of test animals to mount delayed hypersensitivity responses. Faith *et al.* (1979) found that the depression of splenic T-lymphocyte proliferative responses following pre- and postnatal exposure to lead was associated with significantly reduced delayed hypersensitivity reactions to purified protein derivative. A similar lead-induced suppression of delayed-type hypersensitivity to sheep red blood cells in the mouse was reported by Muller *et al.* (1977). Other investigators have chosen to examine responses to the contact sensitizing chemical 2,4,6-trinitro-chlorobenzene (picryl chloride). In a series of experiments performed by Laschi-Loquerie *et al.* (1984), contact sensitization to picryl chloride in mice was assessed by measurement of challenge-induced increases in ear thickness. Exposure to lead acetate before sensitization, during sensitization and challenge or following challenge in each case caused a modest reduction in the strength of the elicitation reactions achieved when compared with sensitized control animals. In a subsequent study by the same group, a similar, but quantitatively more marked, inhibition of contact sensitization associated with lead exposure was recorded (Descotes *et al.*, 1985). The significance of these observations is unclear, as in a separate investigation Descotes *et al.* (1984) found that the intraperitoneal administration of various lead salts had divergent effects on the ability of mice to mount delayed hypersensitivity reactions to sheep red blood cells. While lead oxide, lead nitrate and lead carbonate resulted in a significant impairment of challenge-induced increases in footpad thickness, other lead salts (acetate and chloride) had a potentiating effect. Not only do these data cast some doubt on the biological significance of changes in delayed hypersensitivity associated with lead exposure, but they also pose questions regarding the importance of the anion in studies of lead salt immunotoxicity.

Finally, of relevance to considerations of T-lymphocyte function is a study in which the influence of lead was examined on the synthesis of interleukin-2, a T-cell growth factor necessary for antigen-driven proliferation. Exon *et al.* (1985) reported that exposure of rats to lead caused a reduction in 'endogenous' interleukin-2 synthesis by isolated splenocytes; however, following culture with Con A, spleen cells from lead-treated animals produced levels of interleukin-2 comparable to control values.

On balance, therefore, studies to date suggest that, although some effects have been observed, the case for a substantive influence of lead on T-lymphocyte function and cell-mediated immune responses remains largely unproven.

NATURAL CYTOTOXICITY

In the period since their first description, natural killer (NK) cells have been investigated actively. Of particular interest has been the suggestion, as yet unsubstantiated, that NK cells are the vectors of an innate form of immunosurveillance against malignant disease and viral infection (Kimber, 1985). The functional activity of NK cells is conventionally measured by their capacity to lyse spontaneously a variety of malignant cell types *in vitro*. A number of studies have addressed the question of whether lead influences such NK cell-mediated natural cytotoxicity; the results show that chronic exposure of either rats (Talcott *et al.*, 1985; Kimber *et al.*, 1986a) or mice (Neilan *et al.*, 1983; Exon *et al.*, 1985) to lead fails to affect splenic NK cell function significantly. Neither does lead appear to compromise the capacity of interferon to augment NK cell-mediated cytotoxicity (Neilan *et al.*, 1983; Kimber *et al.*, 1986a).

It is difficult, on the basis of the information reviewed above, to draw firm conclusions regarding the impact of lead on immune function in rodents. Certainly, it is not easy to reconcile the reported increase in susceptibility to infection with the effect of lead on components of the natural and adaptive immune system, and one is forced to speculate that changes in other organ systems may be of importance in this respect. It cannot, however, be concluded that lead is without effect on immune function; sustained high exposure levels certainly cause significant changes in some circumstances. The possibility that exposure to lead at levels below those which have been associated with overt immunotoxicity causes subtle, but potentially important, alterations in immune status clearly warrants further study. Perhaps one approach will be to examine in greater detail the reported influence of lead on mononuclear-cell populations in the bone marrow (Burchiel *et al.*, 1986, 1987). Irrespective of the mechanism(s) through which lead may act, evidence for lead-related changes in the immunological status of man following occupational or environmental exposure to the metal must be examined.

LEAD EXPOSURE AND IMMUNE FUNCTION IN MAN

There are relatively few sources of information available in this area. Ewers *et al.* (1982) examined 72 male employees in a battery plant and in a lead smelter plant who had an average duration of exposure of 10.2 years and blood lead concentrations of 18.6-85.2 µg/100 g (mean, 55.4). Serum IgM, IgG, IgA and complement C3 levels were measured and compared with values derived from a control group of 25 male subjects with a mean blood lead concentration of 12.0 µg/100 g (range, 6.6-20.8). The authors reported a trend towards reduced levels of each of these serum proteins among the lead workers, although, with the exception of IgM, the differences from the control values did not reach statistical significance. In the same study, lead-exposed subjects were also found to have a significant reduction in salivary IgA compared with controls. Among both lead workers and the test population as a whole, there was a negative correlation between blood lead levels and serum concentration of IgG and C3. In a similar study conducted in this laboratory, we were unable to confirm these observations (Kimber *et al.*, 1986b). We examined a group of 39 male workers with occupational exposure to inorganic lead who were employed at a plant manufacturing tetraethyllead, and who had a mean blood lead concentration of 38.4 µg/100 ml (range, 25-53). The mean exposure period to lead (10.3 years) was almost exactly the same as that of the population studied by Ewers *et al.* (1982). In our investigation, the age-matched control population comprised 21 unexposed individuals with blood lead concentrations of 8 and 17 µg/100 ml (mean, 11.8). No difference in the serum concentrations of IgM, IgG or IgA was observed between the populations, and there was no correlation between the concentration of blood lead and serum immunoglobulin levels. In addition, we examined the capacity of peripheral blood mononuclear cells to mount a proliferative response to PHA and to lyse spontaneously cells of the erythroleukaemic cell line K562 , a measure of NK cell function. In neither case was there a difference between exposed and control groups and no association between cellular reactivity and blood lead concentration (Kimber *et al.*, 1986b).

The reasons for these apparently contradictory findings is uncertain. As we failed to find any correlation between blood lead levels and serum immunoglobulin concentrations, it is unlikely that the different results recorded in the two studies are simply attributable to the fact that the population examined by Ewers *et al.* (1982) had somewhat higher blood lead concentrations. The only other information of relevance is a report by Wagnerova *et al.* (1986) in which a group of Czechoslovak children resident in the vicinity of a lead smelting plant were examined. Compared with age-matched controls, these children had elevated levels of blood lead, a downward trend in the serum concentration of IgM and a tendency toward lower levels of secretory IgA.

Thus, the limited human data are somewhat contradictory. Although in our own study we failed to observe changes in any of the parameters measured, this might not prove to be the case with higher blood lead concentrations. Certainly the work of Wagnerova *et al.* (1986) suggests that additional studies on the immunological status of children exposed to lead would be appropriate.

In conclusion, it would appear that, under some conditions of exposure, lead can effect some changes on the immune function of rodents, but it is difficult, in many instances, to reconcile such affects with reported alterations in host resistance. Although the situation in man is presently unresolved, there is no evidence for a substantial depression of immunoglobulin levels or for a serious impairment of immune function following sustained occupational exposure to lead.

REFERENCES

Bick, P.H., Holsapple, M.P. & White, K.L., Jr (1985) Assessment of the effects of chemicals on the immune system. In: Li, A.P., ed., *New Approaches in Toxicity Testing and Their Application in Human Risk Assessment,* New York, Raven Press, pp. 165-178

Blakely, B.R. & Archer, D.L. (1981) The effect of lead acetate on the immune response in mice. *Toxicol. appl. Pharmacol.,* **61:** 18-26

Blakley, B.R., Sisodia, C.S. & Mukkur, T.K. (1980) The effect of methylmercury, tetraethyl lead and sodium arsenite on the humoral immune response in mice. *Toxicol. appl. Pharmacol.,* **52:** 245-254

Burchiel, S.W., Hadley, W.M., Cameron, C.L., Fincher, R.H., Lim, T.-W. & Stewart, C.C. (1986) Flow cytometry coulter volume analysis of lead- and cadmium-induced cellular alterations in bone marrow obtained from young adult and aged Balb/c mice. *Toxicol. Lett.,* **34:** 89-94

Burchiel, S.W., Hadley, W.M., Cameron, C.L., Fincher, R.H., Lim, T.-W., Elias, L. & Steward, C.C. (1987) Analysis of heavy metal immunotoxicity by multi-parameter flow cytometry: correlation of flow cytometry and immune function data in B6CFl mice. *Int. J. Immunopharmacol.,* **9:** 597-610

Cook, J.A. & Di Luzio, N.R. (1973) Protective effect of cysteine and methylprednisolone in lead-endotoxin-induced shock. *Exp. mol. Pathol.,* **19:** 127-138

Cook, J.A., Marconi, E.A. & Di Luzio, N.R. (1974) Lead, cadmium, endotoxin interaction: effect on mortality and hepatic function. *Toxicol. appl. Pharmacol.,* **28:** 292-302

Cook, J.A., Hoffman, E.O. & Di Luzio, N.R. (1975) Influence of lead and cadmium on the susceptibility of rats to bacterial challenge. *Proc. Soc. exp. Biol. Med.,* **150:** 741-747

Dean, J.H. & Adams, D.O. (1985) The effect of environmental agents on cells of the mononuclear phagocyte system. In: Hadden, J.W. & Szentivanyi, A., eds, *The Reticuloendothelial System,* Vol. 8, New York, Plenum, pp. 389-409

Dean, J.H. & Thurmond, L.M. (1987) Immunotoxicology: an overview. *Toxicol. Pathol.,* **15:** 265-271

Dean, J.H., Luster, M.I. & Boorman, G.A. (1982) Immunotoxicology. In: Sirois, P. & Rola-Pleszczynski, M., eds, *Immunopharmacology,* Amsterdam, Elsevier, pp. 349-397

Descotes, J., Evreux, J.C., Laschi-Loquerie, A. & Tachon, P. (1984) Comparative effects of various lead salts on delayed hypersensitivity in mice. *J. appl. Toxicol.,* **4:** 265-266

Descotes, J., Tedone, R. & Evreux, J.C. (1985) Immunotoxicity screening of drugs and chemicals: value of contact hypersenstivity to picryl chloride in the mouse. *Meth. Findings exp. clin. Pharmacol.,* **7:** 303-305

Ewers, U., Stiller-Winkler, R. & Idel, H. (1982) Serum immunoglobulin, complement component C3 and salivary IgA in lead workers. *Environ. Res.*, **29:** 351-357

Exon, J.H., Talcott, P.A. & Koller, L.D. (1985) Effect of lead, polychlorinated biphenyls, and cyclophosphamide on rat natural killer cells, interleukin 2 and antibody synthesis. *Fundam. appl. Toxicol.*, **5:** 158-164

Faith, R.E., Luster, M.I. & Kimmel, C.A. (1979) Effect of chronic developmental lead exposure on cell-mediated immune functions. *Clin. exp. Immunol.*, **35:** 413-420

Filkins, J.P. (1970) Bioassay of endotoxin inactivation in the lead-sensitized rat. *Proc. Soc. exp. Biol. Med.*, **134:** 610-612

Gainer, J.H. (1973) Activation of Rauscher leukaemia virus by metals. *J. natl Cancer Inst.*, **51:** 609-613

Gainer, J.H. (1974) Lead aggravates viral disease and represses the antiviral activity of interferon inducers. *Environ. Health Perspect.*, **7:** 113-119

Gallagher, K., Mattarazzo, W.J. & Gray, I. (1979) Trace metal modification of immunocompetence. II. Effect of Pb^{2+}, Cd^{2+} and Cr^{3+} on RNA turnover, hexokinase activity and blastogensis during B lymphocyte tranformation in vitro. *Clin. Immunol. Immunopathol.*, **13:** 369-377

Gaworski, C.L. & Sharma, R.P. (1978) The effects of heavy metals on [^{3}H] thymidine uptake in lymphocytes. *Toxicol. appl. Pharmacol.*, **46:** 305-313

Hambach, A., Stiller-Winkler, R., Oberbarnscheidt, J. & Ewers, U. (1983) [Suppressor T cells - a sensitive target of lead toxicity.] (in German) *Zbl. Bakt. Hyg.I. Abt. Orig. B*, **178:** 316-328

Hemphill, F.E., Kaeberle, M.L. & Buck, W.B. (1971) Lead suppression of mouse resistance to Salmonella typhimurium. *Science,* **172:** 1031-1032

Hinton, D.E., Lipsky, M.M., Heatfield, B.M. & Trump, B.F. (1979) Opposite effects of lead on chemical carcinogenesis in kidney and liver of rats. *Bull. environ. Contam. Toxicol.*, **23:** 464-469

Holper, K., Trejo, R.A., Brettschneider, L. & Di Luzio, N.R. (1973) Enhancement of endotoxin shock in the lead-sensitized subhuman primate. *Surg. Gynecol. Obstet.*, **136:** 593-601

Kerkvliet, N.I. & Baecher-Steppan, L. (1982) Immunotoxicology studies on lead effects on tumour growth and cell-mediated tumour immunity after syngeneic or allogenic stimulation. *Immunopharmacology,* **4:** 213-224

Kimber, I. (1985) Natural killer cells. *Med. Lab. Sci.*, **42:** 60-77

Kimber, I., Jackson, J.A. & Stonard, M.D. (1986a) Failure of inorganic lead exposure to impair natural killer (NK) cell and T lymphocyte function in rats. *Toxicol. Lett.*, **31:** 211-218

Kimber, I., Stonard, M.D., Gidlow, D.A. & Niewola, Z. (1986b) Influence of chronic low-level exposure to lead on plasma immunoglobulin concentration and cellular immune function in man. *Int. Arch. occup. environ. Health.*, **57:** 117-125

Koller, L.D. (1973) Immunosuppression induced by lead, cadmium and mercury. *Am. J. vet. Res.,* **34:** 1457-1458

Koller, L.D. (1980) Immunotoxicology of heavy metals. *Int. J. Immunopharmacol.*, **2:** 269-279

Koller, L.D. & Brauner, J.A. (1977) Decreased B-lymphocyte response after exposure to lead and cadmium. *Toxicol. appl. Pharmacol.*, **42:** 621-624

Koller, L.D. & Kovacic, S. (1974) Decreased antibody formation in mice exposed to lead. *Nature.*, **250:** 148-150

Koller, L.D. & Roan, J.G. (1977) Effects of lead and cadmium on mouse peritoneal macrophages. *J. Reticuloendothel. Soc.*, **21:** 7-12

Koller, L.D., Exon, J.H. & Roan, J.G. (1976) Humoral antibody response in mice after a single dose exposure to lead or cadmium. *Proc. Soc. exp. Biol. Med.*, **151:** 339-342

Koller, L.D., Roan, J.G. & Kerkvliet, N.I. (1979) Mitogen stimulation of lymphcytes in CBA mice exposed to lead and cadmium. *Environ. Res.*, **19:** 177-188

Laschi-Loquerie, A., Descotes, J., Tachon, P. & Evreux, J.C. (1984) Influence of lead acetate on hypersenstivity. Experimental study. *J. Immunopharmacol.*, **6:** 87-93

Laschi-Loquerie, A., Eyraud, A., Morisset, D., Sanou, A., Tachon, P., Veysseyre, C. & Descotes, J. (1987) Influence of heavy metals on the resistance of mice toward infection. *Immunopharmacol. Immunotoxicol.*, **9:** 235-241

Lawrence, D.A. (1981a) In vivo and in vitro effects of lead on humoral and cell-mediated immunity. *Infect. Immunol.*, **31:** 136-143

Lawrence, D.A. (1981b) Heavy metal modulation of lymphocyte activities. I. In vitro effects of heavy metals on primary humoral immune responses.*Toxicol. appl. Pharmacol.*, **57:** 439-451

Lawrence, D.A. (1981c) Heavy metal modulation of lymphocyte activites. II. Lead, an in vitro mediator of B-cell activation. *Int. J. Immunopharmacol.*, **3:** 153-161

Lawrence, D.A. (1985) Immunotoxicity of heavy metals. In: Dean, J.,Luster, M.I., Munson, A.E. & Amos, H., eds, *Immunotoxicology and Immunopharmacology*, New York, Raven Press, pp. 341-353

Luster, M.I., Faith, R.E. & Kimmel, C.A. (1978) Depression of humoral immunity in rats following chronic developmental lead exposure. *J. environ. Pathol. Toxicol.*, **1:** 397-402

Moore, M.R., Meredith, P.A. & Goldberg, A. (1980) Lead and heme biosynthesis. In: Singhal, L. & Thomas, J.A., eds, *Lead Toxicity*, Baltimore, Urban and Schwarzenberg, pp. 79-117

Mudzinski, S.P., Rudofsky, U.H., Mitchell, D.G. & Lawrence, D.A. (1986) Analysis of lead effects on in vivo antibody-mediated immunity in several mouse strains. *Toxicol. appl. Pharmacol.*, **83**: 321-330

Muller, S., Gillert, K.E., Krause, C.L., Gross, U., Age-Shehr, J.L. & Diamanstein, T. (1977) Suppression of delayed type hypersensitivity of mice by lead. *Experimentia*, **33**: 667-668

Neilan, B.A., O'Neill, K. & Handwerger, B.S. (1983) Effect of low-level lead exposure on antibody-dependent and natural killer cell-mediated cytotoxicity. *Toxicol. appl. Pharmacol.*, **69**: 272-275

Salaki, J., Louria, D.B. & Thind, I.S. (1975) Influence of lead intoxication on experimental infections. *Clin. Res.*, **23**: 417A

Schlick, E. & Friedberg, K.D. (1981) The influence of low lead doses on the reticulo-endothelial system and leukocytes of mice. *Arch. Toxicol.*, **47**: 197-207

Schlipkoter, H.W. & Freiler, L. (1979) The influence of short-term lead exposure on the bacterial clearance. *Zh. Bakt. Hyg. I. Abt. Orig. B.*, **168**: 256-265

Seyberth, H.W., Schmidt-Gayk, H. & Hackenthal, E. (1972) Toxicity, clearance and distribution of endotoxin in mice as influenced by actinomycin D, cycloheximide, α-amanitin and lead acetate. *Toxicon*, **10**: 491 -500

Seyle, H., Tuchweber, B. & Bertok, L. (1966) Effect of lead acetate on susceptibility of rats to bacterial endotoxins. *J. Bacteriol.*, **91**: 884-890

Shenker, B.J., Matarazzo, W.J., Hirsch, R.L. & Gray, I. (1977) Trace metal modification of immunocompetence. I. Effect of trace metals in the cultures on in vitro transformation of B-lymphocytes. *Cell. Immunol.*, **34**: 19-24

Talcott, P.A., Koller, L.D. & Exon, J.H. (1985) The effect of lead and polychlorinated biphenyl exposure on rat natural killer cell cytotoxicity. *Int. J. Immunopharmacol.*, **7**: 255-261

Tam, P.E. & Hinsdill, R.D. (1984) Evaluation of immunomodulatory chemicals: alteration of macrophage function in vitro. *Toxicol. appl. Pharmacol.*, **76**: 183-194

Thind, I.S. & Khan, M.Y. (1978) Potentiation of the neurovirulence of langat virus infection by lead intoxication in mice. *Exp. mol. Pathol.*, **29**: 342-347

Thomas, P.T., Fugmann, R.A., Aranyi, C. & Fenters, J.D. (1985) Development and validation of a panel of host resistance and immune function assays designed to detect chemical-induced immunomodulation. In: Li, A.P., ed., *New Approaches in Toxicity Testing and Their Application in Human Risk Assessment.*, New York, Raven Press, pp. 213-222

Treagan, L. (1975) Metals and the immune response. A review. *Res. Commun. Chem. Pathol. Pharmacol.*, **12**: 189-219

Trejo, R.A. & Di Luzio, N.R. (1971) Impaired detoxification as a mechanism of lead acetate-induced hypersensitivity to endotoxin. *Proc. Soc. exp. Biol. Med.*, **136**: 889-893

Trejo, R.A., Di Luzio, N.R., Loose, L.D. & Hoffman, E.O. (1972) Reticuloendothelial and hepatic functional alterations following lead acetate administration. *Exp. mol. Pathol.*, **17**: 145-158

Truscott, R.B. (1970) Endotoxin studies in chicks: effect of lead acetate. *Can. J. comp. Med.*, **34**: 134-137

Wagnerova, M., Wagner, V., Madlo, Z., Zavazal, V., Wokounova, D., Kriz, J. & Mohyla, 0. (1986) Seasonal variations in the level of immunoglobulins and serum proteins of children differing by exposure to air-borne lead. *J. Hyg. Epidemiol. Microbiol. Immunol.*, **30**: 127-138

ADVERSE EFFECTS OF ZINC ON THE IMMUNE SYSTEM

R.F. Hertel & A. Wibbertmann

Fraunhofer Institute of Toxicology and Aerosol Research
3000 Hanover 61
Federal Republic of Germany

ABSTRACT

Literature was reviewed to document the adverse effects of zinc on the immune response of experimental animals and man. In animals, zinc deficiency affected several metalloenzymes and the activity of the thymus. There is evidence that zinc alters humoral- and cell-mediated immunity, NK-cell activity, immunopathological parameters and host resistance in both experimental animals and humans. In man, an immunotoxic effect of exposure to airborne zinc is suggested, but this requires confirmation due to lack of information on various important exposure parameters.

INTRODUCTION

Dietary zinc deficiency impairs the optimal activity of many metalloenzymes and leads to thymic atrophy, which causes altered immune responses. In 1985, the American Institute of Nutrition organized a symposium dealing with the interrelationships between zinc and immune function, in which experimental and clinical studies were reported that demonstrated the importance of zinc in host defence and immune ontogeny (Fraker *et al.*, 1986). This paper gives further information on the immunotoxic effects of zinc on the basis of a literature review.

EFFECTS ON ANIMALS

Immunopathology

In rats, a deficiency of zinc and essential fatty acids accentuated dermal scores and severely depressed growth. Dietary zinc deficiency (7 ppm zinc) increased the proportion of arachidonic acid in foot skin especially in animals deficient in essential fatty acids (300 ppm). In chicks, polyunsaturated fatty acids aggravated the signs of zinc deficiency (6 ppm zinc in the diet). In both species, a higher than normal proportion of arachidonate was found in the fatty acids of zinc-deficient skin (Bettger *et al.*, 1979, 1980).

Beach *et al.* (1980) fed 2.5, 5, 9 or 100 ppm zinc to young adult, outbred N:NIH(S) female mice at ten weeks of age and investigated the influence of postnatal zinc deprivation upon growth and development. Reductions in body weight and length were noted, but only the relative liver growth was significantly retarded; heart and kidney were affected to a lesser extent. At six weeks of age, neonatal mortality was 100% with the 2.5-ppm treatment. High zinc concentrations in the diet may reduce the uptake of copper, inducing common clinical signs of copper deficiency in many species (Van Campen, 1966). Dietary exposure of adult mink to 1000 ppm zinc, however, did not result in gross toxicity or copper deficiency (Bleavins *et al.*, 1983). In the offspring of treated females, achromotrichia, alopecia, lymphopenia and a reduced rate of growth were observed; and the haematocrit value was significantly decreased at eight weeks of age. In ferrets *(Mustela furo)*, high zinc concentrations (1500 and 3000 ppm) resulted in diffuse kidney nephrosis and severe macrocytic hypochromic anaemia (Straube *et al.*, 1980).

Immunotoxicity of Metals and Immunotoxicology, Edited by
A. D. Dayan *et al.,* Plenum Press, New York, 1990

Two studies have described the effects of inhalation in cattle exposed to fumes of zinc oxide derived from oxyacetylene cutting and arc welding of galvanized pipe: congestion and haemorrhage in the trachea, interstitial emphysema, and interlobular and pulmonary oedema were noted at necropsy (Breeze, 1985). Exposure of guinea-pigs to zinc oxide particles at 5 mg/m^3 by nose for 3 h/day for six days resulted in decreased vital capacity, functional residual capacity, alveolar volume and diffusing capacity for carbon monoxide (DL$_{co}$) following the last exposure, which did not return to normal levels by 72 h; furthermore, lung weights were elevated due to inflammation. These pulmonary changes occurred with relatively few exposures to zinc oxide (Lam et al., 1985). Neither study provides information on aerosol characteristics.

Humoral-, cell-mediated and nonspecific immunity

In a 28-day study, a zinc-deficient diet (0.5-0.6 ppm zinc) had no significant effect on antibody-mediated immune response to sheep red blood cells in five-week old female A/J mice, but the animals showed a pronounced loss of immune capacity. The zinc-deficient symptoms produced were more severe in a 32-day study, and thymus weight and plaquing capacity were affected (Luecke et al., 1978).

Luecke and Fraker (1979) fed 0.7, 3.3, 5.9, 8.2, 11 or 31.4 ppm zinc to growing female outbred Swiss mice for three weeks and to inbred A/J mice for two weeks. Animals attained maximal growth and normal antibody-mediated response (IgM, IgG) after immunization with sheep red blood cells at a dietary zinc level of 5.9 ppm.

Six- to eight-week old A/J, C57Bl/Ks and CBA/H mice showed loss of body weight, low lymphoid tissue weight, and profound involution of the thymus within four to eight weeks of eating a zinc-deficient diet. Approximately 50% developed severe acrodermatitis enteropathica, diarrhoea, a depressed response in the plaque-forming cell assay to immunization with sheep red blood cells in vivo, depressed T killer cell activity against EL-4 tumour cells after immunization in vivo, and low natural killer cell activity. After immunization with EL-4 allogenic lymphoma cells in vitro, no deficiency of T killer cell activity was observed, but a loss of relative increase in cells bearing Fc receptors was seen in spleen and lymph nodes (Fernandes et al., 1979).

In young NZB mice (six weeks of age), zinc deficiency had the most impact when it was instituted early in life and in animals fed the lowest levels of dietary zinc (5 and 2.5 ppm). Mice showed significantly higher packed cell volume and haemoglobin values and significantly reduced incidence and titre of anti-erythrocyte autoantibodies. Serum immuno-globulin levels decreased with advancing age; furthermore, there was an enhanced rate of survival. In older mice (six months of age), a delayed increase in anti-erythrocyte autoantibody and a significant influence on the levels of serum IgG1, IgG2a, and IgG2b contributed to an enhanced rate of survival. The signs of zinc deficiency included alopecia, exfoliative dermatitis, hypopigmentation, corneal opacity, oedema around the eyes and mouth and on the feet, and generally hyperactive behaviour (Beach et al., 1981).

Typical murine lupus characterized by anti-dsDNA antibodies, proteinuria, glomerulonephritis and 50% mortality at nine months of age were observed in young female NZB/W mice (six weeks of age) fed 9 or 100 ppm zinc, while mice fed 2.5 or 5 ppm zinc experienced a significant delay in the appearance and lower titres of antibodies to dsDNA, reduced proteinuria and prolonged life span, with 90% survival at ten months of age. All mice that were entered into the study at six months of age had established disease with initiation of the diets; zinc deprivation induced effects similar to those seen in young mice (Beach et al., 1982a).

Beach et al. (1982b) fed different levels of dietary zinc to female MRL/l mice beginning at either four or ten weeks of age. Mice that were entered into the study at four weeks and were fed 2.5 ppm zinc showed a lower incidence and titre of antibodies to dsDNA, less severe glomerulonephritis, and a better immune response than control animals. Survival was significantly prolonged. When zinc deprivation was induced at ten weeks of age, the beneficial effect on disease progression was small. Zinc deprivation at four or ten weeks of age resulted in a significantly greater reduction of lymphoproliferation.

Dietary exposure of adult mink to 1000 ppm zinc did not result in gross toxicity or copper deficiency (Bleavins et al., 1983). In the offspring of treated females, the blastogenic response of peripheral blood lymphocytes to concanavalin A in vitro was significantly lower than in controls. Approximately 14 weeks after weaning and consuming an unsupplemented basal diet, the lymphocyte response returned to normal.

The offspring of outbred Swiss Webster mice deprived of zinc (5 ppm dietary zinc) between days 7 and 20 of gestation showed an aberrant pattern of development of serum levels of IgG2a and IgA; only at six months of age were these concentrations similar to those in the offspring of control dams. IgG1 and IgG2b levels were within normal ranges by six weeks of age. Cross-fostering of zinc-deprived offspring to dams adequately nourished during pregnancy did little to ameliorate their aberrant pattern of serum immunoglobulin development. In F2 and F3 progeny, the defective maturation of serum IgG2a and IgA did not persist, but the offspring continued to have higher perinatal mortality (Beach et al., 1983).

Administration of zinc-deficient diet (0.6 ppm) to seven-week-old female A/J mice resulted in a decreased delayed-type hypersensitivity (DTH) reaction when the animals were sensitized percutaneously with dinitrofluorobenzene after 26 days. After three weeks of nutritional repletion with an adequate zinc diet (55 ppm), the DTH responses were nearly identical to those of control mice (Fraker et al., 1982).

When A/J mice were fed a zinc-deficient diet (1.6 ppm) on days 5-17 post partum, the suckling pups showed reduced body weights and produced only 44% and 49% as many antibody-producing cells per spleen as control pups in response to T-cell independent antigens (trinitrophenol-lipopolysaccharide and trinitrophenol-Ficoll). The relative avidities of the antibodies produced by pups were significantly lower and the responses to sheep red blood cells were 25-30% of the response of control pups, whether direct (IgM) or indirect (IgG) plaques were enumerated. The antibody-mediated response capacity returned to normal after a short period of zinc supplementation (Fraker et al., 1984).

In guinea-pigs fed a zinc-deficient diet (1.25 ppm), a significantly decreased ability to elicit a DTH response to sheep red blood cells on day 9 of immunization was observed. The animals showed a significant reduction in direct splenic plaque-forming cell response and haemagglutinating antibody titre. Zinc repletion resulted in marked, though incomplete, restoration of immunological responses (Verma et al., 1988).

Rodents made zinc-deficient were found to exhibit reduced levels of 'serum thymic factor', and the mitogenesis of peripheral blood lymphocytes was significantly suppressed in vitro (Depasquale-Jardieu & Fraker, 1979, 1980; Iwata et al., 1979; Chandra et al., 1980; Carlomagno & McMurray, 1983).

Kiremidjian-Schumacher et al. (1981a,b) reported that zinc chloride at a concentration of 1×10^{-3} to 1×10^{-6} M significantly interfered with the interaction between an antigen (ovalbumin) and the surface of sensitized guinea-pig spleen lymphocytes. It also inhibited the ability of sensitized lymphocytes to produce macrophage migration inhibitory factor and the motility of macrophages and decreased the effect of this factor on their migration.

Zinc at concentrations below $10^{-3.5}$ M was not significantly cytotoxic to macrophages from C57Bl/6J and A/J inbred mice, and at concentrations below 10^{-4} M it was not toxic to sarcoma I tumour cells. Macrophages from immunized C57Bl/6J mice were highly toxic to these cells at all zinc concentrations; the cytotoxicity indices were not significantly different from those in the control mice. At a concentration of 1×10^{-3} to 1×10^{-8} M, zinc had no significant effect on the ability of macrophages from immunized animals to kill sarcoma I cells (Nelson et al., 1982).

Splenic lymphocyte blastogenesis in response to concanavalin A and phytohaemagglutinin (PHA)-P was decreased in adult BALB/c mice that received a single intraperitoneal injection of 12 mg/kg body weight of zinc, while responses to lipopolysaccharide and pokeweed mitogen were initially depressed, subsequently increased, and finally declined sharply. Splenic B-cell colony formation decreased linearly in relation to zinc dosage, with 50% suppression observed at approximately 8 mg/kg bw, but bone-marrow granulocyte-macrophage colonies were enhanced at doses ≥ 2.5 mg/kg bw (Murray *et al.*, 1983).

Pretreatment of splenocytes from C3H/HeJ, CBA/Ca and BALB/c-nu/nu mice with non-toxic concentrations of zinc sulfate decreased lytic activity against YAC-1 and RDM4 target cells; the lytic function of non- and poly(I)•poly(C)-activated natural killer cells was similarly inhibited. A significant inhibition of natural killer lysis was noted, which was maximal after 30 min, when the interaction of effector cells with zinc was studied for 5 min. Lysis was completely suppressed after the addition of 10^{-4} M zinc sulfate, while the frequency of target-binding cells was inhibited only partly (Ferry & Donner, 1984).

Host resistance

McMurray and Yetley (1983) vaccinated groups of Hartley strain guinea-pigs with *Mycobacterium bovis* BCG and fed them on purified diets (10 or 30% protein combined with 50 ppm or no added zinc); animals were skin tested with purified protein derivative seven weeks later. Protein- and zinc-deficient animals showed significant growth retardation, and, in the two groups consuming the 10% protein diet, haematocrit, total serum proteins and spleen weight were significantly reduced. Protein deficiency with or without zinc-deficiency resulted in increased tissue levels of *M. bovis* BCG in the inguinal lymph nodes and subcutaneous vaccination nodule, and the DTH reaction was significantly impaired. In protein- and protein-zinc-deficient animals, phytohaemagglutinin polyclonal T-cell blastogenesis *in vitro* was significantly diminished in peripheral lymphocytes at low mitogen doses but only in the protein-zinc-deficient animals with higher doses of PHA. Feeding of a zinc-deficient diet to female Sprague-Dawley rats for eight or ten weeks, followed by experimental infection with *Listeria monocytogenes* five days prior to sacrifice, resulted in thymic atrophy, reduced DTH responses to *Listeria* antigen, and impaired lymphocyte response of spleen cells to PHA. A separate group of zinc-deficient rats was vaccinated with viable *L. monocytogenes* ten days prior to respiratory challenge; this resulted in successful control of bacteria (Carlomagno *et al.*, 1986).

Guinea-pigs were maintained for three weeks on purified diets (30% protein/50 ppm zinc; 10% protein/50 ppm zinc; or 30% protein/0 ppm zinc) and vaccinated with *L. monocytogenes* (2.5×10^3 cells intrapetironeally) after eight days of treatment. Ten days later, all animals received an aerosol challenge of 250 *L. monocytogenes* organisms and were killed four days later. Zinc and protein deficiency resulted in growth retardation, and vaccinated animals had impaired DTH reaction and loss of peripheral antigen-specific T lymphocyte function (Coghlan *et al.*, 1988).

EFFECTS ON HUMANS

Immunopathology

Recent reports describe immunopathological effects in humans following exposure to zinc by inhalation. Most of these lack information on both aerosol characteristics and possible confounding effects of other immunopathological exposures, so that they cannot prove that zinc is the specific causal agent.

Lange and Kirk (1986) reported two cases of bronchial asthma caused by exposure to zinc chloride smoke for approximately 75 min. One of the cases ended fatally, but both were complicated by advanced age and pre-existing heart and lung disease.

Malo and Cartier (1987), Kawane *et al.* (1988) and Weir *et al.* (1989) described cases of occupational asthma due to fumes from galvanized metals, with 'metal fume fever'-like symptoms. Environmental measurements revealed the presence of zinc from soldering on galvanized metal. In persons exposed to metal (zinc) fumes, the release of prostaglandins and leukotrienes from activated neutrophils, airway epithelial damage and release of histamine or histamine-like substances might be responsible for the development of asthma.

A 34-year old man who occasionally welded zinc showed an immediate anaphylactoid reaction and a delayed reaction consisting of urticaria and angioedema to zinc fumes, associated with a 'metal fume fever'-like reaction. On the basis of a challenge test, the conditions of which were not defined, the author concluded that the effect was due to zinc (Farrell, 1987). In general, symptoms occur 4-12 h after inhalation of zinc oxide and are characterized by rapid breathing, shivering, fever, sweating, chest and leg pain and weakness. The symptoms usually abate within 24-48 h and are not exacerbated by subsequent exposure within 48 h of the onset. This phenomenon has been termed 'tachyphylaxis' or 'quick immunity' (Bertholf, 1988).

Zinc deficiency can result in dwarfism, hypogonadism, hepatosplenomegaly and changes in alkaline phosphatase, similar to the effects seen in zinc-deficient animals. Nonspecific skin changes, such as roughened skin and hyperpigmentation on exposed areas, are commonly seen in dwarfs. An adrenal hypofunction may be due to pituitary or hypothalamic hypofunction resulting from zinc deficiency (Prasad et al., 1961, 1963).

Humoral-, cell-mediated and nonspecific immunity

Loss of reactivity in skin tests has been correlated with decreased levels of plasma zinc. Rapid conversion to a positive reaction was accomplished by oral or topical zinc therapy. In seven of ten malnourished children with low serum zinc levels, total anergy to skin test antigens has been reported (McMurray, 1984).

In a 17-year-old, partly decerebrated male with acquired zinc deficiency, skin reaction to dinitrochlorobenzene was negative, and the ability of lymphocytes to undergo blast transformation in response to mitogen stimulation was significantly depressed. Within three weeks after zinc therapy (22.7 mg/day), the patient demonstrated a positive delayed skin reaction to dinitrochlorobenzene and a normal lymphocyte response stimulation index (Pekarek et al., 1979).

Peripheral blood lymphocytes from persons aged 23-38 years stimulated with concanavalin A and PHA showed either no change or an enhancement of the mitogenic response, while blastogenesis by peripheral blood lymphocytes from persons aging 63-72 years was suppressed by zinc chloride at concentrations of 1×10^{-5} to 2×10^{-4} M (Rao et al., 1979).

Zinc sulfate (660 mg) given orally for one month to 83 normal subjects significantly increased the lymphocyte response to PHA and concanavalin A. The lymphocyte response was decreased in high responders and had an enhancing effect on low responders. Preliminary observations indicated that zinc interferes with the binding of transferrin to its specific receptors on lymphocytes. Before and after treatment, no correlation between lymphocyte response and serum zinc concentration was found (Duchateau et al., 1981).

Wagner et al. (1983) described an improved delayed dermal hypersensitivity in five anergic individuals aged 64-76 years following zinc supplementation (55 mg zinc per day for four weeks). Two cases of cutaneous generalized allergy (pruritus, urticaria and itching) due to zinc used in a diluting medium for Monotard® and protamine in an insulin preparation were reported by Bruni et al. (1986) and Gin and Aubertin (1987).

Within a ten-year period, eleven cases of multiple sclerosis occurred in a manufacturing plant where zinc was used, the observed disease incidence being greater than expected on the basis of population data (Stein et al., 1987).

Bogden et al. (1988) treated 103 apparently healthy elderly subjects aged 60-89 years with a placebo, with 15 mg zinc per day, or with 100 mg zinc per day for three months. Only in the 100-mg zinc group was the plasma zinc level significantly increased, but the delayed dermal hypersensitivity to seven antigens (tetanus, diphtheria, Streptococcus, tuberculin, Candida, Proteus and Trichophyton) and in-vitro lymphocyte proliferation responses to PHA, concanavalin A, pokeweed mitogen and antigens were not significantly altered by the treatment.

227

CONCLUSION

Although this review is not complete, it may be concluded from the information compiled that zinc has an immunotoxic impact in experimental animals. It is well documented that a diet deficient in zinc has an important effect on the activity of thymic hormone as well as on various metalloenzymes, whereas supplementation of zinc may interfere with other metals, thus exaggerating or inducing, e.g., copper deficiency. In particular, zinc alters humoral- and cell-mediated immunity, influences natural killer-cell activity, affects immunopathological parameters, and is effective in host resistance challenge models.

Human studies suggest an impact on humoral, cell-mediated and nonspecific immunity. Furthermore, occupational studies suggest an immunotoxic effect of airborne zinc. These studies must be confirmed, as insufficient information was available on the physical and chemical characteristics of the aerosol and on possible confounding effects of other immunotoxic exposures.

REFERENCES

Beach, R.S., Gershwin, M.E. & Hurley, L.S. (1980) Growth and development in postnatally zinc-deprived mice. *J. Nutr.*, **110**: 201-211

Beach, R.S., Gershwin, M.E. & Hurley, L.S. (1981) I. Immunopathology of zinc deprivation in New Zealand mice. *J. Immunol.*, **126**: 1999-2006

Beach, R.S., Gershwin, M.E. & Hurley, L.S. (1982a) II. Prolongation of survival in zinc-deprived NZB/W mice. *J. Immunol.*, **128**: 308-313

Beach, R.S., Gershwin, M.E. & Hurley, L.S. (1982b) III. Zinc deprivation versus restricted food intake in MRL/1 mice - the distinction between interacting dietary influences. *J. Immunol.*, **129**: 2686-2692

Beach, R.S., Gershwin, M.E. & Hurley, L.S. (1983) Persistent immunological consequences of gestation zinc deprivation. *Am. J. clin. Nutr.*, **38**: 579-590

Bertholf, R.L. (1988) Zinc. In: Seiler, H.G., Sigel, H. & Sigel, A., eds, *Handbook on Toxicity of Inorganic Compounds*, New York, Marcel Dekker, pp. 787-800

Bettger, W.J., Reeves, P.G., Moscatelli, E.A., Reynolds, G. & O'Dell, B.L. (1979) Interaction of zinc and essential fatty acids in the rat. *J. Nutr.*, **109**: 480-488

Bettger, W.J., Reeves, P.G., Moscatelli, E.A., Savage, J.E. & O'Dell, B.L. (1980) Interaction of zinc and polyunsaturated fatty acids in the chick. *J. Nutr.*, **110**: 50-58

Bleavins, M.R., Aulerich, R.J., Hochstein, J.R., Hornshaw, T.C. & Napolitano, A.C. (1983) Effects of excessive dietary zinc on the intrauterine and postnatal development of mink. *J. Nutr.*, **113**: 2360-2367

Bogden, J.D., Oleske, J.M., Lavenhar, M.A., Munves, E.M., Kemp, F.W., Bruening, K.S., Holding, K.J., Denny, T.N., Guarino, M.A., Krieger, L.M. & Holland, B.K. (1988) Zinc and immunocompetence in elderly people: effects of zinc supplementation for 3 months. *Am. J. clin. Nutr.*, **48**: 655-663

Breeze, R. (1985) Respiratory disease in adult cattle. *Vet. clin. North Am. Food Anim. Pract.*, **1**: 311-346

Bruni, B., Barolo, P., Gamba, S., Grassi, G. & Blatto, A. (1986) Case of generalized allergy due to zinc and protamine in insulin preparation. *Diabetic Care*, **9**: 552

Carlomagno, M.A. & McMurray, D.N. (1983) Chronic zinc deficiency in rats: its influence on some parameters of humoral and cell-mediated immunity. *Nutr. Res.*, **3**: 69-78

Carlomagno, M.A., Coghlan, L.G. & McMurray, D.N. (1986) Chronic zinc deficiency and listeriosis in rats: acquired cellular resistance and response to vaccination. *Med. Microbiol. Immunol.*, **175**: 271-280

Chandra, R.K., Heresi, G. & Au, B. (1980) Serum thymic factor activity in deficiences of calories, zinc, vitamin A and pyridoxine. *Clin. exp. Immunol.*, **42**: 332-335

Coghlan, L.G., Carlomagno, M.A. & McMurray, D.N. (1988) Effect of protein and zinc deficiencies on vaccine efficacy in guinea pigs following pulmonary infection with Listeria. *Med. Microbiol. Immunol.*, **177**: 255-263

Depasquale-Jardieu, P. & Fraker, P.J. (1979) The role of corticosterone in the loss in immune function in the zinc-deficient A/J mouse. *J. Nutr.*, **109**: 1847-1855

Depasquale-Jardieu, P. & Fraker, P.J. (1980) Further characterization of the role of corticosterone in the loss of humoral immunity in zinc-deficient A/J mice as determined by adrenalectomy. *J. Immunol.*, **124**: 2650-2655

Duchateau, J., Delespesse, G. & Vereecke, P. (1981) Influence of oral zinc supplementation on the lymphocyte response to mitogens of normal subjects. *Am. J. clin. Nutr.*, **34**: 88-93

Farrell, F.J. (1987) Angioedema and urticaria as acute and late phase reactions to zinc fume exposure, with associated metal fume fever-like symptoms. *Am. J. ind. Med.*, **12**: 331-337

Fernandes, G., Nair, M., Onoe, K., Tanaka, T., Floyd, R. & Good, R.A. (1979) Impairment of cell-mediated immunity functions by dietary zinc deficiency in mice. *Proc. natl Acad. Sci. USA*, **76**: 457-461

Ferry, F. & Donner, M. (1984) In vitro modulation of murine natural killer cytotoxicity by zinc. *Scand. J. Immunol.*, **19**: 435-445

Fraker, P. J., Zwickl, C.M. & Luecke, R.W. (1982) Delayed type hypersensitivity in zinc deficient adult mice: impairment and restoration of responsivity to dinitrofluorobenzene. *J. Nutr.*, **112**: 309-313

Fraker, P.J., Hildebrandt, K. & Luecke, R.W. (1984) Alteration of antibody-mediated responses of suckling mice to T-cell-dependent and independent antigens by maternal marginal zinc deficiency: restoration of responsivity by nutritional repletion. *J. Nutr.*, **114**: 170-179

Fraker, P.J., Gershwin, M.E., Good, R.A. & Prasad, A. (1986) Interrelationships between zinc and immune function. *Fed. Proc.*, **45**: 1474-1479

Gin, H. & Aubertin, J. (1987) Generalized allergy due to zinc and protamine in insulin preparation treated with insulin pump. *Diabetic Care.*, **10**: 789

Iwata, T., Incefy, G.S., Tanaka, T., Fernandes, G., Menendez-Botet, C.J., Pih, K. & Good, R.A. (1979) Circulating thymic hormone levels in zinc deficiency. *Cell. Immunol.*, **47**: 100-105

Kawane, H., Soejima, R., Umeki, S. & Niki, Y. (1988) Metal fume fever and asthma. *Chest*, **93**: 1116

Kiremidjian-Schumacher, L., Stotzky, G., Dickstein, R.A. & Schwartz, J. (1981a) Influence of cadmium, lead, and zinc on the ability of guinea pig macrophages to interact with macrophage migration inhibitory factor. *Environ. Res.*, **24**: 106-116

Kiremidjian-Schumacher, L., Stotzky, G., Likhite, V., Schwartz, J. & Dickstein, R.A. (1981b) Influence of cadmium, lead, and zinc on the ability of sensitized guinea pig lymphocytes to interact with specific antigen and to produce lymphokine. *Environ. Res.*, **24**: 96-105

Lam, H.F., Conner, M.W., Rogers, A.E., Fitzgerald, S. & Amdur, M.O. (1985) Functional and morphologic changes in the lungs of guinea pigs exposed to freshly generated ultrafine zinc oxide. *Toxicol. appl. Pharmacol.*, **78**: 29-38

Lange, B. & Kirk, N.U. (1986) Bronchial asthma precipitated by zinc chloride smoke. *Ugeskr-Laeger.*, **148**: 455

Luecke, R.W. & Fraker, P.J. (1979) The effect of varying dietary zinc levels on growth and antibody-mediated response in two strains of mice. *J. Nutr.*, **109**: 1373-1376

Luecke, R.W., Simonel, C.E. & Fraker, P.J. (1978) The effect of restricted dietary intake on the antibody mediated response of the zinc deficient A/J mouse. *J. Nutr.*, **108**: 881-887

Malo, J.-L. & Cartier, A. (1987) Occupational asthma due to fumes of galvanized metal. *Chest*, **92**: 375-377

McMurray, D.N. (1984) Cell-mediated immunity in nutritional deficiency. *Prog. Food nutr. Sci.*, **8**: 193-228

McMurray, D. N. & Yetley, E. A. (1983) Response to mycobacterium bovis BCG vaccination in protein- and zinc-deficient guinea pigs. *Infect. Immun.*, **39**: 755-761

Murray, M.J., Wilson, F.D., Fisher, G.L. & Erickson, K.L. (1983) Modulation of murine lymphocyte and macrophage proliferation by parenteral zinc. *Clin. exp. Immunol.*, **53**: 744-749

Nelson, D.J., Kiremidjian-Schumacher, L. & Stotzky, G. (1982) Effects of cadmium, lead, and zinc on macrophage-mediated cytotoxicity toward tumor cells. *Environ. Res.*, **28**: 154-163

Pekarek, R.S., Sandstead, H.H., Jacob, R.A. & Barcome, D.F. (1979) Abnormal cellular immune responses during acquired zinc deficiency. *Am. J. clin. Nutr.*, **32**: 1466-1471

Prasad, A.S., Halsted, J.A. & Nadimi, M. (1961) Syndrome of iron deficiency anemia, hepatosplenomegaly, hypogonadism, dwarfism and geophagia. *Am. J. Med.*, **31**: 532-546

Prasad, A.S., Miale, A., Jr, Farid, Z., Sandstead, H.H., Schulert, A.R. & Darby, W.J. (1963) Biochemical studies on dwarfism, hypogonadism, and anemia. *Arch. intern. Med.*, **111**: 65-86

Rao, K.M.K., Schwartz, S.A. & Good, R.A. (1979) Age-dependent effects of zinc on the transformation response of human lymphocytes to mitogenes. *Cell. Immunol.*, **42**: 270-278

Stein, E.C., Schiffer, R.B., Hall, W.J. & Young, N. (1987) Multiple sclerosis and the workplace: report of an industry-based cluster. *Neurology.*, **37**: 1672-1677

Straube, E.F., Schuster, N.H. & Sinclair, A.J. (1980) Zinc toxicity in the ferret. *J. comp. Pathol.*, **90**: 355-361

Verma, P.C., Gupta, R.P., Sadana, J.R. & Gupta, R.K.P. (1988) Effect of experimental zinc deficiency and repletion on some immunological variables in guinea-pigs. *Br. J. Nutr.*, **59**: 149-154

Van Campen, D.R. (1966) Effects of zinc, cadmium, silver and mercury on the absorption and distribution of copper-64 in rats. *J. Nutr.*, **88**: 125-130

Wagner, P.A., Jernigan, J.A., Bailey, L.B., Nickens, C. & Brazzi, G.A. (1983) Zinc nutriture and cell-mediated immunity in the aged. *Int. J. Vit. Nutr. Res.*, **53**: 94-101

Weir, D.C., Robertson, A.S., Jones, S. & Burge, P.S. (1989) Occupational asthma due to soft corrosive soldering fluxes containing zinc chloride and ammonium chloride. *Thorax*, **44**: 220-223

INVESTIGATIONS OF IMMUNOTOXICITY

IMMUNOTOXICOLOGY: FUNCTIONAL CHANGES

L.D. Koller

College of Veterinary Medicine, Oregon State University
Corvallis, Oregon 97331-4802, USA

ABSTRACT

The field of immunotoxicology has undergone considerable growth and expansion since its inception in the early 1970s. The discipline was founded by combining knowledge from the areas of immunology and toxicology and by ascertaining the effect xenobiotics exert on the functioning immune system. The field has progressed through a series of stages that include initial identification of immunotoxic chemicals, development of sensitive, quantitative assays to assess chemically induced immunomodulation, and determination of the mechanism by which xenobiotics compromise immune function. Immunoassays have been successfully developed and modified to characterize the immunotoxic properties of xenobiotics. Acceptable immunotoxicological procedures are available to assess modulation of humoral immunity, cell-mediated immunity, macrophage function, natural killer cell cytotoxicity and cytokine activity. These procedures, coupled with recent developments in monoclonal antibody technology and advances in cell culture techniques and immunology, are available to immunotoxicologists to probe the biomolecular actions of drugs and chemicals objectively. Clinical immunologists and immunotoxicologists/pharmacologists must be aware, however, that some immune assays currently employed do not measure immune function. These procedures are used to enumerate cells, identify subpopulations and evaluate the ability of cells to divide, but not to assess the true functional capacity of such cells. The relevance and application of assessing immune function is presented.

IMMUNE SYSTEM

The immune system is extremely complex and sophisticated. It is composed of a network of organs, tissues, cells and cellular products that act in unison to protect the living organism against invasion by infectious and neoplastic agents. This system, which is dispersed throughout the body of living organisms, regulates defence mechanisms by recognizing and subsequently responding to the altered antigenic composition of the body. Therefore, the regulatory events of the immune system identify foreign 'non-self' antigens, such as microorganisms and neoplastic cells, to successfully destroy and eliminate them from the body. A delicate balance must be maintained for optimal performance.

The immune system is regulated by multiple chemical signals that operate at different levels. Antigens trigger the release of local chemical signals, which, in turn, incite a network of responding cells throughout the body. A typical cascade of immunological events following antigenic stimulation might include initial expression of Ia molecules on the surface of macrophages and activation and production of interleukin 1 (IL-1). T Lymphocytes are activated by antigen, Ia and IL-1 to produce IL-2, which mediates the proliferation of T-helper lymphocytes that produce other lymphokines which stimulate B lymphocytes to proliferate and differentiate into antibody-producing plasma cells or memory B lymphocytes. Thus, the overall responsiveness of the system is controlled by modulations of immunocytes and their secretory products.

Immunotoxicity of Metals and Immunotoxicology, Edited by
A. D. Dayan *et al.*, Plenum Press, New York, 1990

Four major classes of immunocytes have been identified to date, including B and T lymphocytes, macrophages and natural killer (NK) cells. The B lymphocytes are the primary effector cells for humoral immunity, i.e., antibody production. They generally require regulation by T helper cells and macrophages for optimal response to most antigens. T Lymphocytes are composed of both effector and regulator subsets, which can be divided into at least two subpopulations on the basis of function and phenotype. These subpopulations include the cytotoxic and delayed-type hypersensitive-reactive T lymphocytes. Effector T cells are responsible for cell-mediated immunity and act *via* cell-to-cell contact. Regulatory T lymphocytes are divided into T helper and T suppressor subsets on the basis of phenotype and regulatory activity. L3T4 (CD4 in humans) and Lyt1$^+$ antigens serve as phenotypic surface markers for the T cells responsible for helper activity, mixed lymphocyte reactions and cutaneous hypersensitivity in mice, whereas Lyt23$^+$ (CD8 in humans) is the surface molecule expressed on T suppressor and cytotoxic T lymphocytes. T Lymphocytes also synthesize and secrete numerous lymphokines, which act as immuno-hormones; two of the most prominent lymphokines are interferon-γ and IL-2.

Macrophages, which are also composed of both effector and regulator subpopulations, phagocytize, process and transfer antigenic information to other immunocytes, particularly T lymphocytes. Macrophages also produce and secrete numerous monokines. Two of the most reactive monokines are IL-1 and prostaglandin E$_2$. These cytokines act on activated effector immunocytes in an interrelated manner to regulate the magnitude of the ongoing immune response.

NK cells are morphologically classified as large granular lymphocytes, but, unlike other lymphocytes, can react immediately without prior antigenic sensitization. Therefore, NK cells serve as a first line of defence against infectious agents and neoplastic events. They also produce and secrete lymphokines, such as interferon and IL-2, which may serve as a feedback mechanism to turn off antibody production of B lymphocytes (Abruzzo & Rowley, 1983).

Another population of immunocytes which has recently received considerable attention are lymphokine activated killer cells. Peripheral blood lymphocytes cultured in the presence of IL-2, in the absence of antigen or mitogen, stimulate predominately CD-16 (Leu 19)-positive lymphocytes to express nonrestrictive cytolytic activity (Ortaldo & Longo, 1988). These cells, of heterogenous phenotype, are defined primarily by their unique cytotoxic function - to lyse tumour cells. These unique killer cells are distinct from cytotoxic lymphocytes and NK cells and possess strong antitumour activity both *in vitro* and *in vivo*. Lymphokine activated killer cells have chemotherapeutic value in the treatment of some tumours.

The immune system is extremely sophisticated and is both intraregulated and interregulated. Immunocytes, orchestrated by their secretory products, act in a network fashion for optimal performance. Although the immune system was long considered to be autonomous in both regulation and action, recent data suggest that a significant reciprocal interaction occurs between the nervous, endocrine and immune systems (Besedovsky *et al.*, 1984; Blalock, 1984a,b; Martin, 1984). For instance, some classical neuroendocrine hormones and neurotransmitters possess immunomodulatory activity, whereas immunocytokine hormones share common receptors with the central nervous system and function as endocrine glands (Blalock, 1984 a,b). These interregulatory patterns confirm the existence of a nervous-endocrine-immune axis, which complicates the researcher's attempt to duplicate whole-body system responses *in vitro*. Therefore, intact animal systems are essential for an accurate assessment of the immunotoxic potential of xenobiotics.

IMMUNOTOXICOLOGY

Immunotoxicology originated in the early 1970s when immunologists and toxicologists began investigating the immunotoxic potential of prominent environmental chemicals such as the polychlorinated biphenyls and lead (Vos, 1977; Koller, 1979). From these early studies, it became apparent that chemicals known to be ubiquitous in the environment could compromise immunity in animals. Thus, the stage was set for a new discipline, presently known as immunotoxicology. The adverse immune effects exerted by chemicals were confirmed when exposure to these agents resulted in increased susceptibility of the host to infectious agents. These initial discoveries provided the foundation for the development of modern immunotoxicology as a prominent discipline shared with immuno-pharmacology.

After it was recognized that chemicals could modulate immunity, conventional immunoassays were adopted to assess chemical-induced immune dysfunction. These assays generally included evaluation of humoral- and cell-mediated immune responses as well as macrophage activity. In addition, animals exposed to chemicals for prolonged periods were frequently challenged with an infectious agent to assess resistance to infections.

During the past decade, a number of immunoassays have been developed and adapted to test for the immunotoxicity of chemical agents. Some of these procedures include responses to mitogens, antibody-producing plaque-forming cells, enzyme-linked immunosorbent assay (ELISA), radioimmunoassay, delayed-type hypersensitivity, mixed lymphocyte reaction, lymphocyte cytotoxicity, T helper:T suppressor-cell ratios, NK cell cytotoxicity, bone-marrow progenitor cells, cytokine activity and several host-resistant assays. The discovery of monoclonal antibodies has stimulated interest in flow cytometry and immunocytochemistry. Many of these procedures have been validated as acceptable assays to assess chemical-induced immune dysfunction (Luster et al., 1988).

Immunotoxicology gained credibility when it was confirmed that some chemicals, such as pentachlorophenol (Kerkvliet et al., 1982), lead (Koller et al., 1983), toxaphene (Allen et al., 1982) and polychlorinated biphenyls (Koller et al., 1983), produce immunosuppression at doses lower than those that alter other known, commonly used toxicological indices. This feature revealed that the immune system was indeed a sensitive indicator of perturbation by chemicals and that the ensuing immunosuppression could not only render an animal susceptible to infectious agents but could also contribute to an increased risk for cancer. There is substantial evidence that immunocompromised individuals are highly susceptible to some forms of cancer. This is exemplified by Kaposi's sarcoma, which occurs in patients with acquired immune deficiency syndrome (Safai et al., 1985).

Most chemicals target a specific organ within the body. Toxicologists, pathologists and clinicians have used this characteristic to diagnose, treat and ascertain the biological mechanism by which a chemical produces toxicosis. Thus, the symptoms and pathology associated with a chemical that is primarily hepatotoxic are expressed in those parameters used to detect injury to the liver. The immune system, however, is distributed throughout the body in cells, tissues, organs and the circulating blood and lymph. Therefore, different components can be exposed to the parent chemical and its metabolite(s) systemically at different sites throughout the body. This factor in itself indicates that the immune system is a highly sensitive organ for detecting toxicosis.

The impact of toxic substances on human immune function is virtually unknown. There is, however, documented evidence that exposure to chemicals such as polychlorinated and polybrominated biphenyls and lead suppresses immune responses in man (Bekesi et al., 1978; Sachs, 1978; Bekesi et al., 1983; Ewers et al., 1984; Lui & Wong, 1984). The continued development of new clinical immunological techniques to assess immune function in man will facilitate accumulation of the data needed to evaluate chemically induced immune dysfunction in man.

MECHANISMS OF IMMUNOTOXICOLOGY

Immunotoxicology is a science that explores the effects of physical and chemical agents and other toxic substances on the immune system. The founding years of the discipline were devoted primarily to identifying immunotoxic chemicals and to developing a battery of sensitive, quantitative immunoassays. Much of the research carried out during the past few years, however, has concentrated on investigating the mechanisms by which immunotoxic chemicals compromise immune function.

Because optimal performance of the immune system is dependent upon a cascade of immune events, disruption of any one of the components of this circuit can alter the immune response. Interference in the early stages of the immune sequence might be suspected to result in a generalized effect on immune function; however, occasionally, a chemical will elicit a more selective response within this chain of events because it exerts a more specific effect directly on an immunocyte or a particular subset of cells. Thus, the response may range from highly selective to generalized. These features account, at least in part, for the lack of the typical linear dose-response curve that is normally observed in standard toxicological procedures.

The mechanisms of immunity are extremely complex. A complete immunological paradigm would include assessment of several compartments of the immune response, including humoral immunity, cell-mediated immunity, macrophage activity, NK cell cytotoxicity, cytokine production/activity and other associated immunoregulators. Chemicals can compromise one or several reactive sites within the immune network. The actual mechanistic effect, however, may occur by an alteration of internal cell structures, membranes, surface antigens and/or a variety of receptors. Chemicals may alter the composition of these structures, bind to or block their activity, or interfere with numerous putative nonimmune regulators required for activation, differentiation, proliferation and normal development of immune responsiveness.

ASSESSMENT OF IMMUNOTOXICITY

Advances in biotechnology and the development of animal models have improved the process of interpreting and extrapolating data from laboratory animals to man. Many of the procedures utilized for immunotoxicity assessment are reproducible, quantitative and highly sensitive for detecting chemically induced immune dysregulation. It is universally accepted that the immune systems of some animals and man are comparable, that animal models are available to assess immune dysfunction objectively, that positive immunosuppressants such as cyclophosphamide and corticosteroids can be used to validate assays, and that data obtained in animals can be verified in man. Although the principles and phenomena in man and animals are basically similar and comparable, it is recognized that variations in these responses can occur between species.

A myriad of immunoassays has been developed to assess the integrity of the immune system both *in vivo* and *in vitro*. Most immunotoxicologists agree that a panel of immunoassays should include procedures to assess humoral immunity, cell-mediated immunity, macrophage function, pathotoxicological examination of lymphoid tissues, and host resistance to an infectious and/or oncogenic agent. More recently, this panel has been expanded to include NK cell cytotoxicity and the production and activity of numerous regulatory cytokines.

Animal models have been used successfully during this century to develop methods of diagnosis, prevention and treatment of human disease. Two laboratory animals, the mouse (Buck *et al.*, 1985) and the rat (Exon *et al.*, 1984, 1989) have been proposed as models for assessing xenobiotic-induced immunotoxicity. Each species has certain advantages and disadvantages; however, this subject deserves considerable attention and will not be discussed here.

Several laboratories have proposed multitiered approaches to evaluating the immunotoxic potential of xenobiotics. The initial tier generally includes nonspecific but quantitative procedures to assess the major compartments of the immune system. Other tiers are designed to evaluate specifically, in greater detail, those compartments of the immune response which, in tier 1, were identified as being affected by the test chemical. Thus, a comprehensive immune profile can be characterized for each agent tested.

IMMUNE FUNCTION

Frequently, basic scientists focus on a narrow subject and attack a problem using a funnel approach, with the ultimate goal of identifying the actual mechanism responsible for the condition. During this process, however, and occasionally when the mechanism is identified, these individuals are unprepared to apply this new-found knowledge. Application of basic information sometimes requires specialized expertise removed from the expertise of the scientist who discovered the actual underlying cause of the condition. Clinical immunologists, immunotoxicologists and pharmacologists are not exempt from this phenomenon. These scientists frequently use, modify and/or adapt immune assays and basic information that is developed by others. Application of this knowledge prevents duplication of effort and provides an avenue for transfer of information that can be used in a pragmatic manner. It is the responsibility of the clinical immunologists, immunotoxicologists and pharmacologists to utilize this new biotechnology in a way that will contribute to the diagnosis, control, prevention, treatment and eventually, eradication of immune-related diseases. In addition, these individuals must continue to advance the state-of-the-art of their respective disciplines not only by using the tools provided by basic science but also by pursuing the discovery process themselves. This collaboration and rapid exchange of knowledge will facilitate success in our conquest of many diseases that are prevalent in our societies today.

The chasm between the basic and applied sciences is occasionally quite large. The clinical immunologist has successfully used much of the information provided from basic research, but in some areas tools are not available to assess immune function in humans. Procedures that are developed in animals or *in vitro* frequently are not adaptable to humans, while others have yet to be developed for humans. These problems have frustrated many clinical immunologists, who have therefore been compelled to use many less-than-ideal immune procedures to evaluate immune reactivity in humans. It is not uncommon for physicians to request an immune profile for a patient. The principal problems that confront the physician regarding the immune status of a patient are: what do the values mean, how can they be interpreted, what is their relevance to the condition in question, are the results reliable, and do they actually measure immune function? The remainder of this article will deal predominantly with the last issue - immune function.

Immune function can be defined as the normal, special or proper action of immunocytes and their secretory products. The principal word in this definition is 'action'. Action may be expressed by a macrophage phagocytizing foreign debris; B lymphocytes producing antibody that neutralizes foreign antigen; T lymphocytes, NK or lmphokine activated killer cells killing tumour cells; or a number of the cytokines catalysing certain segments of immune circuits. Other immune parameters do not, in my opinion, constitute immune function. Some of the commonly used immune assays will be evaluated for characteristics applicable to immune function.

A variety of procedures has been used to assess humoral immunity. Techniques for measuring antibody titres to numerous microorganisms have been used for decades to ascertain the stage of infection as well as degree of immunity. Two procedures commonly utilized by immunotoxicologists are the plaque-forming cell and ELISA. The ELISA detects the amount of specific antibody produced that combines with the inciting antigen to 'neutralize' that antigen. The plaque-forming cell assay, on the other hand, indicates the number of cells that synthesize antibody but does not allow quantification of the amount of specific antibody produced. In many disease processes, the antigen is an infectious agent that frequently requires combination with high-affinity/high-avidity antibody to destroy it effectively.

Two cell-mediated assays used in immunotoxicology include a delayed-type hypersensitivity procedure and the mixed lymphocyte reaction. The first is an in-vivo inflammatory reaction that emulates cellular immunity. Xenobiotics can significantly alter the degree of the reaction. The mixed lymlphatic reaction is an in-vitro reaction that allows an assessment of the ability of a recipient to destroy cells of a donor. 'Like' cells are not be destroyed, while dissimilar, histocompatible cells are killed. The reaction involves T helper and suppressor cells as well as cytotoxic T lymphocytes. The procedure can be used to assess immune function *in vitro*, which may not entirely emulate in-vivo reactions.

Macrophage phagocytosis and most digestion procedures can be used to assess immune function, as can evaluation of cytotoxic macrophage activity. The inherent problem of phagocytic procedures is that the macrophage seems to be able to withstand considerable insult before its ability to engulf foreign material is impaired. Other cytotoxicity testing procedures, such as the NK, lymphokine activated killer and antibody-dependent cell tests are functional assays.

Most cytokines serve as essential catalysts in immune circuits, and, therefore, significant changes in levels of these immunohormones can have a major impact on the ensuing immune response. Many lymphokines (interferon, IL-2, IL-3, IL-4, IL-5, IL-6, etc.) and monokines (IL-1, prostaglandin E_2, tumour necrosis factor) synthesized by their respective immunocytes are necessary for an optimal immune response. Immune dysfunction results if abnormal levels are present. These products are regulatory in nature.

Mitogen assays are probably the most misrepresented immune assays and do not provide a measure of immune function. Mitogens (such as concanavalin A, phytohaemagglutinin and lipopolysaccharide) stimulate cells to divide and do not ascertain the ability of the divided cell to function, i.e., perform its immune function. Further, a specific subpopulation of cells may be affected while others are unaffected. Finally, mitogen responses occasionally do not correlate with the results of other reliable assays representative of the same compartment of immune response. Thus, the validity of mitogen responses as a correlate of immunity is questionable.

Antigens on the surface of immunocytes are usually specific for identifying subpopulations of cells. Immunocytes can be analysed easily in flow cytometers using monoclonal antibodies to count and separate individual cell types. This method permits enumeration of cell types in a given specimen (peripheral blood, spleen, lymph node) and can be used to determine normal ranges of cell populations in various tissues and organs. Although this method can be used to enumerate cells, it does not test their functional capacity.

The catchword today is 'receptors'. Frequently, surface receptors must be expressed for the cell to become activated. For instance, IL-2 receptor (IL-2R) expression is associated with activation of mature T lymphocytes. Expression of the IL-2R promotes T-cell cycle progression, which is vital for an optimal immune response; however, it is not clear at this time if IL-2R expression on lymphocytes reflects immune function. For example, more than 50% of L3T4$^-$/Lyt2$^-$ fetal (immature) thymocytes express IL-2R; T cells from patients with primary or secondary immunodeficiency can be induced to express IL-2R; glucocorticoids prevent IL-2 production but do not prevent IL-2R expression; and cyclosporin A inhibits T-cell IL-2 gene expression (IL-2 production is inhibited) but does not prevent IL-2R expression. These examples indicate that IL-2R expression does not represent, in all instances, functional activity of the lymphocyte. Additional information is necessary to characterize fully and to comprehend the implication of IL-2R expression on lymphocytes.

Clinical immunologists, immunotoxicologists and pharmacologists have many tools available to them but must understand that some of the procedures that are easy to perform (mitogens and flow cytometry) frequently do not yield the information desired. Nevertheless, the value of these procedures lies in the fact that significant, consistent changes should stimulate further interest to substantiate an effect. Should a positive correlation exist between nonfunctional and functional parameters, repetition of the correlation will confirm that the nonfunctional indices actually represent a functional change. This feature is obvious in acquired immunodeficiency syndrome in humans. T Helper cells are destroyed by a retrovirus, resulting in an inverted ratio of helper to suppressor T cells. These values are not necessarily diagnostic in themselves but indicate that an abnormality exists and that further tests should be performed to diagnose the disease.

Dr William E. Paul, in his presidential address to the American Association of Immunologists in 1987, alerted the profession to the void in knowledge concerning immune function. 'And yet, our knowledge of how the immune system actually functions is very primitive. We are only at the very beginning of the understanding of the physiologic rules of immunity.'

REFERENCES

Abruzzo, L.V. & Rowley, D.A. (1983) Homeostasis of the antibody response: immunoregulation by NK cells. *Science*, **222**: 151-155

Allen A.C., Koller, L.D. & Pollock, G.A. (1982) Effect of toxaphene exposure on immune responses in mice. *J. Toxicol. environ. Health*, **11**: 61-69

Bekesi, J.G., Holland, J.F., Anderson, H.A., Fishbein, A., Rom, W., Wolff, M.S. & Selikoff, I.J. (1978) Lymphocyte function of Michigan dairy farmers exposed to polybrominated biphenyls. *Science*, **199**: 1207-1209

Bekesi, J.G., Roboz, J.P., Solomon, S., Fishbein, A., Roboz, J. & Selikoff, I.J. (1983) Altered immune function in Michigan residents exposed to polybrominated biphenyls. In: Gibson, G.G. Hubbard, R. & Parke, D.V., eds, *Immunotoxicology*, London, Academic Press

Besedovsky, H., Del Rey, A. & Sarkin, E. (1984) Immunoregulation by neuroendocrine mechanisms. In: Behan, P. & Spreafico, F., eds, *Neuroimmunology*, New York, Raven Press

Blalock, J.E. (1984a) The immune system as a sensory organ. *J. Immunol.*, **132**: 1067-1070

Blalock, J.E. (1984b) Relationships between neuroendocrine hormones and lymphokines. *Lymphokines*, **9**: 1-13

Buck, P.H., Holsapple, M.P. & White, K.L. (1985) Assessment of the effect of chemicals on the immune system. In: Li, A.P., ed., *New Approaches in Toxicity Testing and Their Application in Human Risk Assessment*, New York, Raven Press

Ewers, U., Stiller-Winkler, R. & Idel, H. (1984) Serum immunoglobulin, complement C3, and salivary IgA levels in lead workers. *Environ. Res.*, **29**: 351-357

Exon, J.H., Koller, L.D., Henningsen, G.M. & Osborne, C.A. (1984) Multiple immunoassay in a single animal: a practical approach to immunotoxicologic testing. *Fundam. appl. Toxicol.*, **4**: 278-283

Exon, J.H., Koller, L.D., Talcott, P.A., O'Reilly, C.A. & Henningsen, G.M. (1989) Immunotoxicity testing: an economical multiple assay approach. *Fundam. appl. Toxicol.* (in press)

Kerkvliet, N.I., Beacher-Steppan, L., Claycomb, A.T., Craig, A.M. & Sheggeby, G.G. (1982) Immunotoxicity of technical pentachlorophenol (PCP-T): depressed hormonal immune responses to T-dependent and T-independent antigen stimulation in PCP-T exposed mice. *Fundam. appl. Toxicol.*, **2**: 90

Koller, L.D. (1979) Effects of environmental chemicals on the immune system. *Adv. vet Sci. comp. Med.*, **23**: 367-395

Koller, L.D., Exon, J.H. & Moore, S.A. (1983) Evaluation of ELISA for detecting *in vivo* chemical immunomodulation. *J. Toxicol. environ. Health*, **11**: 15-22

Lui, Y.-C. & Wong, P.-N. (1984) Dermatological, medical, laboratory findings of patients in Taiwan and their treatments. *Am. J. ind. Med.*, **5**: 81-115

Luster, M.I., Munson, A.E., Thomas, P.T., Holsapple, M.P., Fenters, J.D., White, K.L., Jr, Lauer, J.D., Germolec, D.R., Rosenthal, G.J. & Dean, J.H. (1988) Development of a testing battery to assess chemical-induced immunotoxicity: National Toxicology Program guidelines for immunotoxicity evaluation in mice. *Fundam. appl. Toxicol.*, **10**: 2-19

Martin, J.B. (1984) Neuroendocrine regulatin of the immune response. In: Behan, P. & Spreafico, F., eds, *Neuroimmunology*, New York, Raven Press

Ortaldo, J.R. & Longo, D.L. (1988) Human natural lymphocyte effector cells: definition, analysis of activity, and clinical effectiveness. *J. natl Cancer Inst.*, **80**: 999-1010

Sachs, H.K. (1978) Intercurrent infection in lead poisoning. *Am. J. Dis. Child.*, **132**: 315-316

Safai, B., Johnson, K.G., Myskowski, P.L., *et al.* (1985) The natural history of Kaposis' sarcoma in the acquired immunodeficiency syndrome. *Ann. int. Med.*, **103**: 744-750

Vos, J.G. (1977) Immune suppression as related to toxicology. *CRC crit Rev. Toxicol.*, **5**: 67-101

THE IMMUNE SYSTEM AS A TARGET FOR TOXICITY:
A TIERED APPROACH TO TESTING,
WITH SPECIAL EMPHASIS ON HISTOPATHOLOGY

M.A.M. Krajnc-Franken[1], H. Van Loveren[1], H.J. Schuurman[1,2] & J.G.Vos[1]

[1]Laboratory for Pathology, National Institute of Public Health
and Environmental Protection, 3720 BA Bilthoven; and
[2]Department of Internal Medicine and Pathology
University Hospital, 3508 GA Utrecht, The Netherlands

ABSTRACT

A tiered approach with panels of tests is employed to identify and characterize the immunotoxicity of environmental chemicals in rats. The first-tier screening includes general parameters of the specific and nonspecific defence potential, such as weight and histopathological appearance of the lymphoid organs, and serum immunoglobulin concentrations. When there are indications of immunotoxicity, the compound is further explored in the series of assays of the second tier, which comprises immune function studies of nonspecific defence mechanisms, cellular immunity and humoral immunity, including host-resistance models. Finally, in-vitro test systems may be considered a third tier of screening. In this report, after a short description of the microscopic and biological features of thymus, spleen, lymph nodes and mucosa-associated lymphoid tissues, some examples of immunotoxic compounds are given as assessed in both the first and the second tier. Special emphasis is placed on histopathological alterations induced by such immunotoxicants.

INTRODUCTION

In toxicological studies following subacute or semichronic exposure to xenobiotics, the immune system often turns out to be the target organ. The discipline that is concerned with the study of the events that can lead to undesired effects as a consequence of interaction of xenobiotics with the immune system is designated immunotoxicology and was defined as such at an international workshop held in Luxembourg in autumn 1984. The undesirable effects may result from the direct or indirect action of the xenobiotic or its biotransformation product on the immune system or an immunobiological host response to the compound or its metabolite(s), or host antigens modified by the compounds or its metabolites. The discipline of immunotoxicology can be subdivided into four specialities: (i) study of the altered immunological events associated with exposure of humans or animals to xeno-biotics, including drugs administered to produce immunomodulation; (ii) study of altered immune events that may follow exposure to immunotherapeutic agents; (iii) study of allergy and autoimmunity resulting from exposure to xenobiotics (including drugs); and (iv) development and application of immunological techniques and approaches in toxicology (Berlin et al., 1987).

IMMUNOTOXICITY ASSESSMENT; CHOICE OF ANIMAL SPECIES AND SCREENING TEST PROCEDURES

In general toxicity studies, the toxicological profile of a compound is ascertained in multidose four-week or three-month experiments, yielding a range between a high dose causing overt toxicity and a low dose with no observable effect. This no-effect level for the experimental animal can be used as a first step for human risk assessment. In these studies, the rat is the species most frequently used. Therefore, at our institute, this experimental animal was also selected for immunotoxicity testing, thus enabling comparisons with data on general toxicity. Moreover, in an international workshop held in London in autumn 1986, the rat was recommended as the main experimental animal for immunotoxicity testing (International Programme on Chemical Safety, 1986).

A tiered approach with panels of tests is employed to identify and characterize the immunotoxicity of environmental chemicals, so that the performance and nature of the second-tier panel is determined by the outcome of the preceding panel. Overall, this tiered system consists of three screening test procedures. In the first-tier screening, a set of general parameters of the specific and nonspecific defence potential is used (Table 1). First indications of chemically induced modifications of the immune system may be obtained from weight changes and histopathological alterations of the lymphoid organs. Routine histological staining procedures, such as haematoxylin and eosin staining of formalin-fixed and paraffin-embedded tissue sections, are very useful in assessing the immunotoxicity of a chemical, in particular when histopathological appearances are related to the effect on the weight of the lymphoid organs. Because of the structural separation of spleen and lymphoid nodes into thymus-dependent and thymus-independent areas, indications regarding the relative effects of the chemicals on T- and B-cell compartments can be obtained. Depending on the route of exposure to the test compounds, it may be necessary to examine mucosa-associated lymphoid tissues, including bronchus-associated, gut-associated and the recently described nasal lymphoid tissue (Spit et al., 1989); these tissues also show T-/B-cell compartmentalization.

Since bone marrow constitutes an essential component of the immune system, with pluripotent stem cells capable of differentiating into all types of leukocytes, morphological examination of this tissue is a prerequisite. Microscopy can be performed on tissue sections, marrow smears or cytocentrifuged preparations of cells collected from the marrow. In immunotoxicity assessment, bone-marrow cellularity has been designated as a sensitive indicator of toxicity (Luster et al., 1980).

In inhalation toxicity studies, enumeration and characterization of cells obtained by bronchoalveolar lavage is a good quantitative method (Bingham et al., 1972).

Apart from differential enumeration of white blood cells, tier I includes the analysis of serum. Levels of serum immunoglobulins, notably IgM, IgG and IgA, can be established with the very sensitive 'sandwich' enzyme-linked immunosorbent assay (Vos et al., 1979a, 1982).

When in the first-tier experiment a compound is suspected of having effects on the immune system at a relevant dose, i.e., a dose that causes no overt toxicity, this potential immunotoxicity can be confirmed or further analysed with material from the same experiment by more sophisticated and sensitive techniques such as (immuno)-histochemistry. In general, immunohistochemical methods have the advantage that many antigens can be demonstrated through antigen-antibody reactions using a marker conjugated to the antibody. The aim of these methods is to achieve intense staining with minimal background, and sufficient sensitivity to stain the cells with high dilutions of the antiserum. In immunofluorescence using frozen sections, markers such as isothiocyanates of fluorescein and of tetramethylrhodamine are employed, as these are directly visible under

Table 1. Methods for detecting immunotoxic alterations in the rat: tier-I screening parameters

Routine haematology (differential white blood cell counts)
Serum IgM, IgG and IgA concentrations
Bone-marrow cellularity
Organ weights (thymus, spleen, lymph nodes)
Histopathology (thymus, spleen, lymph nodes, Peyer's
  patches, bronchus-associated lymphoid tissue)
Optional: immunohistochemistry and cytofluorography of
  lymphoid tissues

the fluorescence microscope. Enzyme markers, including horseradish peroxidase, glucose oxidase and alkaline phosphatase, are widely used in paraffin sections of formalin-fixed tissue and in frozen tissue sections; they are visualized by addition of a substrate solution which reacts with the enzyme label to form an insoluble coloured product. Of the enzyme markers mentioned, horseradish peroxidase is by far the most widely used, because it conjugates with immunoglobulins relatively easily without much impairment of activity. Moreover, many chromogenic substrates for peroxidase are available (e.g., diaminobenzidine and aminoethylcarbazole). Various immunoperoxidase techniques are accessible, including the peroxidase-labelled antibody method, of which there are both direct and indirect versions (Nakane & Pierce, 1966), the unlabelled antibody method of peroxidase-antiperoxidase (Sternberger, 1979) and the avidin-biotin-peroxidase complex method (Hsu *et al.*, 1981). Apart from these, immunogold-silver staining (Holgate *et al.*, 1983) can be used, based on a combination of the immunogold staining procedure in electron microscopy and the detection of gold particles in histological preparations by a silver precipitation reaction (Danscher, 1981).

The indirect peroxidase-labelled antibody method is most commonly used in our toxicity studies with rats. Most cytoplasmic antigens, e.g., immunoglobulins in plasma cells and lysozyme in macrophages, can readily be localized in paraffin sections. Cell surface antigens, which are present only at low density, e.g., surface markers on lymphocyte subpopulations and stromal cells, are better demonstrated in frozen sections. A problem for the toxicological pathologist in evaluating often subtle changes is designing an objective classification. By randomizing and coding the slides of control and treated animals, reader's bias can be avoided. In immunohistochemistry, semiquantitative reading is thus possible. A semiquantitative method may be followed by quantitative techniques on cells in suspension using cytofluorography (Vos *et al.*, 1984). For these purposes, monoclonal antibodies have been developed that specifically recognize markers on subpopulations of rat lymphocytes and other leukocytes (Vaessen *et al.*, 1986) and which are useful tools in immunotoxicology. For a review of the characteristics of these antibodies, see Schuurman *et al.* (1990).

One should be aware, however, that the changes in the immune system found in the first tier of screening may represent indirect effects, e.g., as a consequence of undernutrition, impaired protein synthesis or stress. As an illustration, the starry sky appearance in the thymus of stress-vulnerable rats after subcutaneous injection can be mentioned. This phenomenon does not occur as a direct result of the substance injected or other manipulation of the immune system, but from stress-induced adrenocortical hyperactivity leading to focal disintegration of cortical thymocytes (Fig. 1).

If the first tier of screening provides indications that the test compound is immunotoxic, the second tier, with immune function tests, should be initiated. This comprises various immunological in-vivo and ex-vivo/in-vitro tests on cell-mediated immunity, humoral immunity, macrophage function, natural killer cell function and host resistance (Table 2). Depending on the observations in the first-tier studies, tests will be chosen from the second tier. For example, if the humoral aspects of defence mechanisms are affected by the compound, B-cell function tests should be performed; and if the first-tier data indicate changes in thymus-dependent immunity, cell-mediated immune function tests should be carried out. Most of the host resistance models cover more than one aspect of immunity and nonspecific defence mechanisms. In our institute, two infection models are now available to measure host resistance, i.e., the ability to respond adequately to opportunistic pathogens whether or not this is influenced by environmental chemicals. Apart from functional endpoint alterations, these models also include histopathological lesions, which makes it possible not only to evaluate quantitative differences, but also to make a qualitative discrimination. In the context of this paper, only the latter two tier-II tests are explained. For a detailed description of all test procedures of the second tier, the reader is referred to Vos and Van Loveren (1987 and Van Loveren and Vos (1989).

Effects of exposure to environmental chemicals on the cellular immune response are examined *in vivo* in the host resistance model that involves infection with *Listeria monocytogenes*. Defence mechanisms to Listeria infection are based on phagocytic activity of macrophages and T cell-mediated lymphokine production that aggravates phagocytosis

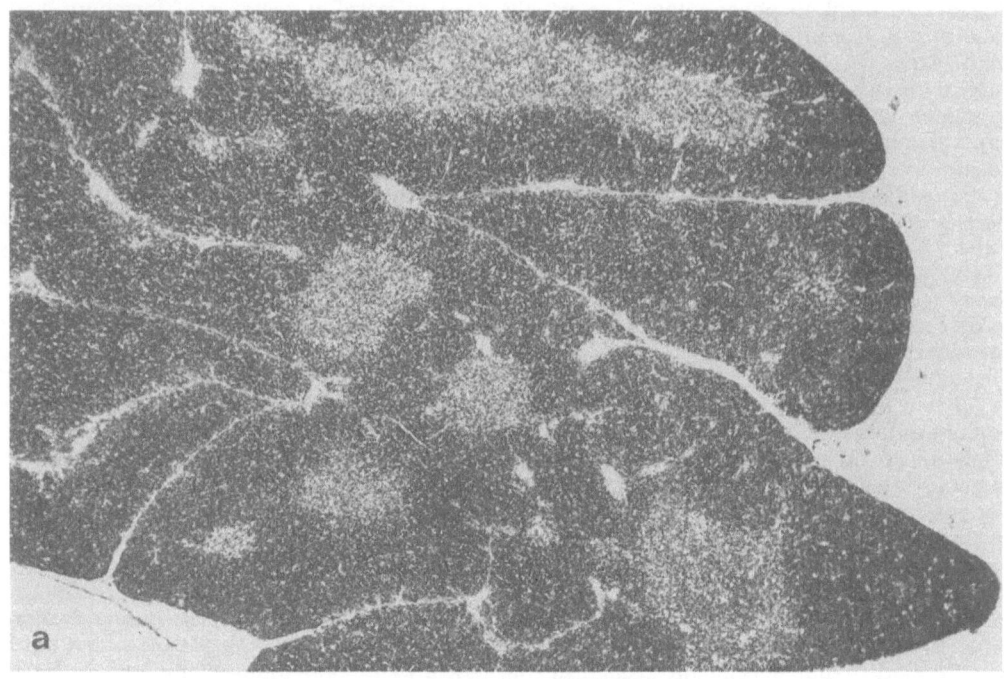

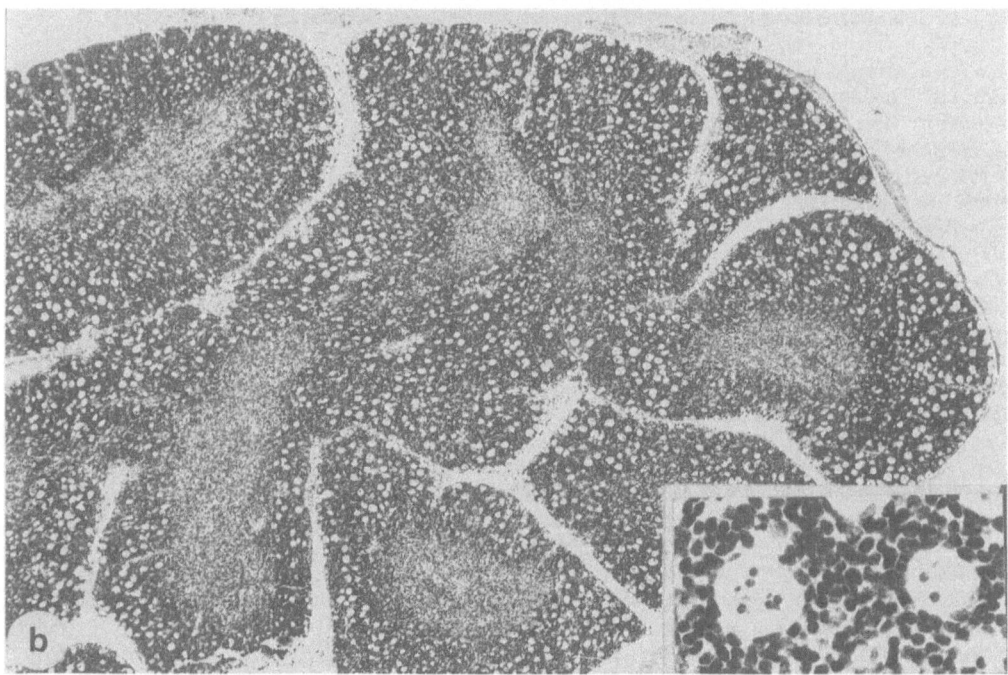

Fig. 1. Thymus, Wistar rat: (a) from untreated rat and (b) from rat after daily subcutaneous injection of physiological saline for 4 days; note thymic atrophy in the cortex giving a typical starry sky appearance. H & E, x45. Inset shows higher magnification of focal disintegration of cortical thymocytes, x425.

Table 2. Methods for detecting immunotoxic alterations in the rat: tier-II function assays

Category	Parameters
Cell-mediated immunity	Sensitization to T-cell dependent antigens (e.g. ovalbumin, tuberculin, Listeria) and delayed-type hypersensitivity response Lymphoproliferative responses to specific antigens (Listeria) and T-cell mitogens (concanavalin A, phytohaemagglutinin) *in vitro*
Humoral immunity	Serum titration of IgM, IgG, IgA, IgE responses to T cell-dependent antigens (ovalbumin, tetanus toxoid, sheep red blood cells, *Trichinella spiralis*) Serum titration of the T cell-independent IgM response to *Escherichia coli* lipopolysaccharide Lymphoproliferative response to the B-cell mitogen lipopolysaccharide *in vitro*
Macrophage function	Phagocytosis and killing of *Listeria monocytogenes* by adherent spleen and peritoneal cells *in vitro* Cytolysis of YAC-1 lymphoma cells by adherent spleen and peritoneal cells *in vitro*
Natural killer cell function	Cytolysis of YAC-1 lymphoma cells by non-adherent spleen and peritoneal cells *in vitro*
Host resistance and autoimmunity	*Trichinella spiralis* challenge (muscle larvae counts and worm expulsion) *Listeria monocytogenes* challenge (spleen and lung clearance) Adjuvant arthritis

(Mackaness, 1964). Apparently, there is no interference with humoral immunity. Listeria is administered intravenously or intratracheally to investigate systemic and respiratory defence, respectively. Clearance of Listeria, as evidenced by the number of viable bacteria in homogenates of spleen or lung on day 1 and 2, reflects macrophage function; on day 4 and 6, and even later after infection with a sublethal dose of bacteria, it is indicative of acquired resistance to Listeria (Takeya *et al.*, 1977). When host animals are immunized subcutaneously or intratracheally and subsequently challenged *via* the same or other routes, the number of viable bacteria in the organs mentioned can be determined earlier and is indicative of cellular immunity to Listeria. The influence of chemical compounds on the morphological lesions caused by a Listeria infection can be investigated by histopathology.

The model that involves oral infection with the nematode *Trichinella spiralis* yields an even more comprehensive insight into responses of the immune system. Infectious muscle larvae administered orally to rats develop in the gastrointestinal tract, enter the small intestinal mucosa and produce so-called newborn larvae. These in their turn migrate from the intestine, enter the lymph and blood circulation and penetrate the musculature elsewhere in the body. In this model, various parameters of resistance to the infection can be studied. In the infected intestine, both T cell-dependent immune responses (such as infiltration of inflammatory cells) and humoral responses (T cell-dependent production of IgM, IgG, IgE and IgA) occur against adult worms; this sequence of events results in expulsion of the worms. With respect to newborn larvae in the infected musculature, the response by inflammatory reactions around the encysted larvae is T cell-dependent (Vos *et al.*, 1983a). Thus, apart from the effect of environmental chemicals on the expulsion of adult worms from the small intestine, on the yield of muscle larvae and on immunoglobulin levels in serum and intestine, the effect of these compounds on the inflammatory response around muscle larvae can be investigated histopathologically.

Finally, after identification and characterization of immunotoxic chemicals *in vivo*, application of in-vitro test systems to elucidate the mechanism of action of these compounds may then be considered as a third tier of screening.

MICROSCOPIC AND BIOLOGICAL FEATURES OF LYMPHOID STRUCTURES

The immune system is lodged in central or primary lymphoid tissues, such as bone marrow and thymus, and in peripheral or secondary lymphoid tissues, such as spleen, lymph nodes and mucosa-associated lymphoid tissues in the respiratory and intestinal tract. The primary organs contain the microenvironment for antigen-independent differentiation of precursor cells into functional lymphocytes that can initiate and effect antigen-specific responses. The generation of functional T lymphocytes from bone marrow-derived precursors occurs in the thymus. Four main distinct subtypes of T cell exist: T helper/inducer cells, which, after activation by antigen, regulate the subsequent activation and proliferation of B lymphocytes into antibody-producing plasma cells and of precursor cytotoxic T cells into effector cytotoxic cells; T suppressor cells, which have a down-regulatory effect by their action on T helper lymphocytes; T cytotoxic cells, which kill targets after antigen-specific recognition; and T delayed-type hypersensitivity cells, which after antigen contact secrete lymphokines to attract and activate macrophages. The primary lymphoid organ that facilitates the maturation of immature B cells is the bone marrow. After antigen recognition and subsequent activation and proliferation, these cells become antibody-producing plasma cells. The process of antigen presentation, followed by activation and differentiation of mature lymphocyte populations into effector cells and regulatory events in this reaction, occurs in the secondary lymphoid tissue. Non-antigen-specific resistance also occurs, which includes cell types such as macrophages, neutrophilic granulocytes and cells exhibiting natural killer activity, which act in the first line of defence.

In this paper, after a short description of the microscopic and biological features of the thymus, spleen, lymph nodes and mucosa-associated lymphoid tissues, some examples of immunotoxic compounds are given, as assessed in both first- and second-tier tests, with special emphasis on histopathology.

Thymus

The thymus is a primary or central lymphoid organ situated in the mediastinum. During embryogenesis, the thymus arises from the invagination of epithelial cells of the third and fourth pharyngeal pouches into the underlying mesenchyme. The organ reaches its maximal size and cellularity during neonatal life, after which it gradually involutes; apart from this age-associated involution, acute involution can be generated by the action of, e.g., corticosteroids and sex hormones. Unlike the lymph nodes, the thymus has no afferent lymphatics, but efferent lymphatics are present. In rats and other laboratory animals, the thymus consists of two lobes, each formed by several lobules, which are partially separated by septa. These septa are foldings of the inner layer of the capsule of connective tissue enveloping the thymus. In contrast to other lymphoid structures, which are exclusively of mesenchymal origin, the framework of the thymus is formed by epithelial reticular cells. Within this framework, the bone marrow-derived lymphocytes (thymocytes) and non-lymphoid cells (macrophages and dendritic cells) occur. Each lobule has an outer zone (cortex) of dense lymphoid tissue with a high density of thymocytes and a lightly stained central zone (medulla) in which lymphocytes are less frequent. Between the cortex and medulla is the corticomedullary region, containing many blood vessels. In the medulla, some of the epithelial reticular cells are arranged in concentric layers, forming Hassall's corpuscles, the function of which is not known.

Precursor cells migrate from the bone marrow to the thymus and develop into immunocompetent T lymphocytes. This process involves the rearrangement of genes that encode for T-cell antigen receptors, followed by positive selection of cells that can recognize putative antigen in the context of products of the major histocompatibility complex (self-major histocompatibility complex restriction) and negative selection of cells that can recognize self antigen (self-tolerance) (Schuurman, 1988). This rearrangement and selection takes place in close interaction with the microenvironment of epithelial cells in the cortex and the epithelial and dendritic cells in the medulla. Ultrastructurally, contacts between the cytoplasmic processes of epithelial cells and thymocytes can be seen in the cortical membrane and even a complete surrounding of thymocytes by the cytoplasm of one distinct epithelial cell (so-called thymic nurse cell). In addition, epithelial cells, especially in the medulla, secrete thymic hormones (humoral factors) that promote T lymphocyte maturation in the thymus and at other sites in the body. Examples of these hormones are the nonapeptide thymulin and the polypeptide thymosin α1. During T-cell education, the thymocytes migrate from the cortex to the medulla, from which they then migrate to the peripheral lymphoid system as mature cells. It is still a matter of discussion whether the thymus functions in T-cell education after the full T-cell repertoire is reached. The T cells in the medulla have the immunological phenotype of mature T cells in peripheral lymphoid organs. As antigens can penetrate the medulla and antigen-presenting dendritic cells are present at this location, the medulla may also be partly a secondary lymphoid organ. Scattered B cells are also found in the medulla.

Spleen

The spleen of the rat is a parenchymatous organ. It is surrounded by a capsule of connective tissue from which trabeculae emerge which divide the parenchyma into incomplete compartments. Like the lymph nodes, the spleen is constructed of a reticular stromal network. It does not contain afferent lymphatics, but arteries and nerves penetrate it at the hilus through a number of trabeculae. Through the hilus also leave the veins that emerge from the parenchyma and the lymphatics which extend from the trabeculae. The spleen is arranged in two major regions, which can be easily identified in sectioning, i.e., the white pulp, representing the lymphatic tissue of the spleen, and the red pulp which is rich in blood. The white pulp comprises the lymphoid tissue and can be divided into three compartments, namely the periarteriolar lymphocyte sheath (PALS), the follicles and the marginal zone. Within these compartments, T and B cells occur. The PALS immediately surrounds the central arteriole and can be further subdivided into an inner and an outer PALS. In the inner PALS, T cells are found almost exclusively, while the outer PALS contains both T and B cells. The adjacent follicle consists of a mantle or corona containing exclusively B cells and the germinal centre, in which a few T lymphocytes are also present. The marginal zone surrounds both the PALS and the follicle and is separated from them by a marginal sinus. It contains B lymphocytes and some T lymphocytes. The marginal zone is a special microenvironment not found at other locations of the body. In this B-cell area, T lymphocyte-independent activation of B cells occurs. Examples of so-called T-independent antigens are repeating polysaccharide units occurring on encapsulated bacteria such as *Pneumococcus*. This kind of T-independent B-cell activation differs from that in lymphoid follicles where T-dependent B-cell activation occurs.

The spleen is a lymphoid organ with special characteristics. Its function is formation of lymphocytes which pass into the blood, clearance of particulate materials from the blood and concentration of blood-borne antigens. It is also the site of erythrocyte storage and of removal of effete erythrocytes and leukocytes (red pulp). Non-lymphoid cells also play an important role in host defence. The different compartments of the spleen contain their own types of non-lymphoid cells: in the PALS, the interdigitating cells are the most conspicuous ones; in the follicle, the follicular dendritic cells and tingible body macrophages. This compartmentalization of non-lymphoid cells is similar to that in other peripheral lymphoid tissue. In the marginal zone, a special type of macrophage occurs, known as marginal zone macrophages. Moreover, at the side of the PALS and the follicle, the marginal zone is bordered with a rim of marginal metallophilic macrophages. Finally, macrophages constitute the majority of cells in the red pulp, playing an important role of defence against microorganisms and inert particles which penetrate the circulation.

Lymph nodes

Lymph nodes are encapsulated organs dispersed throughout the body, always along the circuit of the lymph vessels. Many variations exist with regard to shape and internal structure, depending on the state of activation and characteristics of the response. The general architecture of the lymph nodes is similar, however, and comprises a capsule, a cortex with a paracortex and follicles, and a medulla. The lymph is received *via* afferent lymphatics, which penetrate the node at the convex edge and communicate with the subcapsular sinuses lying just beyond the capsule. These subcapsular sinuses are connected with the medullary sinuses through the cortical peritrabecular sinuses. Thus, lymph flows through the cortex, paracortex and medulla towards the efferent lymphatics at the concave side (the hilus) of the lymph node. From the capsule, with dense connective tissue, trabeculae extend inwards to the node. These structures are joined by reticular fibres, giving rise to a three-dimensional reticular network in which lymphocytes are freely suspended. In the superficial cortical region, follicles are present, which are either primary follicles consisting of a mature B-lymphocyte aggregate or secondary follicles with a lymphocyte corona and a germinal centre. Germinal centres are easily identified as they are more lightly stained than lymphocyte corona and primary follicles and contain large activated cells, called centrocytes and centroblasts. Follicles are the main B-cell areas. In primary follicles and the lymphocyte corona of secondary follicles there are almost no T cells, but some occur in germinal centres. The interfollicular areas contain intermingled B and T cells. The paracortex is the principal localization of T lymphocytes in the lymph nodes. This area is further characterized by the presence of postcapillary venules, which are lined by cuboidal or even cylindrical endothelial cells. Through these so-called high endothelial venules, lymphocytes enter the node from the circulation, and this is the main site at which blood lymphocytes enter the lymphatic circulation, enabling continuous recirculation from blood to lymph and back. In the medullary region, medullary cords lie between the medullary sinuses, with plasma cells, macrophages and some myeloid cells as the main leukocyte populations.

As in the spleen, characteristic non-lymphoid cells are present in the different compartments of the lymph nodes.The subsinusoidal macrophages occur immediately under the subcapsular sinus. The follicles contain the follicular dendritic cells, together with the tingible body macrophages. Between the follicles are specific macrophage-like cells. The paracortex comprises the interdigitating cells, with cytoplasmic processes lying in between the T lymphocytes. These interdigitating cells are a macrophage subset closely related to Langerhans cells in skin and to 'veiled' macrophages in the afferent lymph, and function as antigen-presenting cells (to T helper cells). Finally, many macrophages are present in both the medullary cords and sinuses.

Lymph nodes serve as the site of reactivity following stimulation of antigen entering the node *via* the lymph or the blood. In a stimulated lymph node, primary follicles enlarge to secondary follicles with germinal centres as the response to B-cell stimulation. B-Cell stimulation is evidenced by the presence of centrocytes and centroblasts, often accompanied by frequent mitotic figures. Finally, plasmablasts with a pyroninophilic cytoplasm are seen, which become antibody-producing plasma cells in the medullary cords. Following stimulation with an antigen that evokes a T cell-mediated response, the paracortical area enlarges, with lymphoblasts becoming evident.

Mucosa-associated lymphoid tissues

A way of categorizing lymphoid tissue other than as central or peripheral is into external and internal systems. The external system operates just underneath the epithelial surface of the respiratory and gastrointestinal tracts. Apart from lymphoid aggregates just beneath the mucosal layer, draining lymph nodes, like mesenteric lymph nodes, contribute to the external immune system. This functions in a more or less separate way from the internal secondary immune system (including spleen, bone marrow and part of the lymph nodes).

The mucosa-associated lymphoid tissues represent a mucosal defence mechanism which secretes IgA antibody against pathogens and antigenic material to which the respiratory and gastrointestinal tracts are exposed. It is organized along the mucosal surface into nonencapsulated accumulations of lymphocytes or diffuse collections of lymphocytes. In the intestinal tract, these lymphoid structures are called Peyer's patches and are separated into B-cell (follicles) and T-cell areas, which can be easily demonstrated by light microscopy and immunohistochemistry (Fig. 2). A proper evaluation of intestinal lymphoid tissue can be facilitated by preparing so-called Swiss rolls of the intestinal tract (Moolenbeek & Ruitenberg, 1981). In the gastrointestinal tract, the tissue is designated gut-associated lymphoid tissue; in the lower respiratory tract, it is called bronchus-associated lymphoid tissue, and the lymphoid aggregates located at the entrance of the pharyngeal duct were recently denoted nasal lymphoid tissue (Spit *et al.*, 1989). The common

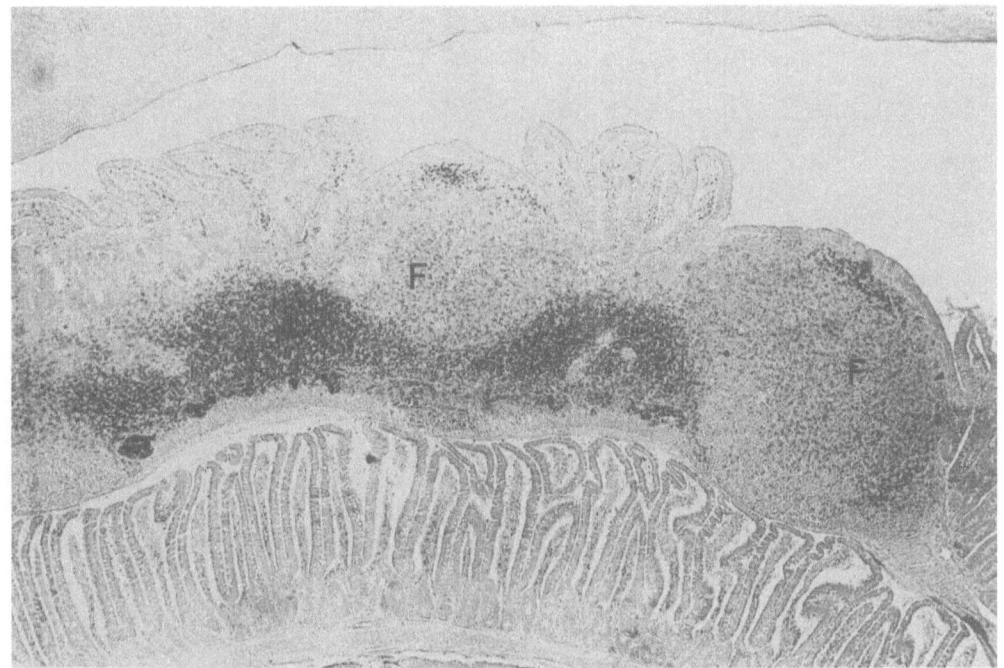

Fig. 2. Immunohistochemical staining for T lymphocytes using monoclonal W3/13 mouse-anti-rat antibodies in Peyer's patches of the jejunum of a Wistar rat showing T cells in the interfollicular area. F (follicle). x110. [Reproduced from Vos *et al.* (1983a), with permission.]

designation of mucosa-associated lymphoid tissue stems from observations that there is a close interaction between lymphoid organs at different secretory sites, e.g., by homing in of (activated) lymphocytes from one to another mucosal site, separated from homing in on the internal immune system. Mucosa-associated lymphoid tissue is characterized by a specialized epithelium overlaying the lymphoid structures. This epithelium contains membranous epithelial or M cells which are claimed to be antigen-presenting cells.

IMMUNOTOXICITY OF ENVIRONMENTAL COMPOUNDS

Bis(tri-*n*-butyltin)oxide

Pronounced effects on rat thymus morphology and thymus-dependent immune function are found in short-term toxicity experiments with the environmental contaminant bis(tri-*n*-butyltin)oxide (TBTO) (Krajnc *et al.*, 1984; Vos *et al.*, 1984). Dietary administration of TBTO to rats for four weeks elicited a conspicuous atrophy of the thymic cortex due to lymphocyte depletion, and leading to disappearance of distinct corticomedullary differentiation (Fig. 3). Administration of TBTO not only affects the thymus but also causes morphological alterations in the spleen. The effects observed are atrophy of both the PALS and the follicles. Analogous to the histopathologically observed lymphocyte depletion in the PALS, a marked decrease in the number of lymphocytes bearing the T immunophenotype is seen in the PALS of rats treated with TBTO (Fig. 4). Lymphocyte depletion is also induced by TBTO in the thymus-dependent area of the lymph nodes. It affects not only the paracortex of the mesenteric lymph node but also decreases the size of the follicles (Fig. 5). A decrease in the number of T lymphocytes in the paracortex of TBTO-treated animals has been demonstrated by immunohistochemical staining.

To evaluate the functional significance of the effects of exposure to TBTO on the lymphoid system, function studies of cell-mediated immunity, humoral immunity and mononuclear phagocyte system have been carried out *in vivo* (Vos *et al.*, 1984). The results

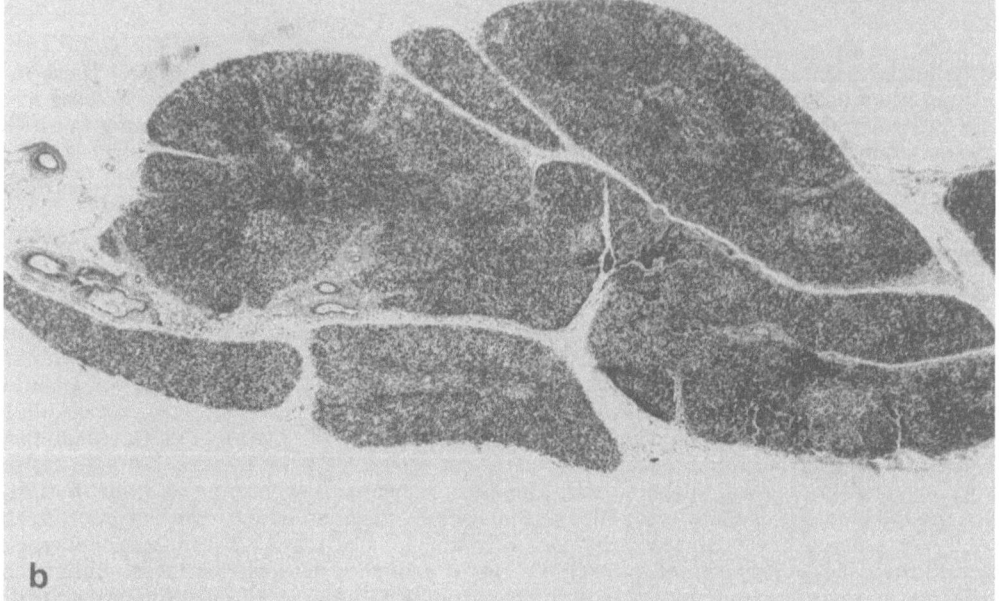

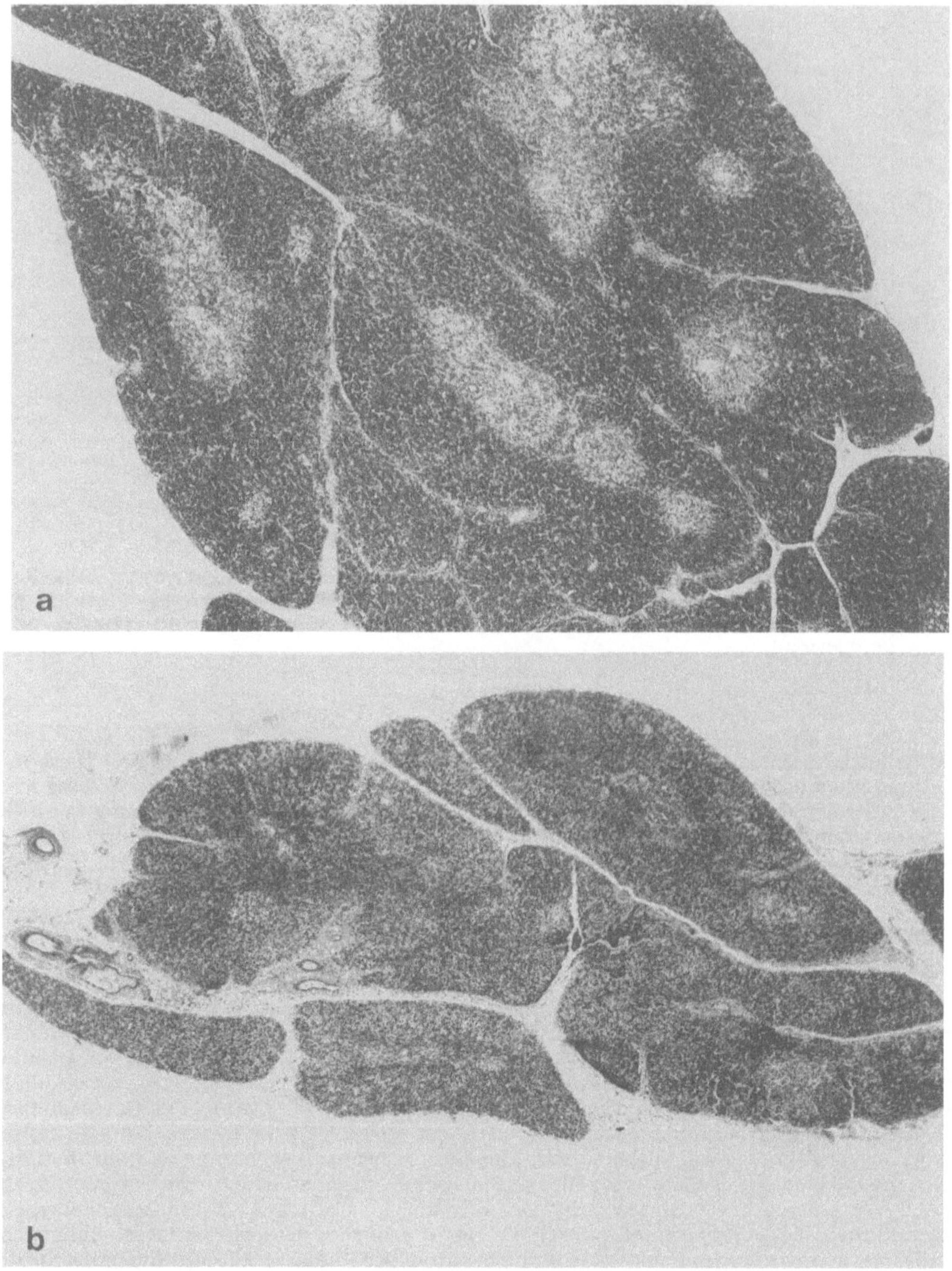

Fig. 3. Thymus, Wistar rat: (a) from control rat and (b) from rat fed bis(tri-*n*-butyltin)oxide at 320 mg/kg diet for 4 weeks; note atrophy of the cortex due to lymphocyte depletion, leading to disappearance of distinct corticomedullary junctions. H & E, x45.

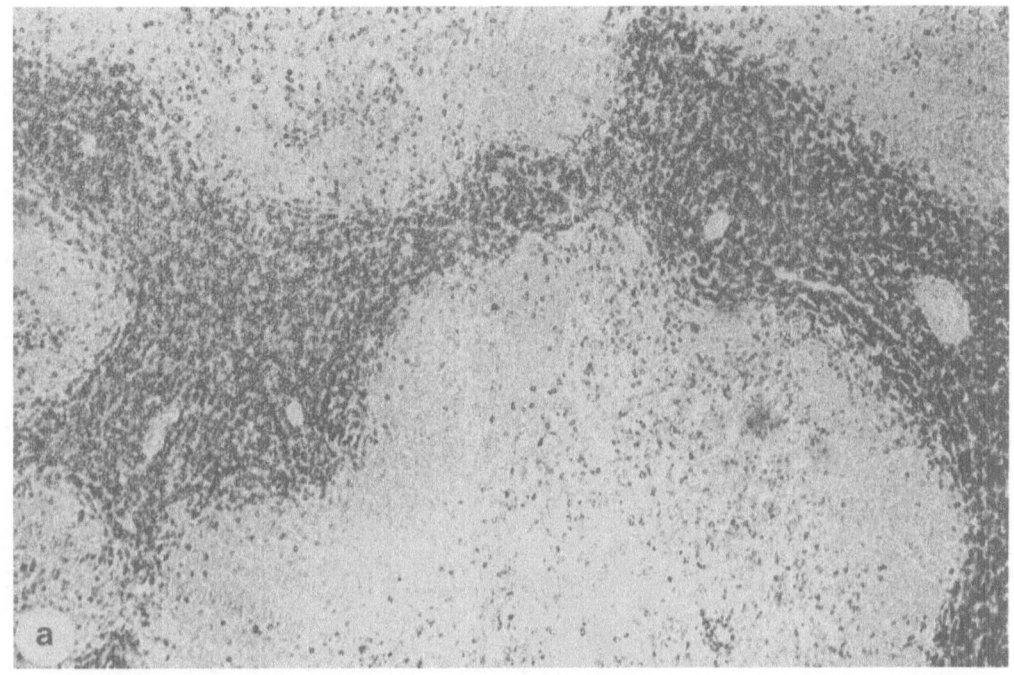

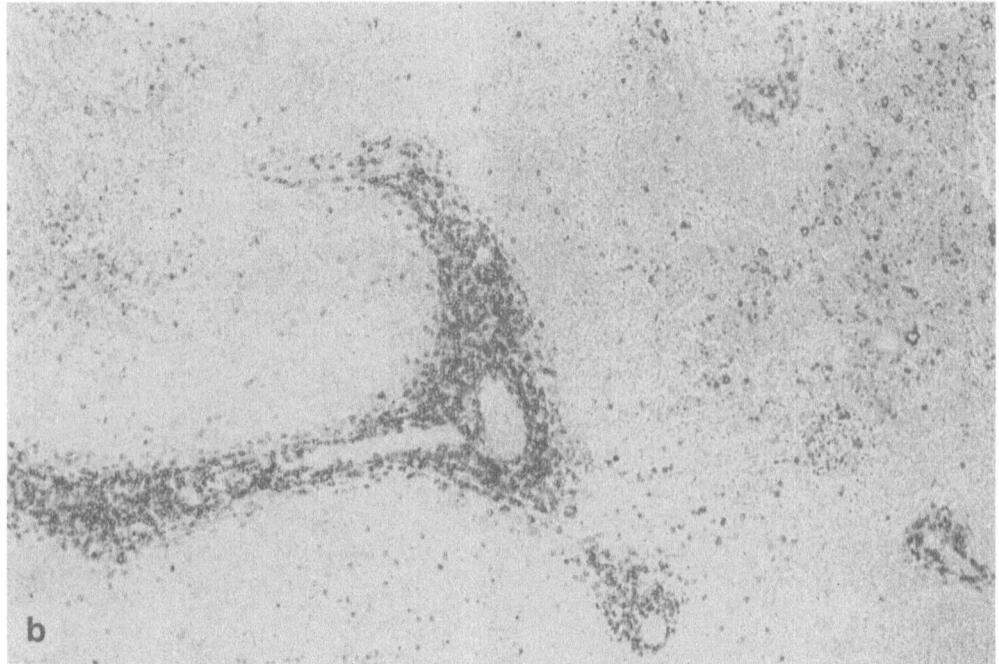

Fig. 4. Immunohistochemical staining for T lymphocytes using monoclonal W3/13 mouse-anti-rat antibodies in the spleen (a) from control Wistar rat showing T cells in periarteriolar lymphocyte sheaths and (b) from Wistar rat fed bis(tri-*n*-butyltin)oxide at 320 mg/kg diet for 4 weeks; note severe T-lymphocyte depletion. x110. [Reproduced from Krajnc *et al.* (1984), with permission.

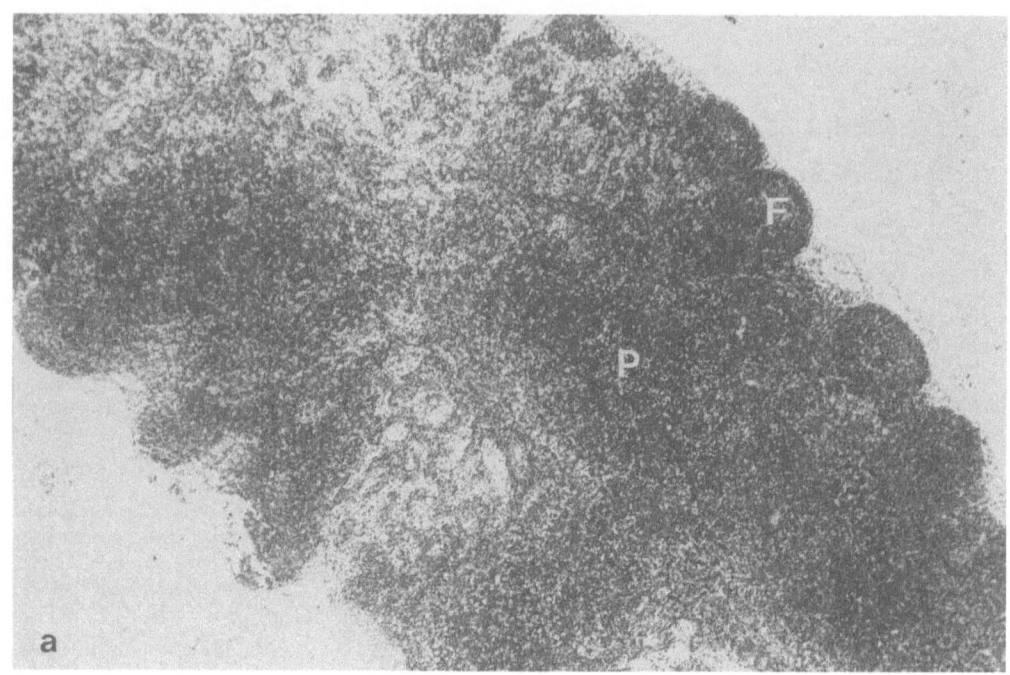

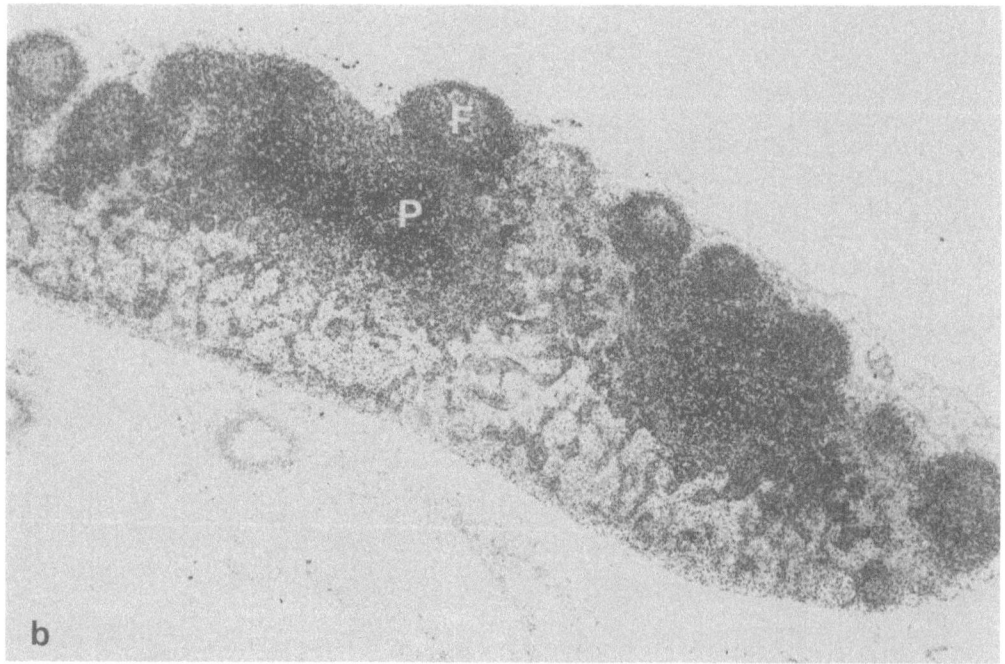

Fig. 5. Mesenteric lymph node, Wistar rat; (a) from control rat with normally developed follicles (F) and paracortex (P) and (b) from rat fed bis(tri-n-butyltin)oxide at 320 mg/kg diet for 4 weeks, showing atrophy of the paracortex. H & E, x45.

of this study are further indicative of the immunotoxic potential of TBTO. Resistance to the nematode *Trichinella spiralis* is impaired by exposure to TBTO in a dose-related way, as demonstrated by a retarded expulsion of adult worms from the small intestine, an increased yield of muscle larvae and a suppression of the IgE antibody response. Histopathologically, in sections of parasitized tongues of control animals, the inflammatory reaction around nurse cells (larva-containing muscle cells) consists of mononuclear cells and eosinophilic granulocytes; in rats treated with TBTO, this inflammatory reaction is strongly reduced (Fig. 6).

Hexachlorobenzene

In contrast to TBTO, hexachlorobenzene stimulates the lymphoid system of exposed rats (Vos *et al.*, 1979b, 1983b). After dietary admin-istration of hexachlorobenzene for three weeks, the weight of the spleen and lymph nodes was increased. The splenomegaly is characterized by an increase in size of marginal zones, follicles, and possibly PALS, as a result of lymphocyte hyperplasia (Fig. 7). In the paracortex of mesenteric and popliteal lymph nodes, an effect on the postcapillary venules is observed, consisting of proliferation of the high endothelial venules, and an increased number of recirculating lymphocytes migrating through the endothelium (Fig. 8). This effect of hexachlorobenzene on endothelial cells is not restricted to the lymphoid organs, as hypertrophy and proliferation of the endothelial cells lining the lung venules also occur (Fig. 9). Hexachlorobenzene also seems to interact with the mononuclear phagocyte system. Accumulation of mononuclear cells is observed focally in the alveolar lumina around venules. The macrophage nature of these cells is evident in immunohistochemistry with a polyclonal antibody against rat lysozyme (Fig. 10). Thus, first-tier screening of hexachlorobenzene shows a stimulatory effect on the immune system; pathological data from second-tier studies with hexachlorobenzene are not yet available.

Morphine and methadone

Opiates cause a striking alteration in lymph node morphology. Oral exposure of rats to methadone and, in particular, morphine for six weeks evoked enlargement of the medullary cords in the mesenteric lymph nodes, together with an increased serum IgG concentration (Van der Laan *et al.*, 1988; Fig. 11). The increased cellularity represents an increase in the number of plasma cells and may indicate an effect on humoral immunity. Immune function tests are currently under way to explore the relevance of this finding *in vivo*.

Ozone

After exposure of rats to ozone, a dose-dependent effect on mononuclear phagocytes is found in the lung, characterized morphologically by an increase in the number of alveolar macrophages (Fig. 12). With immunohistochemistry for lysozyme-positive cells, an increase in free alveolar lysozyme-containing cells is seen, particularly in the centroacinar region; these represent mainly macrophages and occasionally other inflammatory cells (Fig. 13; J.A.M.A. Dormans, P.J.A. Rombout & H. Van Loveren, unpublished observations).

The effects of ozone on defence mechanisms to respiratory infection with *L. mono-cytogenes* in rats have been investigated by functional assessment (Van Loveren *et al.*, 1988). Nonspecific resistance appears to be impaired, since in ozone-exposed rats the capacity of alveolar macrophages to ingest and kill Listeria is diminished. Specific cellular immune responses to a pulmonary Listeria infection are affected by ozone exposure, as evidenced by a decrease in T:B-cell ratios in the lung-draining lymph nodes, in delayed-type hypersensitivity responses to Listeria in the ears and in lymphoproliferative responses to Listeria antigens in spleen and lung-draining lymph nodes. Pulmonary infection with Listeria elicits pathological lesions in the lung, comprising multiple foci of lymphoid cells and histiocytes sometimes exhibiting a granulomatous appearance. If rats are exposed to ozone for one week prior to infection, the lesions are much more pronounced, with granulomatous characteristics (Fig. 14). The increased severity of these lesions is probably the consequence of a synergistic effect between a diminished phagocytic activity of macrophages and a diminished cellular immunity to Listeria, both of which result from ozone exposure. Thus, these studies provide evidence that ozone suppresses nonspecific defence mechanisms as well as specific cellular immune responses.

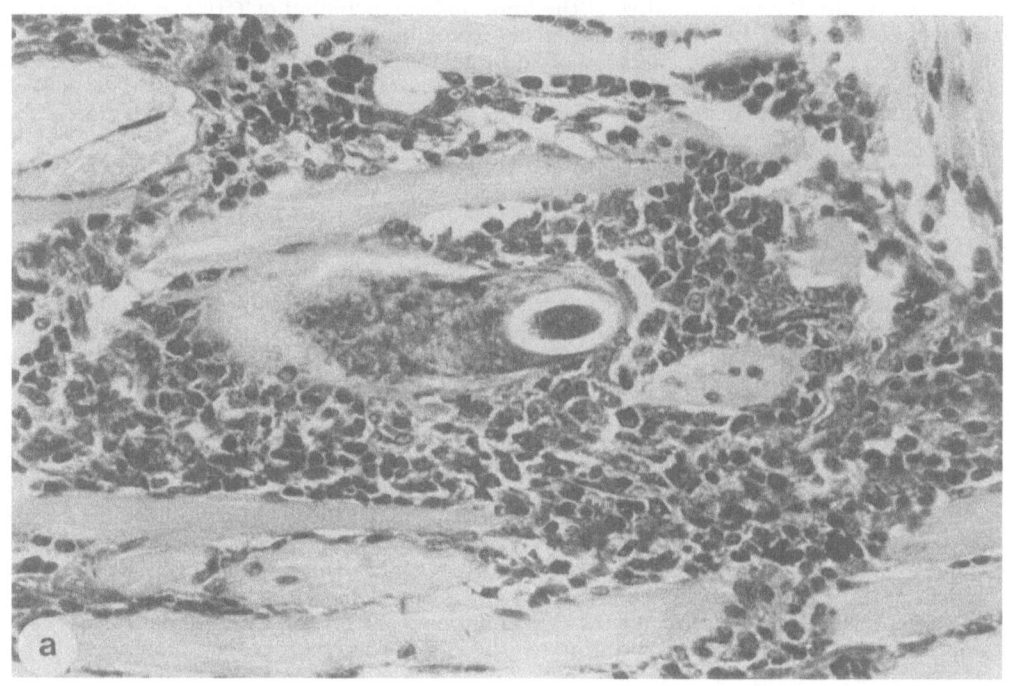

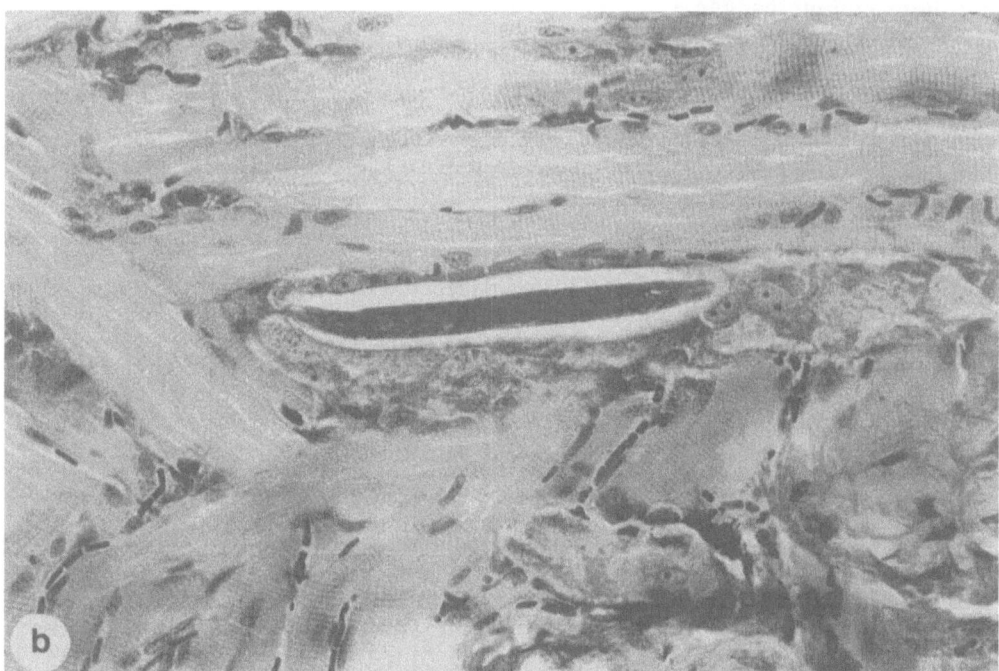

Fig. 6. Inflammatory reaction around nurse cell (larva-containing muscle cell) in tongue 14 days after oral infection with *Trichinella spiralis* (a) from control Wistar rat showing an extensive reaction consisting of many mononuclear cells and eosinophilic granulocytes and (b) from Wistar rat fed bis(tri-*n*-butyltin)oxide at 80 mg for 7 weeks, in which the reaction is strongly reduced. Giemsa stain, x425.

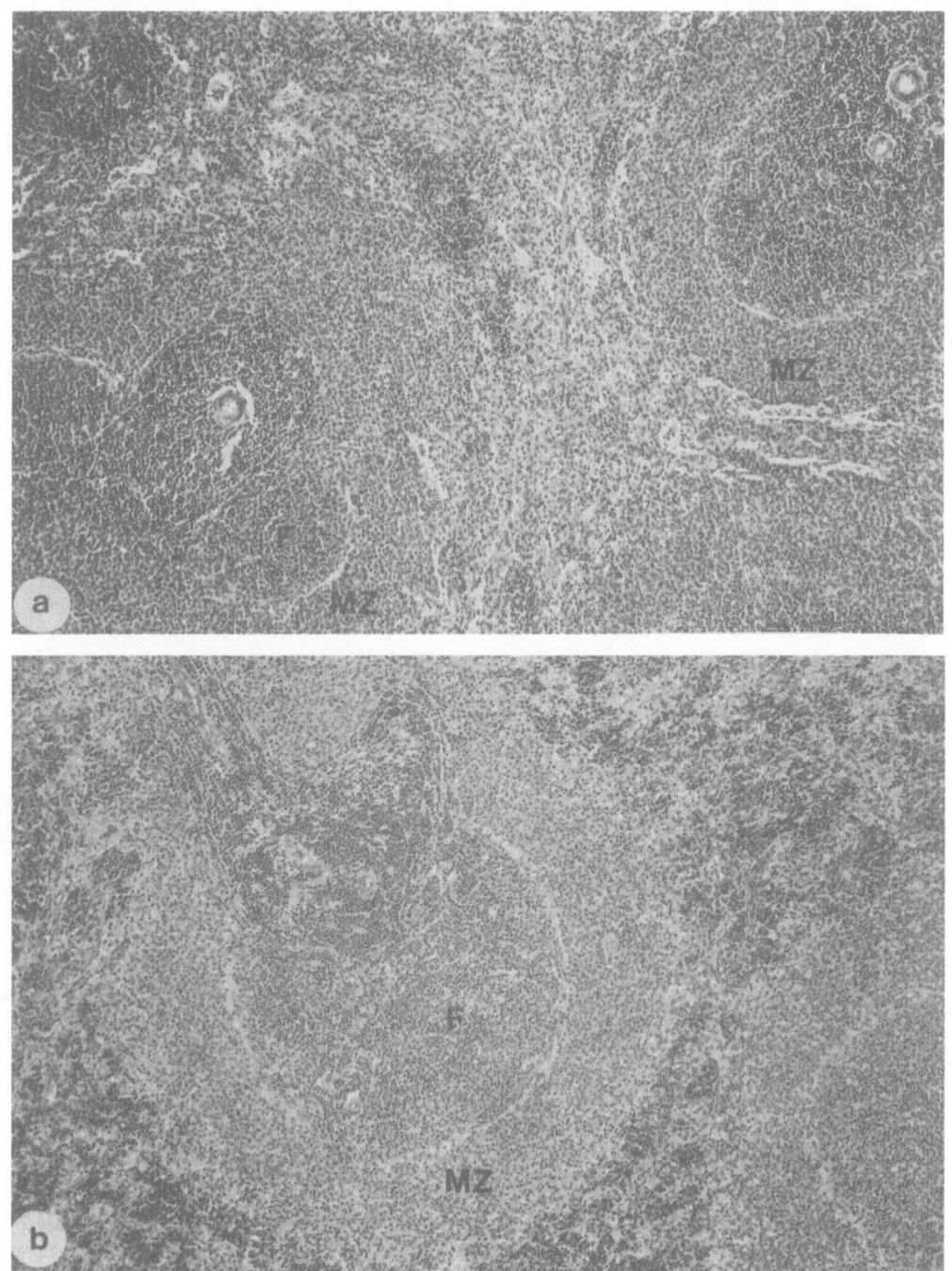

Fig. 7. Spleen, Wistar rat; (a) from control rat showing normally developed follicles (F) with marginal zones (MZ) and (b) from rat fed hexachlorobenzene at 1000 mg/kg diet for 3 weeks; note the enlargement of follicles and marginal zones. H & E, x110.

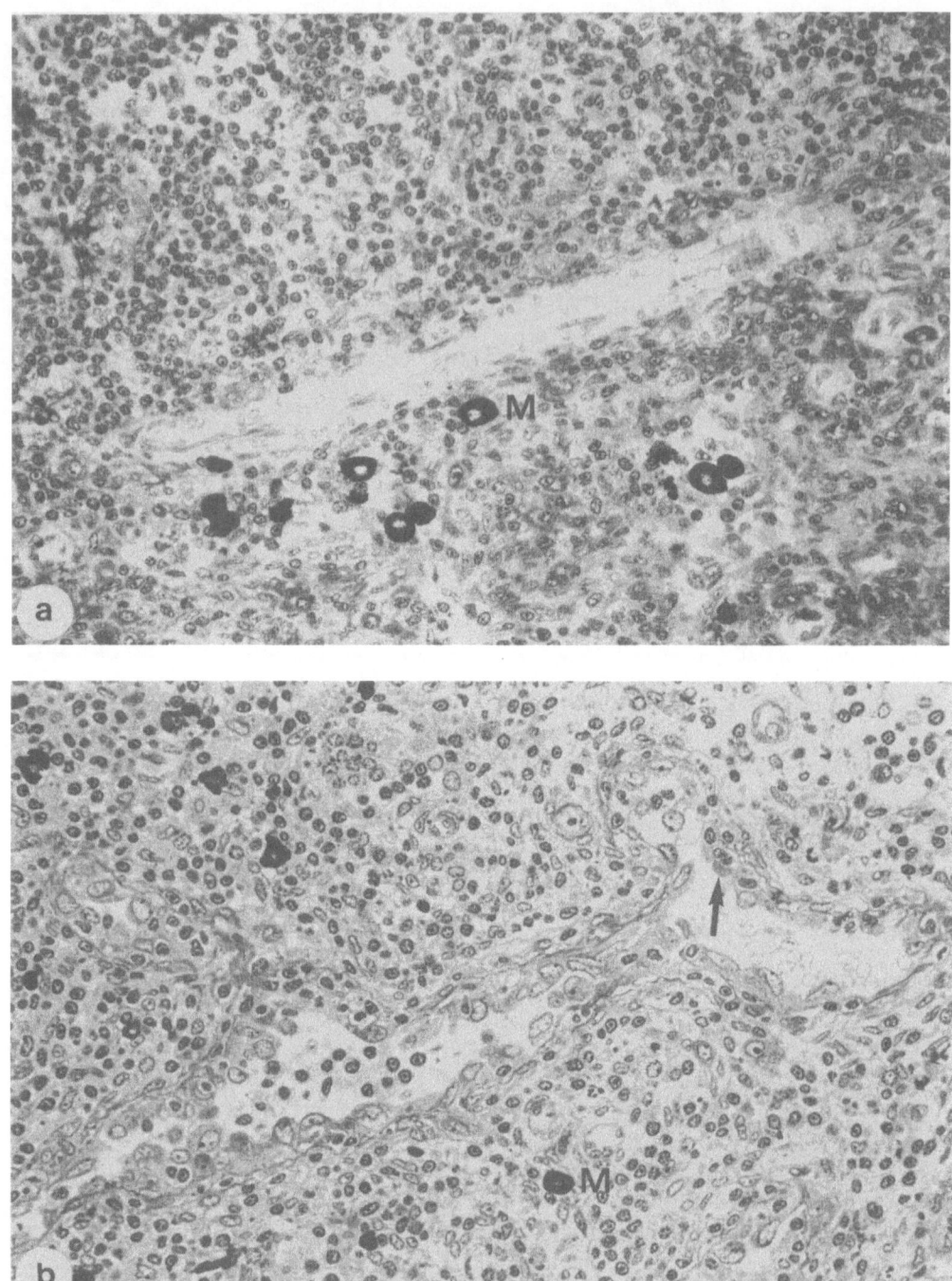

Fig. 8. Popliteal lymph node, Lewis rat; (a) from control rat and (b) from rat fed hexachlorobenzene at 450 mg/kg diet for 6 weeks, showing proliferation of a high endothelial
venule, with an increased number of recirculating lymphocytes migrating through the
endothelium (arrow). (In the popliteal lymph node, mast cells (M) are abundant.)
Glycolmethacrylate embedding, Giemsa, x425.

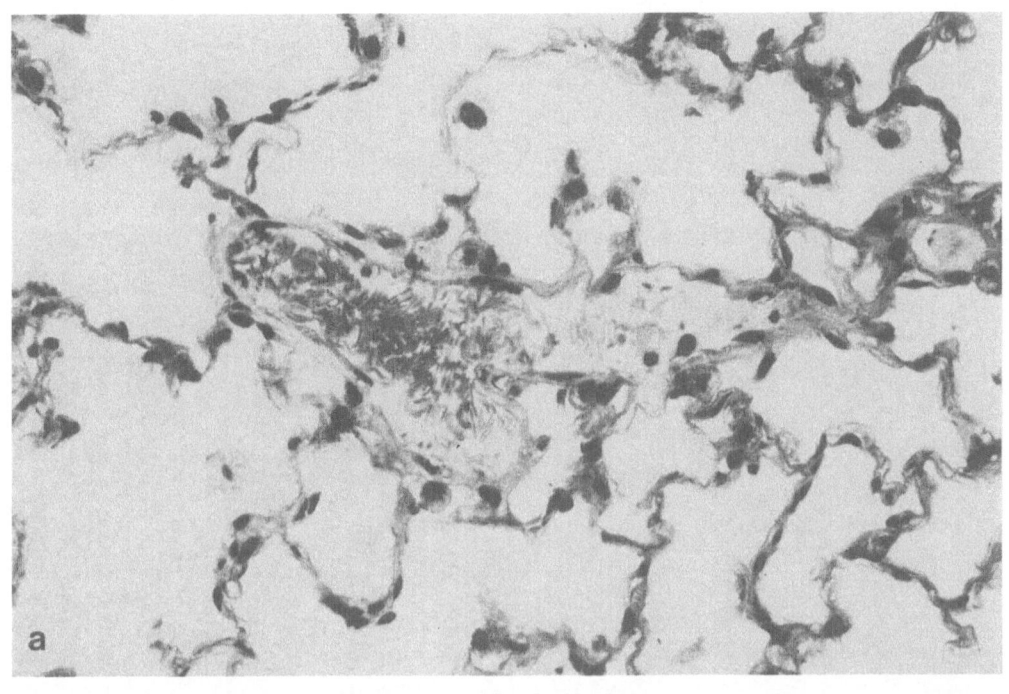

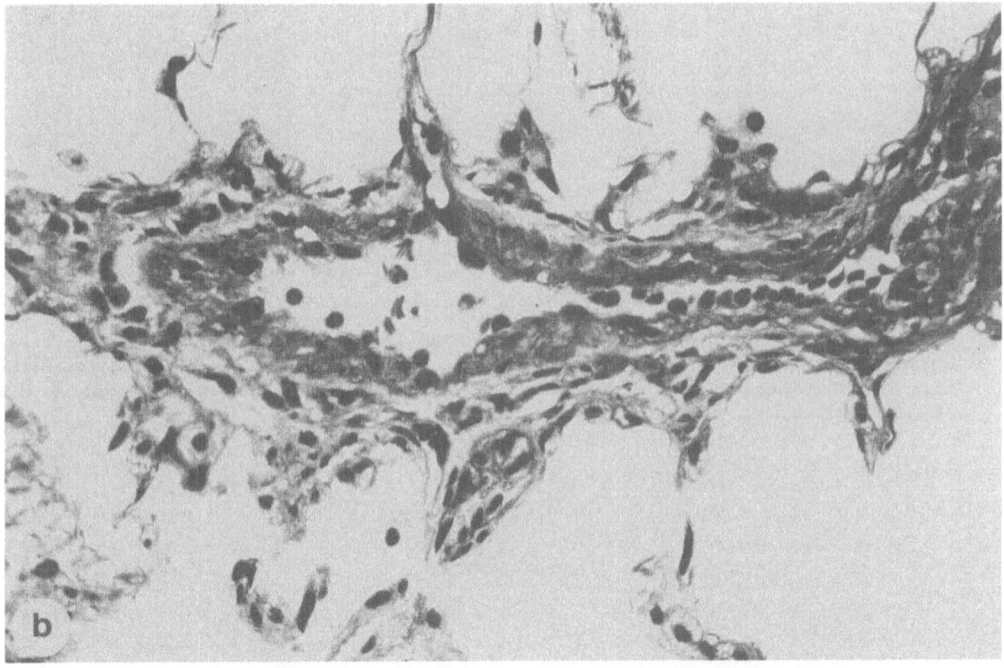

Fig. 9. Lung, Lewis rat; (a) from control rat and (b) from rat fed hexachlorobenzene at 450 mg/
kg diet for 6 weeks, showing hypertrophy and proliferation of the lining endothelial cells
of the venules. Glycolmethacrylate embedding, Giemsa, x425.

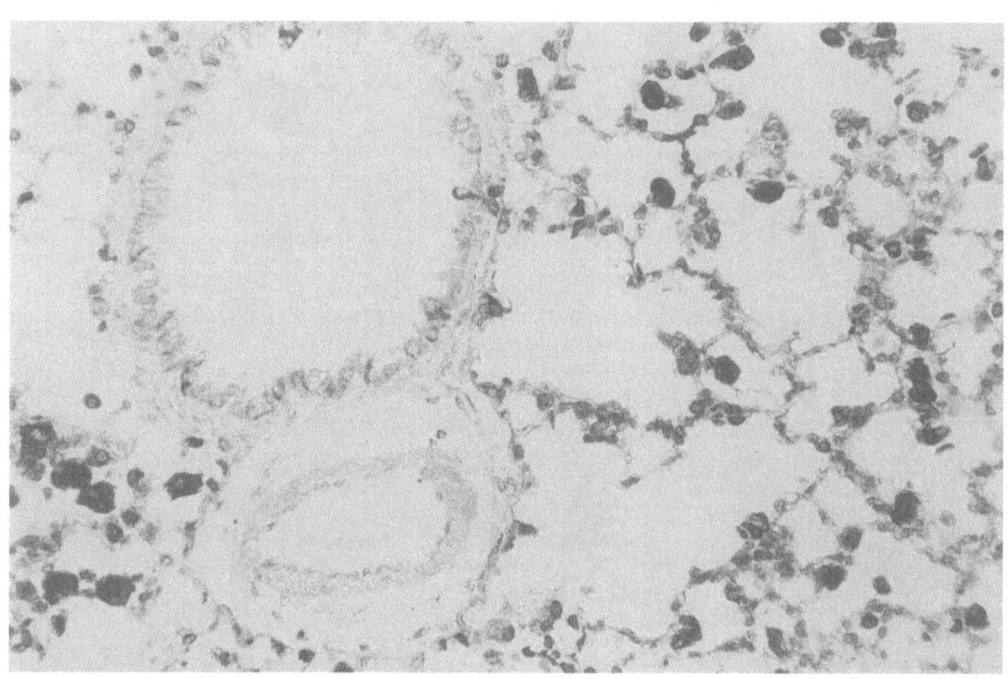

Fig. 10. Immunohistochemical staining for lysozyme in lung from Wistar rat fed hexachlorobenzene at 150 mg/kg diet for 6 weeks following combined pre- and postnatal
exposure, showing the macrophage nature of the accumulated mononuclear cells in the
alveolar lumina around venules. x270.

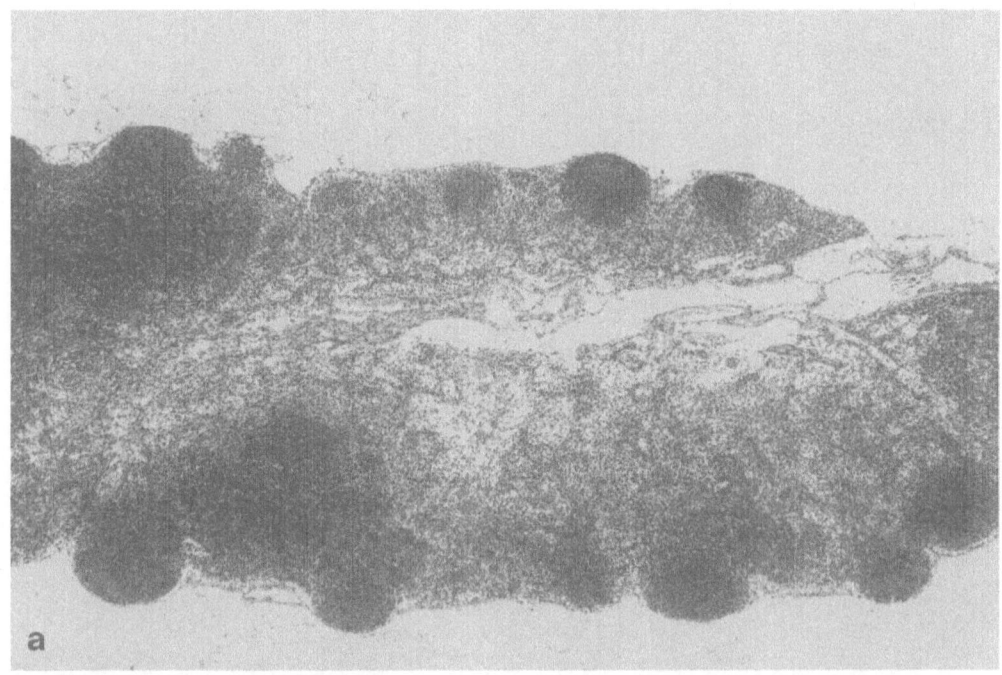

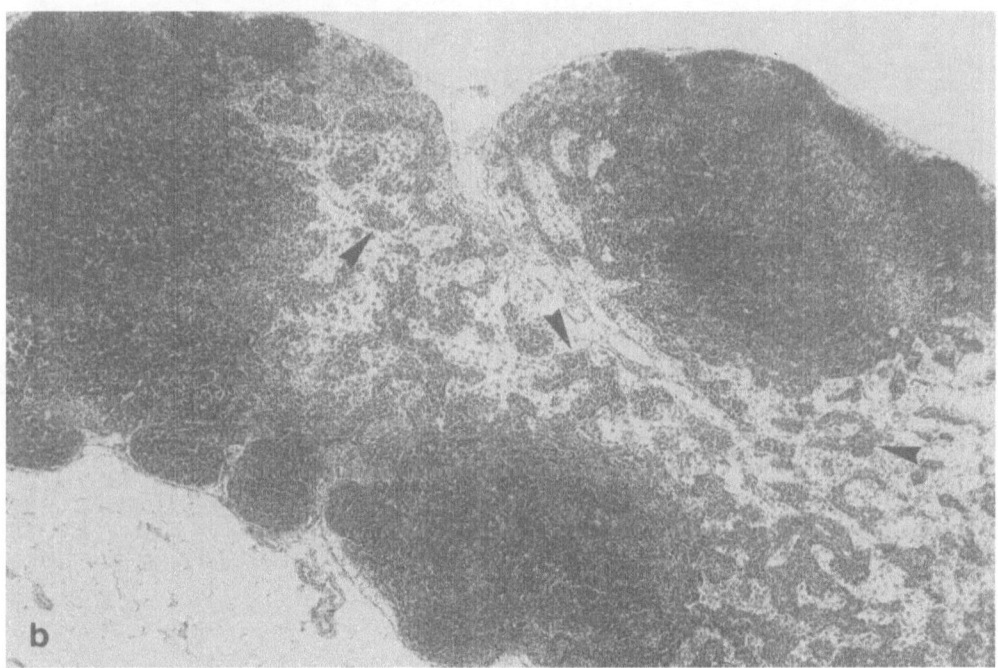

Fig. 11. Mesenteric lymph node, Wistar rat; (a) from control rat and (b) from rat fed morphine at
1 g/kg diet for 6 weeks, showing increased cellularity of the medullary cords (arrows). H &
E, x45. [Reproduced from Vos & Krajnc-Franken (1990), with permission.]

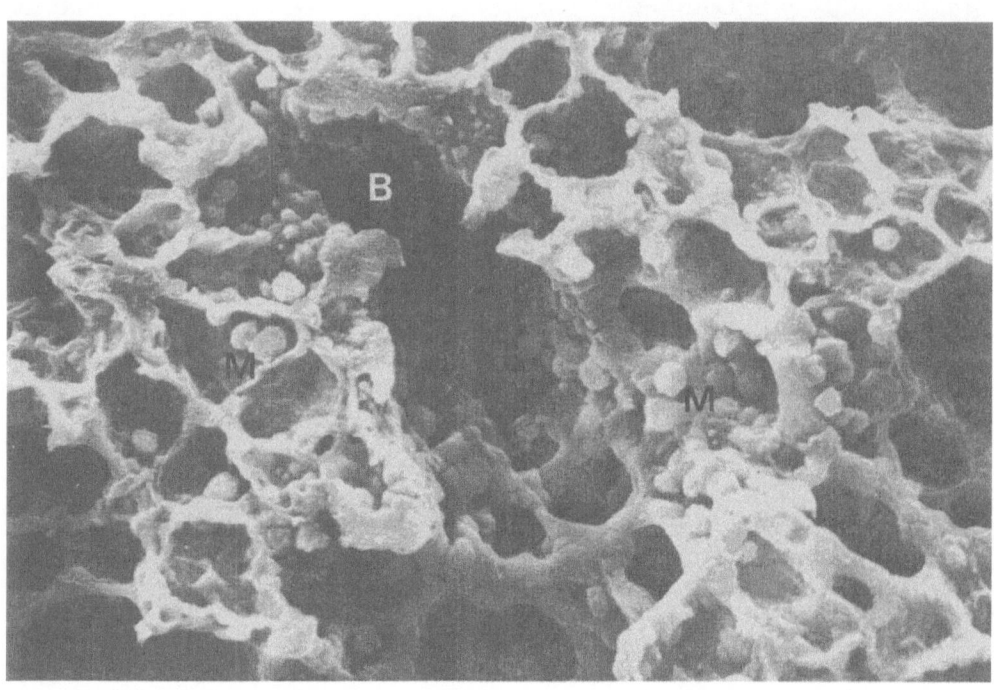

Fig.12. Scanning electron photomicrograph of the lung from a Wistar rat exposed to ozone at 600 µg/m³ for 3 days, showing accumulation of macrophages (M) within alveoli. B, bronchioductular junction. x480. [Courtesy of J.A.M.A. Dormans, National Institute of Public Health and Environmental Protection, The Netherlands]

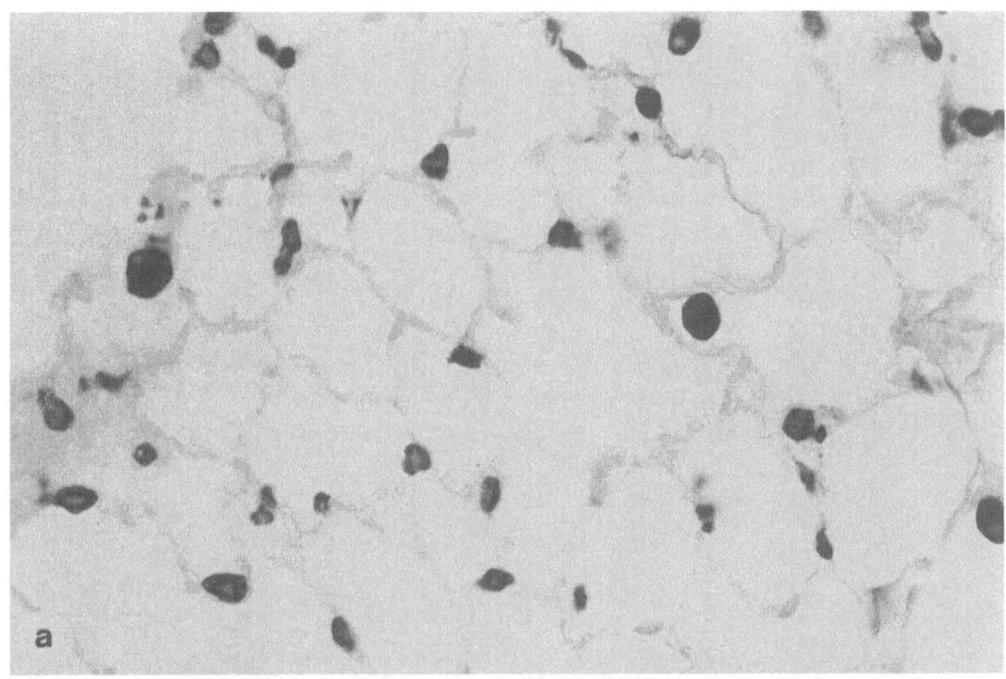

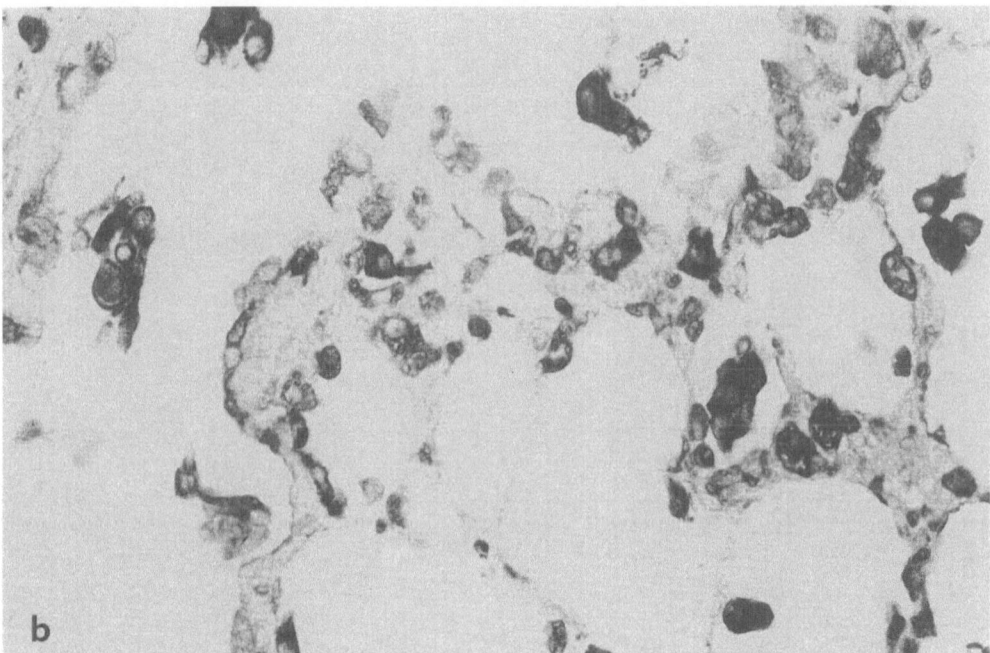

Fig. 13. Immunohistochemical staining for lysozyme in the lung (a) from control Wistar rat, showing lysozyme-containing macrophages in the alveolar lumina, and (b) from rat exposed to ozone at 1.5 mg/m³ for 7 days with an accumulation of macrophages in the centroacinar region, x425.

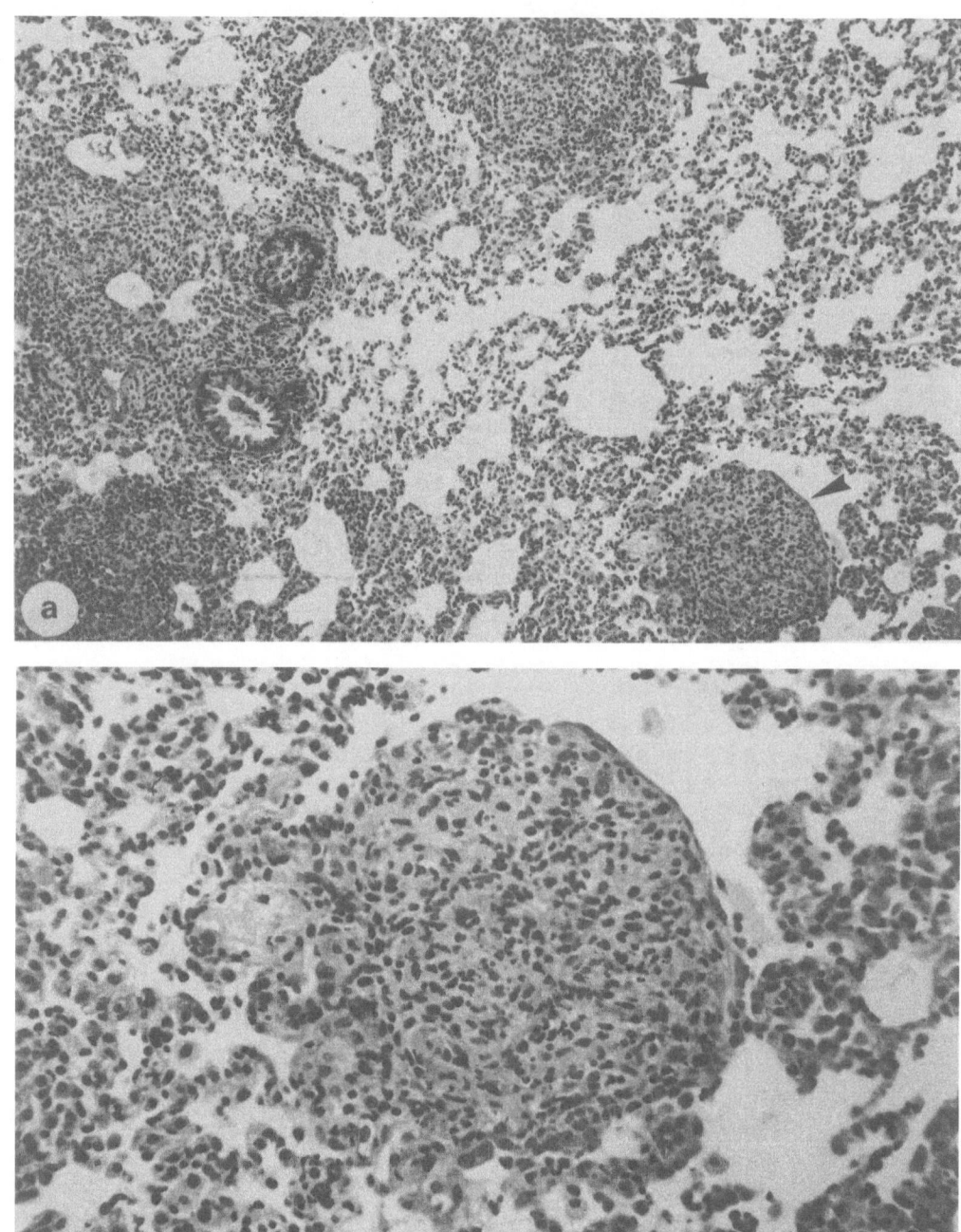

Fig.14. Lung from Wistar rat 5 days after continuous exposure to ozone at 1.5 mg/m³ for 1 week and subsequent respiratory infection with 10⁸ *Listeria monocytogenes*. Inflammatory infiltrates have granulomatous characteristics (arrows). H & E, (a) x110, (b) x425. [Reproduced from Van Loveren *et al.* (1988), with permission.]

REFERENCES

Berlin, A., Dean, J., Draper, M.H., Smith, E.M.B. & Spreafico, F., eds (1987) *Immunotoxicology*, Dordrecht, Martinus Nijhoff

Bingham, E., Barkle, W., Zerwas, M., Stemner, K. & Taylor, P. (1972) Responses of alveolar macrophages to metals. I. Inhalation of lead and nickel. *Arch. environ. Health*, **25**: 406-414

Danscher, G. (1981) Localization of gold in biological tissue. A photochemical method for light and electron microscopy. *Histochemistry*, **71**: 81-88

Holgate, C.S., Jackson, P., Cowen, P.N. & Bird, C.C. (1983) Immunogold-silver staining: new method of immunostaining with enhanced sensitivity. *J. Histochem. Cytochem.*, **31**: 938-944

Hsu, S.M., Raine, L. & Fanger, H. (1981) The use of avidin-biotin-peroxidase complex (ABC) in immunoperoxidase techniques: a comparison between ABC and unlabeled antibody (PAP) method. *J. Histochem. Cytochem.*, **29**, 577-580

International Programme on Chemical Safety (1986) *Immunotoxicology. Development of Predictive Testing for Determining the Immunotoxic Potential of Chemicals*. Report of a technical review meeting, London, 2-5 November 1986

Krajnc, E.I., Wester, P.W., Loeber, J.G., Van Leeuwen, F.X.R., Vos, J.G., Vaessen, H.A.M.G. & Van der Heijden, C.A. (1984) Toxicity of bis(tri-n-butyltin)oxide in the rat. I. Short-term effects on general parameters and on the endocrine and lymphoid systems. *Toxicol. appl. Pharmacol.*, **75**: 363-386

Luster, M.I., Boorman, G.A., Dean, J.H., Harris, M.W., Luebke, R.W., Padarathsingh, M.I. & Moore, J.A. (1980) Examination of bone marrow, immunologic parameters and host susceptibility following pre- and postnatal exposure to 2,3,7,8-tetrachlorodibenzo-p-dioxin (TCDD). *Int. J. Immunopharmacol.*, **2**: 301-310

Mackaness, G.B. (1964) The influence of immunologically committed lymphoid cells in macrophage activity in vivo. *J. exp. Med.*, **129**: 973-992

Moolenbeek, C. & Ruitenberg, E.J. (1981) The 'Swiss roll': a simple technique for histological studies of the rodent intestine. *Lab. Anim.*, **15**: 57-59

Nakane, P.K. & Pierce, J.B., Jr (1966) Enzyme-labelled antibodies: preparation and application for localization of antigens. *J. Histochem. Cytochem.*, **14**: 929-931

Schuurman, H.J. (1988) Biological functions of the thymic microenvironment. *Thymus Update*, **1**: 67-99

Schuurman, H.J., De Weger, R.A., Van Loveren, H., Krajnc-Franken, M.A.M. & Vos, J.G. (1990) Histopathological approaches. In: Miller, K. & Nicklin, S., eds, *Principles and Practice of Immunotoxicology* (in press)

Spit, B.J., Hendriksen, E.G.J., Bruijntjes, J.P. & Kuper, C.F. (1989) Nasal lymphoid tissue in the rat. *Cell Tissue Res.*, **255**: 193-198

Sternberger, L.A., ed. (1979) *Immunocytochemistry*, New York, Wiley, pp. 104-169

Takeya, K., Shimotori, S., Taniguchi, T. & Nomoto, K. (1977) Cellular mechanisms in the protection against infection by Listeria monocytogenes in mice. *J. gen. Microbiol.*, **100**: 373-379

Vaessen, L.M.B., Broekhuizen, R., Rozing, J., Vos, J.G. & Schuurman, H.J.F. (1986) T-Cell development in congenitally athymic (nude) rats. *Scand. J. Immunol.*, **24**: 223-235

Van der Laan, J.W., Van Loveren, H., Krajnc-Franken, M.A.M., De Groot, G., Loeber, J.G. & Krajnc, E.I. (1988) [Influence of morphine and methadone on the immune system. Results of a six-week study in the Riv:TOX rat.] (in Dutch) Report from the National Institute of Public Health and Environmental Protection; RIVM Report no. 318705001

Van Loveren, H. & Vos, J.G. (1989) Immunotoxicological considerations: a practical approach to immunotoxicity testing in the rat. In: Dayan, A.D. & Paine, A.J.K., eds, *Advances in Applied Toxicology*, London, Taylor & Francis, pp. 143-163

Van Loveren, H., Rombout, P.J.A., Wagenaar, S.S., Walvoort, H.C. & Vos, J.G. (1988) Effects of ozone on the defense to a respiratory *Listeria monocytogenes* infection in the rat. Suppression of macrophage function and cellular immunity and aggravation of histopathology in lung and liver during infection. *Toxicol. appl. Pharmacol.*, **94**: 374-393

Vos, J.G. & Krajnc-Franken, M.A.M. (1990) Toxic effects on the immune system, rat. In: Jones, T.C., Mohr, U. & Hunt, R.D., eds, *Hemopoietic System (Monographs on Pathology of Laboratory Animals)*, New York, Springer (in press)

Vos, J.G. & Van Loveren, H. (1987) Immunotoxicity testing in the rat. In: Burger, E.J., Tardiff, R.G. & Bellanti, J.A., eds, *Environmental Chemical Exposure, and Immune System Integrity*, Vol. 13, Princeton, NJ, Princeton Scientific Publishing Co., pp. 167-180

Vos, J.G., Buys, J., Beekhof, P. & Hagenaars, A.M. (1979a) Quantification of total IgM and IgG to a thymus-independent (LPS) and a thymus-dependent (tetanus-toxoid) antigen in the rat by enzyme-linked immunosorbent assay (ELISA). *Ann. N. Y. Acad. Sci.*, **320**: 518-534

Vos, J.G., Van Logten, M.J., Kreeftenberg, J.G. & Kruizinga, W. (1979b) Hexachlorobenzene-induced stimulation of the humoral immune response in rats. *Ann. N.Y. Acad. Sci.*, **320**: 535-550

Vos, J.G., Krajnc, E.I. & Beekhof, P. (1982) Use of the enzyme-linked immunosorbent assay (ELISA) in immunotoxicity testing. *Environ. Health Perspect.*, **43**: 115-121

Vos, J.G., Ruitenberg, E.J., Van Basten, N., Buys, J., Elgersma, A. & Kruizinga, W. (1983a) The athymic nude rat. IV. Immunocytochemical study to detect T-cells, and immunological and histopathological reactions against *Trichinella spiralis*. *Parasite Immunol.*, **5**: 195-215

Vos, J.G., Brouwer, G.M.J., Van Leeuwen, F.X.R. & Wagenaar, S. (1983b) Toxicity of hexachlorobenzene in the rat following combined pre- and post-natal exposure: comparison of effects on immune system, liver and lung. In: Gibson, G.G., Hubbard, R. & Parke, D.V., eds, *Immunotoxicology*, London, Academic Press, pp. 219-235

Vos, J.G., De Klerk, A., Krajnc, E.I., Kruizinga, W., Van Ommen, B. & Rozing, J. (1984) Toxicity of bis(tri-*n*-butyltin)oxide in the rat. II. Suppression of thymus-dependent immune responses and of parameters of nonspecific resistance after short-term exposure. *Toxicol. appl. Pharmacol.*, **75**: 387-408

INVESTIGATIVE METHODS:
CLASSICAL TECHNIQUES

R. Hess, T. Maurer & M. Germer

Central Product Safety
CIBA GEIGY Limited
CH-4002 Basel, Switzerland

ABSTRACT

In the context of conventional rodent studies, immunotoxicity is best assessed in sequence: by establishing the toxicological profile, by determining effects on the constitutive parts of the system (defence potential) and by studying specific immune functions. The first-tier screening in subchronic (28 or 90 days) studies in rats relies heavily on immuno-pathology. Histopathology thus becomes the major parameter for comparative assessment and for defining the toxicological parameters for further investigations. In an expanded tier, quantitative assessment of cellularity and immunocompetent cell types may be added. In subsequent tiers, the action of chemicals is tested (antibody- and cell-mediated immune response) using special host and tumour resistance models, and the effect, if confirmed, is subsequently verified in specific functional tests.

INTRODUCTION

In recent years, the immune system has been identified as a target of direct toxic effects of chemicals. Apart from the limited number of immunosuppressive or immunostimulant drugs used therapeutically, environmental chemicals that may pose a risk to human health by altering the immune system have been little studied epidemiologically. Certain chemicals can induce immunotoxicity, i.e., immune dysfunction and altered host resistance in laboratory animals, although only a few reports indicating immunotoxicity following human exposure are available (Dean *et al.*, 1989).

In his first comprehensive review of immunotoxicology, Vos (1977) suggested that a probable reason that only a limited number of chemicals have been shown to have immunosuppressive properties was that the current procedures for toxicity testing underestimated the importance of the immune system, and the lymphoid organs were poorly examined. It is doubtful whether this statement is true, however, since the lymphoreticular and haematopoietic systems are generally screened in traditional toxicity tests. The particular purpose of subchronic studies is to determine any target organ toxicity under exaggerated conditions of exposure.

The practical importance of immunotoxicology is, however, not restricted to recognition of the most severe effects. In order to assess health risks, adverse immune events will have to be characterized in both qualitative and quantitative terms, taking into account the type of immune dysfunction produced and its relationship to dose and time. This goal is achieved only if the actual endpoint - immunopathology - is duly incorporated into routine safety evaluations.

Immunotoxicity of Metals and Immunotoxicology, Edited by
A. D. Dayan *et al.,* Plenum Press, New York, 1990

OBJECTIVES OF TESTING FOR IMMUNE-RELATED TOXICITY

Immune dysfunction induced by chemicals may result in immunosuppression and in immunopotentiation, i.e., autoimmunity, and types I-IV allergy. These adverse effects may result from the direct action of the chemical (or its metabolites) on the immune system or from an immunomediated response of the host to the agents acting as a hapten, antigen or tolerogen.

Traditional testing can be used, in principle, to determine immunosuppression, but it is inefficient for evaluating most clinically important immunotoxic effects, such as autoimmunity and types I-III allergies. The recognition of antibody- and cell-mediated hypersensitivity reactions in pathological material requires specialized laboratory techniques which are outside the scope of routine toxicity testing (Lebish et al., 1986). In order to investigate substances with yet unkown properties, the toxicologist must work with validated methods in conditions that are as close as possible to the human exposure. Because of the potential diversity of probable effects (Sharma, 1981), it is unlikely that only a few procedures will be sufficient to identify those parts of the highly complex immune system that will be altered by a given toxicant. A practical approach would be to simulate exposure in optimized whole-animal test systems, such as those used for predicting contact allergy (Maurer, 1983).

Immunosuppression after systemic exposure is well documented in animals for a wide variety of compounds, including alkylating agents, hormones, corticosteroids, immune modulating drugs, aromatic hydrocarbons and metals. In these cases, whole-animal toxicology provides the background data for the appraisal of human risk. Examples of the adequacy of the rodent model are provided by cyclosporin A (Ryffel et al., 1983) and the dialkyltins (Seinen et al., 1977).

The first regulatory guidelines for immunotoxicty testing appear to have been drafted by the US Environmental Protection Agency (1985). The US Food and Drug Administration and other agencies recommend handling potentially immunotoxic drugs (e.g., antiviral drugs) on a case-by-case basis. In Annex I of Recommendation 83/751/EEC, the European Community suggested inclusion of the immune system in the pathology protocol of standard toxicity studies, in order to evaluate potential immunotoxicity of drugs. New draft guidelines of the Japan Ministry of Health and Welfare (1988) on drug toxicity studies include a comprehensive proposal for 'antigenicity testing'.

As for other forms of toxicity, immunological hazards should be identified first by feasible, effective means and then evaluated in tests capable of defining the functional defect produced. In order to integrate the procedures, a tiered approach with multiple assays is generally recommended.

Safety evaluation of recombinant DNA products may differ substantially from the testing of environmental chemicals. Species specificity and host interactions require very special testing profiles which cannot be defined in the context of standard protocols.

THE US NATIONAL TOXICOLOGY PROGRAM GUIDELINES PROPOSAL

A number of schedules and assays with emphasis mainly on detecting immunosuppression or immune modulation have been proposed in the USA (Dean et al., 1985) and in Europe (European Chemical Industry Ecology and Toxicology Centre, 1987; Vos & Van Loveren, 1987; Dayan, 1988), which, in part, have already been incorporated into interlaboratory validation programmes.

The general scheme of a tiered procedure is outlined in Figure 1. Tier I usually comprises extended immunopathology as well as tests for antibody-mediated immunity (specific immunoglobulins, plaque-forming cells). Tier II consists of assays for host resistance and cell-mediated immunity. If tier I is conducted in the rat there is a change of species to the mouse in tier II.

The most advanced panel has been developed by the US National Toxicology Program in B6C3F$_1$ female mice, i.e., the strain frequently used by that Program for toxicity and

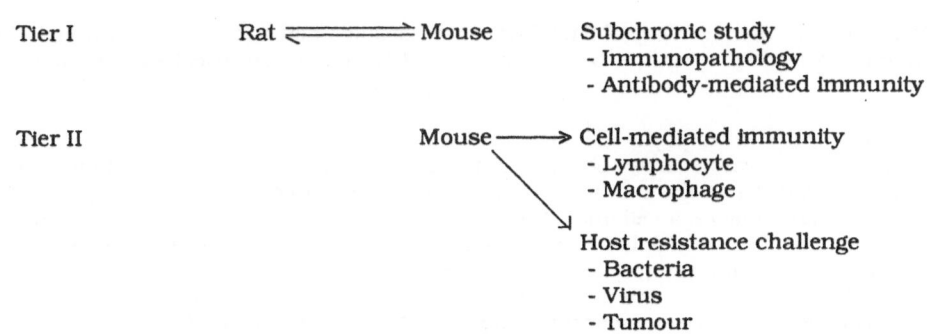

Fig. 1. Immunitoxicological safety evaluation

carcinogenicity testing. It is now being evaluated in several laboratories with a number of known immunotoxicants, including diethylstilboestrol, cadmium, cyclophosphamide, dexamethasone Fig. 1. Immunotoxicological safety evaluation and benzo[a]pyrene. A summary account of the data has been published (Luster *et al.*, 1988). Since probably the most relevant parameter for immunotoxicity is altered host resistance (Bradley, 1985), it was considered significant in the National Toxicology Program configuration to correlate immune dysfunction with infectivity models. Table 1 summarizes results of interlaboratory assays indicating the relationship between altered immune function and challenge parameters (Luster *et al.*, 1988).

The National Toxicology Program screen was developed primarily to assess immunosuppression after treatment with repeated doses. None of the compounds studied showed an effect in tier II without changing some parameter in tier 1. Furthermore, gross histopathological changes of lymphoid organs evaluated in tier I were heavily relied upon and yielded supportive evidence for further investigation.

THE US NATIONAL AGRICULTURAL CHEMICALS ASSOCIATION PROPOSAL

A modified approach to immunotoxicity testing was recently proposed by the US National Agricultural Chemicals Association (1988), with the purpose of placing immunotoxicity assays in line with standard toxicity testing procedures. It is expected that chemicals with potential immunotoxic effects will be identified in the standard 90-day subchronic study in rats, as tier 1. Analysis of the data should indicate whether the immunological effects are secondary (due to systemic toxicity) or primary. In order to confirm the probable immunotoxicity and any dose-response relationship, another subchronic study of at least 28 days' exposure is conducted (tier I A).

In the National Agricultural Chemicals Association panel, the significance of a suspected primary immunotoxic effect is determined ultimately in host defence and tumour

Table 1. Correlation between host susceptibility and depressed immune function[a]

Challenge model	NK cytotoxicity	Proliferation[b]		Antibody[c]		
		MLR	PHA	LPS	PFC	DHR
PYB6 sarcoma	0.45*	0.46*	0.20	0.02	0.22	0.61*
B16F10 melanoma	0.54*	0.02	0.15	0.16	0.15	-
Listeria	0.01	0.47**	0.37*	0.08	0.01	0.19
Influenza	0.11	0.78*	0.03	0.70*	0.83**	-
Plasmodium	0.24	0.59	0.67*	0.64*	0.78**	-

[a]Correlation coefficient as determined by Spearman's rank correlation test; significant correlation at *$p<0.05$, **$p<0.01$; from Luster *et al.* (1988).
[b]MLR, mixed lymphocyte reaction; PHA, phytohaemagglutinin.
[c]LPS, lipopolysaccharide; PFC, plaque-forming cells; DHR, delayed hypersensitivity reaction.

resistance models (tier II). Only if data from these studies demonstrate unequivocal effects will attempts be made to confirm the nature of the immunological defect by specific in-vitro assays (tier III).

In the tier-II studies of the modified approach, rats should be used whenever possible, although various strains may be required. The Wistar Furth transplantable tumour (C58NT)D is proposed as the tumour resistance model to evoke a cytotoxic T-cell response, and the mammary adenoma cell line (MADB106) may be used as a host-resistance model to test the function of natural killer cells in syngeneic Fischer 344 rats. It is suggested that antibody-mediated immune response be checked with streptococcus or influenza virus (Vireligier, 1975; Bradley & Morahan, 1982; Hoshino *et al.*, 1983) and cellular mediated immune response in a *Listeria monocytogenes* infection model (North, 1973).

The purpose of the extended subchronic study protocol is to provide adequate screening for immunotoxicity, to determine dose-related effects and at the same time to form the background upon which the subsequent tiers are based. Therefore, the design of the subchronic study is of paramount importance. Some points to consider are listed in Table 2. In principle, it should be possible to measure multiple functional parameters in single animals, in addition to the more conventional parameters. Exon *et al.* (1986) proposed a multiple immunoassay-single rat model to measure humoral immunity, cell-mediated immunity and macrophage function in rats exposed to antigen-treatment regimens.

If properly defined, with expanded histopathology and immune parameters, the subchronic study in rats should suffice to determine the essential qualities of an immunotoxic effect and its dose-response relationship, and thus obviate the necessity of a time-consuming tier IA repeat experiment. A Science Analysis and Coordination Branch review suggested substituting the tier-IA rat study with a subchronic study in mouse (Sjoblad, 1989). Changing the animal species at this stage would facilitate the use of a possibly more appropriate model for further evaluations. Moreover, it is considered premature to specify a designated series of immunotoxicity studies at the higher tier levels, which, in any case, should be based on the nature of the screening effects.

IMMUNOPATHOLOGY

The guidelines of the Organisation for Economic Co-operation and Development (1981) for testing chemicals address lymphoreticular and haematopoietic tissues; however, for evaluation of immune alterations, routine histopathology must be expanded. All the lymphoid organs are examined grossly, and the weights of thymus and spleen are

Table 2. Design of tier-1 subchronic study protocol

Aim: generation of comparative toxicity data

Chemical: type, identity, analytical assay, toxicokinetics

Animal: species, strain, sex, age, genetic background (e.g., Ah-receptor expression)

Husbandry: environment, caging, food quality, feeding pattern (*ad libitum*, pair-feeding)

Exposure: route, vehicle, expression, dose, duration (single, intermittent, continuous, recovery)

Control data: concomitant, positive, historical

Baseline toxicity data: body weight, food consumption, mortality, signs, clinical chemistry, haematology

Expanded pathology: organ weights, tissue selection, processing mode(s), staining, histochemistry

Selection of appropriate immunological parameters: tier IA, 'key' animals

Statistics

determined: the size of lymph nodes is better estimated during gross examination than at histopathology. The importance of histopathology is qualitative. Morphology provides a detailed picture of altered architecture and changes in the distribution of various populations of cells. Pathologist can identify changes associated with cellular structure, tissue organization, or growth (atrophy, hyperplasia).

In the context of screening studies, routine histopathological examination of lymphoid tissues, together with haematology data, constitute the most straightforward approach to identifying potentially immunotoxic compounds. Cellularity (cell number) is claimed to be a more sensitive parameter than histopathology (Irons, 1985), although the yield may not be quantitative and the important architectural organization is lost. The cellularity of lymphoid organs can be determined by counting the number of nucleated cells in suspension (e.g., by electronic particle counter or flow cytometry).

The primary and secondary lymphoid organs (Table 3) are processed in the context of expanded pathology. Both the peripheral lymph nodes (axillary and popliteal) should be examined, together with the lymphoid tissues associated with the gastrointestinal tract (mesenteric nodes, Peyer's patches). By intergroup comparison, evidence should be obtained about the distribution and cellularity of thymus-independent and thymus-dependent areas. If feasible, morphometric techniques may be used to substantiate suspected changes. Attention should be paid to the mononuclear phagocyte system, especially in areas where the location of macrophages is associated with their interaction with xenobiotics entering the organism *via* the skin or the intestinal or respiratory tract, or when distributed by the blood. Inflammation or tissue damage may result in macrophage-mediated responses.

Morphological examination of the bone marrow is essential for immunotoxicity assessment, as it contains multipotent stem cells that differentiate into B and T cells and macrophages, apart from the haematopoietic parenchyma. Microscopic evaluation is possible on tissue sections, marrow smears or cell suspensions collected from the marrow (Luster *et al.*, 1980). For special purposes, e.g., classification, it may be necessary to examine plastic-embedded bone-marrow and lymphoid tissues in semi-thin section or by electron microscopy. Functional markers (enzymes) and antigen markers may be used in histochemical techniques. Monoclonal antibodies are available for a number of rodent haematopoietic cell antigens (Ward *et al.*, 1989).

At present, there is no internationally agreed set of criteria for the diagnosis of lymphoid and haematopoietic lesions in laboratory animals. Comprehensive descriptions are available for mice (Frith *et al.*, 1985); for rats, representative lesions are usually described in the literature on particular immunotoxicants. Cell migration and homing criteria can be used for spleen and lymph node morphology in rats, such as those proposed by Sainte Marie *et al.* (1982). On the basis of comparative data, patterns of thymus-dependent and thymus-independent responses may be defined, provided that optimized technical procedures are used (Table 4).

Table 3. Primary and secondary lymphoid tissue

Stem-cell pool
 - bone marrow
 - fetal liver

Primary lymphoid organs
 - thymus
 - adult bone marrow

Secondary lymphoid organs
 - lymph nodes
 - spleen
 - bronchus-associated lymphoid tissue
 - gut-associated lymphoid tissue

Table 4. Localization of humoral immune response in spleen and lymph nodes[a]

Cellular event	Spleen	Lymph node
Entry of B lymphocytes	Marginal zone	Extrafollicular zone of peripheral cortex, afferent lymph vessels and marginal sinus, or *via* high endothelial vessels
Antigen-presenting macrophages in thymus-independent response	Marginal zone	Extrafollicular zone of peripheral cortex
Interdigitating T-lymphocyte interaction in thymus-dependent response	Inner periarteriolar lymphocyte sheath (PALS)	Deep cortex unit
T- and B-lymphocyte interaction in thymus-dependent response	Outer PALS	Border between extrafollicular zone of peripheral cortex and deep cortex unit
Differentiation of antigen-reactive B cells into antibody-forming plasma cells	Outer PALS and lymphocyte sheaths around terminal arterioles	Periphery of deep cortex unit
Accumulation of mature antibody-forming plasma cells	Lymphocyte sheaths around terminal arterioles and cords of Billroth in red pulp	Cords of the medulla
Departure	Sinuses of red pulp, circulation	Sinuses of medulla, efferent lymph vessels, circulation

[a]From van Rooijen (1987).

INTERPRETATION OF PATHOLOGY TEST RESULTS

Since toxic dose levels are used in the subchronic study (at or beyond the maximum tolerated dose), indirect effects may occur in the immune system. Atrophy of the lymphoid tissue, especially the thymus, may be due to systemic stress, resulting in reduced food intake and body weight induced by stimulation of pituitary and gonadal hormones, adrenal corticosteroids, catecholamines and other physiological transmitters. Stimulation of haematopoietic activity may follow necrotic tissue changes or toxic anaemia. Serum protein loss, e.g., *via* the intestinal tract or the kidneys, may reduce humoral responses. Furthermore, reactive B-cell stimulation may result from toxic injury to nonimmune tissues.

Possible specific immunotoxic effects are suggested by dose-related changes in total and differential leukocyte counts (lymphocytes, monocytes, eosinophils), by alteration of total globulin or immunoglobulin levels, by changes in specific thymus or spleen weight, as well as by morphological evidence of effects on immunocompetent cell populations and on haematopoietic differentiation in the bone marrow - if such effects are not associated with other relevent systematic or organ-related toxicity.

A word of caution is appropriate, however. Although usually applicable to ascertain the immune system as a target for chemical toxicity, the standard histopathological technique will not usually suffice to differentiate between general effects on the constitutive immune system and changes in its component parts which regulate cell-mediated and humoral immunity (T-cell subsets, B lymphocytes and plasma cells, macrophages). Furthermore, the time of exposure may be critical, as the effect of an immunotoxicant may vary for pharmacokinetic reasons and depend on the turnover rate of the immunocompetent cells. For instance, 90 days of exposure may induce tolerance or may mask an effect in the case of short-lived metabolites. There may be considerable variation in the response of different rodent species and strains because of immunogenetic differences (Foster et al., 1983). The age of the animal may be critical, as immunosuppressive effects are usually enhanced upon exposure during immune-ontogenesis. For dose-response comparisons, it is important to consider the potentially profound influence of such modifying factors.

Moreover, the results of first-tier studies are not sufficient to assess their functional importance. Due to the complex proliferative and compensatory mechanisms that operate in the integrated immune system, there is a large physiological reserve capacity. The reversibility of a given effect may be determined in suitable recovery studies. However, to investigate the importance of compensatory mechanisms, the immunopathology as determined in tier I should be related to changes in the resistance of the host to microbial and tumour challenges (tier II). Although it is appreciated that such changes do not regularly equate with other parameters of immune function and do not necessarily determine its full reserve capacity, it is the ultimate effect on defence mechanisms that is of toxicological significance (Vos & Van Loveren, 1987).

In the absence of information on the consequences of immune impairment, extrapolation to man will remain limited to the dose-response data obtained in the most sensitive model system. In this way, risk assessment may be conducted according to the criteria established for other forms of target organ toxicity.

REFERENCES

Bradley, S.G. (1985) Immunologic mechanisms of host resistance to bacterial and viruses. In: Dean, J.H., Luster, M.I., Munson, A.E. & Amos, H., eds, *Immunotoxicology and Immunopharmacology,* New York, Raven Press, pp. 45-54

Bradley, S.G. & Morahan, P.S. (1982) Approaches to assessing host resistance. *Environ. Health Perspect.,* **43**: 66-19

Dayan, A.D. (1988) *International Collaborative Immunotoxicity Programme,* London, Department of Toxicology, St Bartholomew's Hospital Medical College

Dean, J.H., Luster, M.I., Munson, A.E. & Amos, H., eds, (1985) *Immunotoxicology and Immunopharmacology,* New York, Raven Press

Dean, J.H., Cornacoff, J.B., Rosenthal, G.J. & Luster, M.I. (1989) Immune system: evaluation of injury. In: Hayes, A.W., ed., *Principles and Methods of Toxicology,* 2nd ed., New York, Raven Press, pp. 741-760

European Chemical Industry Ecology and Toxicology Centre (1987) *Identification of Immunotoxic Effects of Chemicals and Assessment of their Relevance to Man (Monograph No. 10),* Brussels

Exon, J.H., Koller, L.D., Talcott, P.A., O'Reilly, C.A. & Henningsen, G.M. (1986) Immunotoxicity testing: an economical multiple-assay approach. *Fundam. appl. Toxicol.,* **7**: 387-397

Foster, H.L., Small, J.D. & Fox, J.G., eds (1983) *The Mouse in Biomedical Research,* Vol. III, *Normative Biology, Immunology and Husbandry,* New York, Academic Press

Frith, C.H., Pattengale, P.K. & Ward, J.M. (1985) *A Color Atlas of Hematopoietic Pathology of Mice,* Little Rock, Arkansas, Toxicology Pathology Associates

Hoshino, A., Takenaka, H., Mizukoshi, O., Imanishi, J., Kishida, T. & Tovey, M. (1983) Effect of anti-interferon serum on influenza virus infection in mice. *Antiviral Res.,* **3**: 59-68

Irons, R.D. (1985) Histology of the immune system: structure and function. In: Dean, J.H., Luster, M.I., Munson, A.A. & Amos, H., eds, *Immunotoxicology and Immunopharmacology,* New York, Raven Press, pp. 10-22

Japan Ministry of Health and Welfare (1988) *Information on the Guidelines (Draft) of Toxicity Studies. The First Section of Evaluation,* Tokyo, Evaluation and Registration Division, Pharmaceutical Affairs Bureau

Lebish, I.J., Hurwitz, A., Lewis, R.M., Cramer, D.V. & Krakowka, S. (1986) Immunopathology of laboratory animals. *Toxicol. Pathol.,* **14**: 129-134

Luster, M.I., Boorman, G.A., Dean, J.H., Harris, M.W., Luebke, R.W., Padarathsingh, M.L. & Moore, J.A. (1980) Examination of bone marrow, immunologic parameters and host susceptibility following pre- and postnatal exposure to 2,3,7,8-tetrachlorodibenzo-p-dioxin (TCDD). *Int. J. Immunopharmacol.,* **2**: 301-310

Luster, M.I., Munson, A.E., Thomas, P.T., Holsapple, M.P., Fenters, J.D., White, K.L., Jr, Lauer, L.D., Germolec, D.R., Rosenthal, G.J. & Dean, J.H. (1988) Methods evaluation, development of a testing battery to assess chemical-induced immunotoxicity: National Toxicology Program's guidelines for immunotoxicity evaluation in mice. *Fundam. appl. Toxicol.,* **10**: 2-19

Maurer, T. (1983) *Contact and Photocontact Allergens, a Manual of Predictive Test Methods,* New York, Marcel Dekker

National Agricultural Chemicals Association (1988) *Proposal for Immunotoxicity Testing* Washington DC

North, R. (1973) Importance of thymus-derived lymphocytes in cell-mediated immunity to infection. *Cell Immunol.*, **7**: 166-176

Organisation for Economic Co-operation and Development (1981) *Guidelines for Testing of Chemicals, Section 4: Health Effects*, Paris

Ryffel, B., Donatsch, P., Madorin, M., Matter, B., Ruttiman, G., Schon, H., Stoll, R. & Wilson, J. (1983) Toxicological evaluation of cyclosporin A. *Arch. Toxicol.*, **53**: 107-141

Sainte-Marie, G., Peng, F.S., & Belisle, C. (1982) Overall architecture and pattern of lymph flow in the rat lymph node. *Am. J. Anat.*, **164**: 275-309

Seinen, W., Vos, J.G., Van Spanje, 1., Snoek, M., Brands, R. & Hooykaas, H. (1977) Toxicity of organotin compounds. II. Comparative in vivo and in vitro studies with various organotin and organolead compounds in different animal species with special emphasis on lymphocytotoxicity. *Toxicol. appl. Pharmacol.*, **42**: 197-212

Sharma, R.P., ed. (1981) *Immunologic Considerations in Toxicology*, Vol. 1, Boca Raton, FL, CRC Press

Sjoblad, R.D. (1989) *SACB Consideration of Proposal from National Agricultural Chemicals Association (NACA) for Immunotoxicity Evaluation of Chemicals*, Washington DC, Office of Pesticides and Toxic Substances, US Environmental Protection Agency

US Environmental Protection Agency (1985) *Final Draft of Subdivision M Guidelines on Immunotoxicity Testing of Biochemical Pest Control Agents*. Washington DC, Office of Pesticide Programs

Van Rooijen, N. (1987) The 'in situ' immune response in lymph nodes: a review. *Anat Rec.*, **218**: 359-364

Vireligier, J. (1975) Host defenses against influenza virus: the role of anti-hemagglutinin antibody. *J. Immunol.*,**115**: 434-446

Vos, J.G. (1977) Immune suppression as related to toxicology. *CRC crit. Rev. Toxicol.*, **5**: 67-101

Vos, J.G. & Van Loveren, H. (1987) Immunotoxicity testing in the rat. In: Burger, E.J., Tardiff, R.G. & Bellanti, J.A., eds, *Environmental Chemical Exposures and Immune System Integrity*, Vol. 13, Princeton, NJ, Princeton Scientific Publishing, pp. 167-180

Ward, J.M., Rehm, S. & Reynolds, C.W. (1989) Tumours of the haematopoietic system. In: Turusov, V.S., ed., *Tumours of the Rat, Pathology of Tumours in Laboratory Animals*, 2nd ed., Lyon, International Agency for Research on Cancer (in press)

REDUCED IMMUNOCOMPETENCE AND RELATIONSHIPS
TO HISTOPATHOLOGY OF THE LYMPHOID SYSTEM

W.E. Parish

Environmental Research Laboratory, Unilever Research
Sharnbrook, Bedford MK44 1LQ, UK

ABSTRACT

Reduced immunocompetence is a potential toxicological hazard; however, demonstration that a chemical induces this effect is not evidence of potential harm. To illustrate this concept, two original studies are described. In one, harmless fatty acids much reduced lymphocyte responsiveness to antigen and mitogen and reduced antibody formation to some antigens in guinea-pigs and mice, without inducing changes in histology or haematology. There was no susceptibility to ill health, and the mice were not more susceptible to experimental infection by three microbial organisms. In the second, rats with severely depleted lymphocytes in the mesenteric lymph node and slight changes in the spleen showed no change in the ability to form antibodies to two antigens. Lymphoid cells with bound antibody to the specific antigen were not found in the affected lymph nodes.

INTRODUCTION

The main applications of immunology to toxicology have been in predictive tests for delayed hypersensitivity (allergic contact dermatitis), for cytotoxicity, particularly in adverse reactions to drugs, and, to a lesser degree, for anaphylactic sensitivity. Recently, with the increasing concern that chemicals, particularly metals, reduce immunocompetence, laboratory techniques are being adapted to detect this adverse effect. Proposals have been made to introduce complex tier systems to test for immune competence during routine screening of chemicals (Vos & Van Loveren, 1987; Luster *et al.*, 1988), but without considering whether such tests will improve the safety of the general population. There is some justification for detailed examination of therapeutic drugs which may be administered for a long time and induce insidious depression of the immune system as a side-effect, but no justification has been seen for applying tests for reduced immunocompetence to the wide range of industrial chemicals. If chemicals have this property, few have selective toxic activity on the immune system. Metals are reported to reduce immunocompetence, but they induce other toxic activities at concentrations relevant to human exposure, which dictate the precautions necessary for safe handling. Reduced immunocompetence is usually a secondary change following damage to or dysfunction of other organs. A true immunotoxicant is selective for the immune system.

Immunotoxicology is the study of adverse effects of substances that are selective for the lymphoid system, including macrophages and dendritic cells as antigen-presenting cells, manifested as enhancement or depression of the immune response, or cytotoxic change.

By definition, toxicity refers to adverse effects, and the initiating stimulus should be selective for the immune system and not a secondary change following damage to other organs or systemic dysfunction. Enhanced activity refers mainly to allergy, e.g., anaphylactic, delayed hypersensitivity or formation of tissue-damaging immune complexes. Depression of the immune response or decreased immunocompetence may not, of itself, be an adverse change but may predispose to other harmful effects, e.g., infection. Toxic reduced immunocompetence may differ only in origin from congenital immunodeficiency or that acquired by viral infection or malnutrition.

Evidence of functional reduced immunocompetence in man or laboratory animals detected by changes in antibody synthesis or lymphocyte function is not of itself reliable evidence of susceptibility to infection, autoimmune disease or cancer. A reduction of 30-50% in antibody formation may represent a drop of only one or two dilutions in antibody titre. Individuals also have a very significant reserve of immune function, as is shown by the difficulties often encountered in therapeutic immunosuppression to protect grafts or to suppress graft-*versus*-host disorders. Protocols to investigate the significance of reduced immunocompetence in animals treated with chemicals, by challenge with infectious agents, have theoretical and practical limitations. Any reduced immunocompetence may be associated with some other undetected dysfunction, e.g., adverse effects on endocrine glands, liver or pancreatic function, or neutrophil mobilization and phagocytosis, which is the underlying cause of the increased susceptibility and distinct from immune function. The practical limitation is the selection of infective agents. Not all laboratories have the barrier facilities necessary for infecting animals with *Listeria monocytogenes*, *Streptococcus pneumoniae*, *Trichinella spiralis* or viruses such as influenza. With the increased regulatory requirements for safety and health of laboratory staff in the UK and Europe, it becomes increasingly difficult to justify the use of such infective agents as routine procedure. Furthermore, at a time when greater efforts are being made to reduce the numbers of animals used in routine toxicology, challenge by infection will re-introduce LD_{50}-type tests, at a time when regulatory authorities have begun to accept limit tests or past experience. Occasional studies in which challenge by infection is necessary to obtain evidence of the fundamental processes of host resistance are generally regarded as acceptable, but use of these techniques as routine procedures could not be justified.

Instead of making a general review, and in order to present the perspective that evidence of significantly reduced immunocompetence in laboratory tests may not indicate hazard to man and that significant histopathological changes in lymph nodes may not be associated with reduced immunocompetence, two laboratory studies are summarized. The first example is that a food substance (fat) to which people are exposed every day reduces immunocompetence in laboratory animals but is harmless and does not predispose them to spontaneous disease or experimental infection. The second example is that a microbial product, aminoglycan, which is representative of a range of substances that are poorly or slowly degraded by macrophages, may induce histiocytosis and depletion of lymphoid follicles in lymph nodes without inducing significantly reduced immunocompetence. These data are discussed in relation to routine toxicological examination of industrial chemicals.

Toxic reduced immunocompetence

A toxic substance that reduces immunocompetence with a selective effect on the immune system should be differentiated from those substances which exert this effect secondarily through damage to other organs, as may occur in routine toxicological tests, as follows:

(1) Reduced immune competence may be nonselective for the immune system, as part of a generalized toxic change or as occurs in man in the case of malnutrition or post-infection.

(2) Selective toxic effects on the lymphoid system may be cytotoxic or functional, without overt cytotoxicity.

(3) These effects may be selective, therapeutic or intentionally cytotoxic in order to greatly depress or abolish the immune response; the term 'immunosuppression' is appropriate for this purpose.

FUNCTIONAL REDUCED IMMUNOCOMPETENCE WITHOUT ADVERSE EFFECT OR CHANGED SUSCEPTIBILITY TO DISEASE

Fatty acids, particularly polyunsaturated fatty acids, reduce cell-mediated immunity by inhibiting lymphocyte responsiveness to antigens and mitogens *in vitro* (Offner & Clausen, 1974; Mertin & Hughes, 1975; Tsang *et al.*, 1977) and increasing the survival time of allografts in rodents (Mertin, 1976). We examined this phenomenon in several studies on guinea-pigs and mice. The results showed that polyunsaturated fats and, to a lesser degree, saturated fats reduced cell-mediated immunity and antibody formation but did not predispose the animals to spontaneous disorders or to experimental infection. The investigations provide a laboratory model for induced depression of immune responsiveness that does not predict hazard to man.

Reduced antibody formation and lymphocyte responsiveness in guinea-pigs fed fats

Guinea-pigs weaned from dams fed 20% polyunsaturated or saturated fats and maintained on the same diets were sensitized to two antigens. Antibody formation was observed by in-vivo skin tests and by two in-vitro techniques and passive cutaneous anaphylaxis; lymphocyte responsiveness was examined *in vivo* by skin tests and *in vitro* by lymphocyte transformation (incorporation of tritiated thymidine) induced by antigen and mitogens and by macrophage migration inhibition (Friend *et al.*, 1980).

Three groups, each of 12 Colworth albino guinea-pigs, derived from the Hartley strain and maintained as a disease-free inbred colony for over 15 years, were fed one of three diets. They were housed in pens with one male to six virgin females. Offspring were maintained on the same diet as their parents; only male offspring from first-litter pregnancies were used for the tests. The number of animals born, sex, birth weight, health and weekly body weight were recorded, and after death a full post-mortem examination was made on all animals, with haematology and histopathology.

The test diets were all standard laboratory BOCM/Silcock Rll pelleted diets on which full details of composition and analytical examination for metals was obtained. The saturated fat (SAFA) was beef tallow, fed at 20%, which contains a small amount of polyunsaturated fat (PUFA). The PUFA was maize oil, also fed at 20%. The fats were analysed for impurities, including heavy metals, and for constituents of the fatty acids by carbon atom chain length and number of double bonds (see Friend *et al.*, 1980). Diets were freshly prepared and stored under conditions to prevent peroxidation, and this was confirmed by analysis.

Healthy male offspring, weaned onto and maintained on their mother's diet, were sensitized at the age of three months to keyhole limpet haemocyanin (KLH) and to tuberculin. KLH was injected in saline solution at 500 µg intramuscularly into the hind leg and 50 µg subcutaneously in the neck. Seven days later, the animals were sensitized to tuberculin by injection of 0.6 ml of Freund's complete adjuvant containing tubercle bacilli (Difco) intramuscularly in the neck.

Tests for immune responsiveness. Tests for antibody formation were made *in vivo* and *in vitro*. *In vivo*, animals were challenged by skin tests with KLH on days 14 and 21 by intradermal injection into the clipped flank with 0.1 ml saline containing 50 µg KLH and with 0.1 ml saline alone at an adjacent site as a control. Challenge responses were assessed at 2, 4, 6, 24 and 48 h. After the challenge responses to both antigens, the animals were bled and serum antibody to KLH was determined *in vitro* by three methods: (i) haemagglutination with KLH-coated erythrocytes; (ii) passive cutaneous anaphylaxis with a challenge 4 h after passive sensitization; and (iii) comple-ment fixation.

Tests for cell-mediated immunity (delayed hypersensitivity) were also made *in vivo* and *in vitro*. *In vivo*, animals were challenqed 14 days after sensitization to tubercle antigen by intradermal injection of 5, 2.5 and 1.25 µg purified protein derivative of tuberculin in 0.1 ml volume, with 0.1 ml saline as control. The sites were examined at 4, 6 and 24 h.

In vitro, two techniques were used - macrophage migration inhibition and lymphocyte transformation by tritiated thymidine incorporation. Macrophage migration inhibition was examined essentially by the technique of David *et al.* (1964), using peritoneal exudate cells elicited by injection with liquid paraffin. The cells were tested in the presence of 20% serum from guinea-pigs fed either normal or high-fat diet in the absence or presence of purified protein derivative of tuberculin antigen (PPD) and the percent inhibition of migration in the presence of antigen was calculated. Lymphocyte transformation was examined essentially by the technique of Levis *et al.* (1974a,b) on suspensions of lymphocytes from lymph nodes

1972), rats (Filkin, 1970; Trejo & Di Luzio, 1971; Trejo *et al.*, 1972; Cook & Di Luzio, 1973; Cook et al., 1974), chickens (Truscott, 1970) and baboons (Holper *et al.*, 1973). Moreover, lead also appears to increase the susceptibility of animals to bacterial infection. Thus, Hemphill *et al.* (1971) found that chronic administration of lead reduced the resistance of mice to *Salmonella typhimurium.* Cook *et al.* (1975) observed a similar phenomenon in rats and reported that the intravenous administration of lead as lead acetate resulted in an approximately 1000-fold increase in susceptibility to *Escherichia coli.* Selected references summarizing the evidence for an impairment of host resistance to pathogens associated with exposure to lead are listed in Table 1.

The influence of lead on viral infection has been ascribed to the capacity of the metal to inhibit interferon production (Gainer, 1974). With respect to bacterial infection, it was originally proposed that increased susceptibility was the result of changes in the reticuloendothelial system and the functional activity of mononuclear phagocytes (Seyle *et al.*, 1966). Although Tam and Hinsdill (1984) reported that culture of murine peritoneal macrophages with noncytotoxic concentrations of lead acetate reduced the proportion of cells capable of ingesting yeast, other studies *in vivo* suggest that lead acetate fails to influence or even potentiates macrophage phagocytosis (Koller & Roan, 1977; Schlick & Friedberg, 1981; Dean & Adams, 1985). It may therefore be difficult to resolve the issue of lead and bacterial resistance in terms of phagocyte function alone. The situation may in fact be complex and involve changes in other organ systems, including hepatic parenchymal cell function (Cook *et al.*, 1974).

Exposure to lead has also been shown to enhance the growth and/or incidence of tumours in rodents (Hinton *et al.*, 1979; Kerkvliet & Baecher-Steppan, 1982), a phenomenon which may or may not be wholly attributable to the putative immunosuppressive properties of the metal.

The difficulties associated with the analysis of lead-induced changes in host resistance have recently been further emphasized by the report of Laschi-Loquerie *et al.* (1987), in which it was observed that the susceptibility of mice to *Klebsiella* was either enhanced or depressed by lead acetate according to the time of administration relative to infectious challenge. The authors argue that the variable influence of lead on *Klebsiella* infection is compatible with the natural history of resistance to this bacterium. Thus, exposure to lead prior to infection enhanced protection through potentiation of phagocytosis. At later stages of the infectious cycle, antibodies are elaborated, and if lead was administered 5 h following bacterial challenge the resultant enhancement of phagocytosis was no longer decisive and the observed increase in susceptibility was secondary to an impairment of humoral immunity (Laschi-Loquerie *et al.*, 1987). It is therefore relevant to consider the influence of lead on components of the adaptive immune system.

HUMORAL IMMUNITY

Antibody responses can be measured in a variety of ways, the most popular of which in immunotoxicology studies is currently the Jerne plaque assay, in which the frequency of

Table 1. **Impairment of host resistance to infectious microorganisms following exposure to lead**

Species	Pathogen	Reference
Mouse	*Salmonella typhimurium*	Hemphill *et al.* (1971)
Mouse	Rauscher leukaemia virus	Gainer (1973)
Mouse	Encephalomyocarditis virus	Gainer (1974)
Mouse	*Staphylococcus aureus*	Salaki *et al.* (1975)
Mouse	Langat virus	Thind & Khan (1978)
Mouse	*Serratia marcescens*	Schlipkoter & Freiler (1979)
Mouse	*Listeria monocytogenes*	Lawrence (1981a)
Rat	*Escherichia coli*	Cook *et al.* (1975)

Table 2. Mean stimulation index of lymphocytes from normal and sensitized animals fed high-fat or normal diet[a]

Diet of cell donor	Diet of serum donor[b]	Average 'stimulation index' in presence of[c]	
		PPD	PHA
Normal	Normal	19.0[d]	100.0[e]
Normal	SAFA	0.7[f] $p = 0.001$	0.6[g] $p = 0.001$
Normal	PUFA	0.5[f] $p = 0.001$	0.5[g] $p = 0.001$
SAFA	Normal	19.0[d]	173.0[e] $p = 0.05$
PUFA	Normal	17.0[d]	155.0[e] $p = 0.05$
PUFA	PUFA	0.5[f] $p = 0.001$	0.2[g] $p = 0.001$

[a]From Friend *et al.* (1980).
[b]SAFA, saturated fat; PUFA, polyunsaturated fat.
[c]PPD, purified protein derivative (cells harvested from tuberculin-sensitized animals); PHA phyto-haemagglutinin; *p* values are for means that differ significantly from those of normal controls.
[d]cpm in media containing PPD and normal serum /cpm in media containing normal serum.
[e]cpm in media containing PHA and normal serum /cpm in media containing normal serum.
[f]cpm in media containing PPD and serum from animals fed either the SAFA or PUFA diet / cpm in media containing PPD and serum from animals fed normal diet.
[g]cpm in media containing PHA and serum from animals fed either the SAFA or PUFA diet / cpm in media containing PHA and serum from animals fed normal diet.

There was no difference in the numbers of blood leukocytes, the differential counts, or leukocyte morphology in the fat-fed animals compared to the controls. The dams and the offspring weaned from them remained healthy. In other tests, three generations of guinea-pigs were maintained on these diets without effects on their health, fertility or life span. Thus, the very significant reduction in immunocompetence was not associated with any disorder or susceptibility to spontaneous infection. The inhibitory effect is due to a factor in the serum which either blocks lymphocyte receptors or membrane responses to stimuli. There is evidence that the factor may be the apoprotein E in fat chylomicrons (De Deckere *et al.*, 1988).

Reduced antibody formation, lymphocyte responsiveness and tests for susceptibility to infection in mice fed fats

In order to investigate the effects of dietary fat on susceptibility to infection, sufficiently large numbers of animals are required to obtain significant results; the mouse is an appropriate species. Before infection tests could be made, it was necessary to establish if the immune response in the mouse was modified in the same manner as that of guinea-pigs fed fat-enriched diets.

Male littermates six to eight weeks of age from an inbred colony of C57Bl mice were allocated randomly to groups fed 20% PUFA, 5% PUFA, 20% SAFA or standard laboratory diet, which was rigorously controlled for content and stability. All tests were made after the mice had been fed the diets for at least ten weeks. Groups of mice were then injected with Freund's adjuvant containing tubercle bacilli to test for delayed hypersensitivity, and with the T-dependent antigens, sheep red blood cells, *Salmonella typhimurium* vaccine and ovalbumin, and the T-independent antigen *Escherichia coli* lipopolysaccharide for antibody formation. Peripheral blood counts were made, and macrophage function examinef at ten weeks and six months (Crevel *et al.*, 1990). The main findings were as follows:

Body weights and health. As the diets were designed to give a similar caloric intake,and the animals adjusted their food intake according to dietary caloric density, very similar body weights were seen in all groups. All mice thrived and remained healthy.

Delayed hypersensitivity. Mice treated with Freund's adjuvant were challenged by injection of tuberculin into the pinna of one ear, which was measured for thickness. The 20% PUFA diet was associated with the weakest reaction, which was about half that of the sensitized mice on the controlled diets. Those on the SAFA diet also had a much reduced response. The 5% PUFA diet slightly reduced the immune response with a dose-response relationship.

Antibody formation. There was no significant difference among the fat-fed animals and the controls after one, two or three injections of the *Salmonella* vaccine (IgG and IgM), of the sheep red cells or of ovalbumin (IgG or IgE, no IgM detected). There was a significantly decreased titre to *E. coli* lipopolysaccharide (IgM) on days 3 and 5 in the 20% PUFA group, but no significant decrease in the other two test groups.

Macrophage function. Macrophages harvested from the peritoneal cavity of mice by saline lavage without elicitation by other substances showed no morphological difference between the test groups and controls. Suspensions of the cells were treated with a toxic (quartz DQ12) and a nontoxic (TiO_2) particulate material and the supernatant fluid assayed for release of lactate dehydrogenase and β-glucuronidase for evidence of cell death or damage. Macrophages from each test group were equally able to ingest the particles. There was no difference in the spontaneous release of the enzymes or that following phagocytosis of the toxic or nontoxic particles. Moreover, there was no difference in macrophage function as determined by the above tests in cells from mice at 10-15 weeks or at six months.

Haematology. Total and differential white blood cell counts revealed no significant difference between mice on the various diets. There was a slight increase in the number of monocytes in the mice on the three fat diets, but this was considered not to be significant as the counts were within the normal range for mice of the colony.

Post-mortem examination. There was no evidence of deviations from the normal in any of the groups.

It is concluded that the mice fed the high-fat diets had significantly reduced delayed hypersensitivity, which was dose-related for the PUFA-fed groups at 20 and 5%. Antibody formation in response to *E. coli* lipopolysaccharide was reduced transiently, but response to the three T-dependent antigens was unaffected. Macrophage phagocytic function was normal and blood leukocyte counts unchanged.

Infection studies. The same groups of mice provided the controls for animals tested for resistance to infection. This study was done concomitantly with mice from the same colony, fed the same food and maintained in the same unit. Mice maintained on the test diets of 20% PUFA, 5% PUFA and 20% SAFA were inoculated with approximately LD_{50} doses of *S. typhimurium* (160 animals), *Staphylococcus aureus* (200 animals) and *Candida albicans* (240 animals). These organisms were selected as representative of a gram-negative and a gram-positive bacterium and a yeast, respectively (Friend *et al.*, 1990). Reasons for not using more pathogenic organisms, such as *Listeria monocytogenes*, are stated in the introduction. There was no difference in susceptibility to infection, as determined by the percentage of deaths and by time of onset of sickness, in the fat-fed animals compared to the controls in groups large enough to show any significant difference.

It is evident that, although the feeding of fats to mice for 12 weeks much reduced lymphocyte responsiveness, together with a transient depression of antibody to a T cell-independent bacterial antigen, they did not increase susceptibity to experimental infection. Furthermore, mice maintained on the diets for six months showed no susceptibility to spontaneous disorders. These studies on mice demonstrate that it is possible to induce a functional decrease in immunity, as judged by standard laboratory tests, without histological change and without significance in terms of infection or general health.

HISTOPATHOLOGICAL CHANGES IN THE LYMPHOID SYSTEM WITHOUT REDUCED IMMUNOCOMPETENCE

Current concerns in interpretation of toxicological studies are (i) the feasibility of detecting disorders of immunity from data of routine studies; and (ii) whether histopathology provides sufficient evidence to indicate immunological disturbance. The opposite also applies: change in the histology of lymph nodes may not be associated with changes in immune function. The following summary of laboratory investigations shows that significant histological changes may occur in lymph nodes in the absence of functional change in immunity. The changes may be severe but confined to local draining nodes, or milder and more widely dispersed. We give a brief description of variations in the histology of lymph nodes that influence interpretation of test results, based on experiments in normal rats and rabbits in a colony at the Lister Institute of Preventive Medicine, and two examples of investigations in which histological changes in lymph node and spleen were not associated with changes in immune function. The examples are taken from control groups of rats and rabbits used in studies of vasculitis induced by immune complexes containing persistent, nondegradable antigens. The tests for immune function were concomitant observations and not the main objective of the experiments.

Spontaneous variations in lymph nodes of normal rats and rabbits

Lister hooded rats and New Zealand white rabbits were maintained in clean but not pathogen-free conditions. There was no history of ill health in the colonies. Animals were fed commercial standard diets that were not changed from the time of weaning. The description concerns rats aged eight weeks and rabbits aged ten weeks.

Lymph nodes continually filter substances absorbed through the mucous membranes or skin and are in a dynamic state of change, determined by the amount and route of entry of the foreign substances or components of damaged tissues. Nonantigenic substances induce acute inflammatory change or chronic histiocytosis and granulomatous change, which may be persistent or even progressive. Antigens stimulate formation of antibody, inducing increased numbers of B lymphocytes and plasma cells or delayed hypersensitivity with increased numbers of T lymphocytes and macrophages and more evident dendritic cells. Acute changes occur within hours.

Lymph nodes of normal animals show considerable variation in histology between individuals within a colony, and between colonies of animals. This 'spontaneous' variation is most evident in mesenteric, cervical and hilar (bronchial) lymph nodes, which are most heavily exposed to substances absorbed through mucous membranes. There is less variability in the histology of the popliteal lymph nodes, less so in the inguinal nodes draining the skin, and least variation in the iliac lymph nodes (Table 3). The iliac lymph nodes have other lymph nodes as partial filters between them and the environment, reducing the likelihood of extraneous stimulation, and are thus suitable lymphoid tissues for studying systemic effects of infectious agents or toxic chemicals.

Apart from spontaneous variation, there is also variability within different portions of the larger lymph nodes, especially the mesenteric chain of nodules and the cervical nodes. This variation occurs in both the stimulated and nonstimulated states. One histological section may show features of a nonstimulated or resting phase, with compact primary follicles, defined paracortex and relatively empty sinuses. Deeper sections from the same

Table 3. Spontaneous variations in lymph node histology in normal, healthy rats in one colony[a]

Lymph node	Secondary follicles	Plasma cells	Macrophages in medulla	Mast cells	Reticulin	Neutrophils
Mesenteric	+++	++	++	+	+	+
Cervical	++	+	+	-	+	-
Hilar (bronchial)	++	++	+	-	-	-
Popliteal	+	+	+	+	+	-
Superficial inguinal	+	-	+	-	-	-
Internal iliac	-	-	-	-	-	-

[a] +, 1.5-fold; ++, 2-fold; +++, 3-fold variation in sections from different animals above and below the mean for the feature in the colony.

block may show areas of stimulation, with large secondary follicles, germinal centres, increased mitoses and small- and medium-sized lymphocytes filling the sinuses. In contrast, chronic changes, as manifested by histiocytosis and decreased numbers of lymphoid follicles, are usually present throughout most of a node when they occur.

Chronic histological changes in draining lymph nodes without change in immune function

In studies of cutaneous vasculitis induced by immune complexes in man, streptococcal, staphylococcal, mycobacterial and *Candida* antigens were found with immunoglobulin in recent lesions (Parish & Rhodes, 1967; Parish, 1971, 1980). These antigens were degradation products, not whole organisms. Animal experiments indicated that bacterial antigens that were not readily degraded by macrophages were more potent than protein antigens in complexes that induce persistent vasculitis (Parish & Rhodes, 1967). Investigations to examine this property were made by administering an aminoglycan extract of *Candida albicans* orally, to represent absorption of *Candida* products by the intestine to stimulate antibody synthesis and formulation of immune complexes. The fermenter-prepared batch of *Candida* aminoglycan was antigenic, but the glycan moiety persisted in macrophages, stimulating release of β-glucuronidase and synthesis of proteases and complement fragment C3, but was not toxic. The macrophages survived in culture. Although microbial extracts were used in these studies, they are representative of a wide range of substances of plant and synthetic origin that are used in industry - e.g., hemicelluloses, carrageenans, cross-linked starches, ditallows and polymers.

Oral doses in rats, with changes in mesenteric lymph nodes

Although the investigation was designed to mimic the uptake of yeast antigens from the intestine and formation of immune complexes *in vivo*, features of the test are relevant to techniques for examining reduced immunocompetence. In the experiment on rats, animals were dosed orally with the aminoglycan extract. Subsequently, they were injected with bovine serum albumin (BSA) to sensitize them to form IgE. They were then challenged by intravenous injection to induce nonfatal anaphylaxis, and the serum examined for immune complexes containing *Candida* antigen.

The design of the protocol is presented in Table 4. Groups of rats were dosed orally with 15 mg (or with 10 and 5 mg) on five days a week for two weeks. On day 28, nine rats were sensitized to BSA in alum to form IgE antibody; 18 rats were also injected with 5 mg BSA intravenously to stimulate formation of precipitating-type IgG and IgM antibodies. The rats injected to form IgE were challenged on day 5 after sensitization; rats injected to form IgG antibody were killed on day 5, on day 8 and on day 14 after the intravenous injection.

Among the tissues examined histologically were the mesenteric, cervical and internal iliac lymph nodes and the spleen. Sera were examined for antibody to all *Candida* antigen, and the BSA for IgE (e.g., passive cutaneous anaphylaxis), for IgG and IgM (e.g., by enzyme-linked immunosorbent assay and by haemagglutination of sheep red cell-coated particles) and for immune complexes containing *Candida* antigen or BSA. Sera were also examined for total globulin and for total IgG and IgM by radial immunodiffusion

Instead of the standard plaque-forming cell assay, cells that formed or had membrane-bound antibody to the aminoglycan or the BSA were detected by cross-linking the antigen to rat erythrocytes and using the mixed-cell agglutination technique (McConnell *et al.*, 1969), based on that of Jonas *et al.* (1965). Suspensions of separated mesenteric lymph node or spleen cells were centrifuged with antigen-treated rat erythrocytes and resuspended, and cells with three or more adherent erythrocytes were counted. Although rat erythrocytes are less discriminating than sheep erythrocytes as carrier particles, any background spontaneous antibody for the foreign species is avoided in this way.

Histopathology. The mesenteric lymph nodes were much enlarged, having a mean of 2.8-fold greater weight than those of the controls. The essential feature was histiocytosis, with numerous macrophages filling the paracortex and extending into the cortex, which contained a few irregular follicles compressed against the capsule. In the paracortex, some

Table 4. Protocol for groups of rats dosed orally with aminoglycan extract of *Candida albicans*, some of which were sensitized to bovine serum albumin (BSA)

Group	No. of animals	Treatment	Tests			
			Tissue examination	Haematology	Antibody formation	Presence of complexes
A	9	Nil	Histology; mixed-cell agglutination; mesenteric node; spleen	+	-	-
B	9	BSA IV/IgG	Histology; mixed-cell agglutination; mesenteric node; spleen	+	+	+
C	9	BSA for IgE	Histology; mixed-cell agglutination; mesenteric node; spleen	+	+	+
D	9	Aminoglycan	Histology only	+	+	+
E	9	Aminoglycan; BSA for IgE	Histology; mixed-cell agglutination; mesenteric node; spleen	+	+	+
F	18	Aminoglycan (9)	Histology; mixed-cell agglutination; mesenteric node; spleen	+	+	+
		BSA IV/IgG (9)	Histology only			

of the macrophages had formed small syncytia, and there were a few scattered epithelial cells. No plasma cell could be detected in the perivascular or perilymphatic cuffs. The spleens of two animals in Group D showed discrete aggregates of histiocytes, and two others had increased numbers of small mononuclear cells, probably lymphocytes, in the white pulp. The spleens of three animals in Group F showed decreased areas of white pulp, and in another two there were a few giant cells. The other lymph nodes examined showed no histiocytosis and little change in the lymphoid follicles.

The histiocytosis is believed to result when macrophages ingest a substance that is poorly degraded but is a potent stimulus to macrophage synthesis of inflammatory mediators, recruiting more macrophages and eventually activating fibroblasts.

Haematology. The essential results are that the aminoglycan induced little change in numbers of lymphocytes or monocytes but a significant increase in the numbers of neutrophils. Intravenous injection of BSA stimulated a very significant increase in the numbers of neutrophils. Injection of BSA in alum resulted in little change relative to the aminoglycan-treated controls.

Total globulins and IgG. There was no statistically significant change in the amounts of total globulins in the groups treated with aminoglycan (Groups D, E and F), and the levels were little different from those in the control Group A. Although the amounts of total globulin in Group F (treated with aminoglycan and BSA intravenously) remained unchanged, there was a significant increase in total IgG. In Group B (injected intravenously with BSA without the aminoglycan), there was an increase in total globulins and total IgG and IgM.

Antibody formation. The animals with severe histiocytosis of the mesenteric lymph nodes (Group F) tended to have higher mean titres to the BSA than did animals not previously treated with the aminoglycan (Group B). Similarly, the titre of anaphylactic antibody in the groups stimulated to form IgE tended to be greater in the group also treated with the aminoglycan (Group E) than in the group without (Group C) (Table 5).

The results of assays for immune complexes are not relevant to considerations of reduced immunocompetence.

Spleen and lymph node cells with bound antibody. The numbers of mononuclear cells forming rosettes of agglutination (equivalent to plaque-forming cells) was greatly reduced or almost abolished in the mesenteric lymph nodes of animals dosed with the aminoglycan and BSA and examined for antibodies to both antigens. The numbers of sensitized cells in the spleen showed no change or some increase. The mean numbers of cells with antibody to BSA are presented in Table 5; there was considerable individual variation. The untreated Group A showed some cells with natural bound antibody to the BSA.

Mitogenic stimulation. Portions of mesenteric lymph nodes from animals of each group were examined for responsiveness to the mitogen phytohaemagglutinin. The samples were the unused longitudinal half of the nodes used for histology or the remaining portions of the samples used for the mixed-cell agglutination tests. The tritiated tissue was incubated on columns of fine glass beads to separate the macrophages and the enriched lymphocyte preparation treated with phytohaemagglutinin, followed by 4-h incubation with ³H-thymidine. Using the counts per minute of Group A as a control base line, the values for the two animals in groups B and C were seen to be increased. In contrast, there were very low counts in cells from the nodes of animals in Groups D, E and F. This is unlikely, however, to represent decreased responsiveness of the lymphocytes, because the numbers of cells recovered were so small that it was difficult to match them with those of Groups A, B and C.

Conclusion. These findings are relevant to studies of test methods to detect immunocompetence. As the mesenteric lymph node is large and easily removed, it tends to be the node taken for histological examination and for assay of plaque-forming cells. In the study summarized above, rats treated with the aminoglycan had severe chronic changes in the mesenteric lymph nodes, with depletion of the lymphoid follicles and other lymphoid elements. The paracortex was vestigial. The changes were so severe that none of the small numbers of lymphocytes isolated had bound antibody to the BSA antigen, present spontaneously in a few cells of the control Group A and in significant number in Groups B and C, which were sensitized to BSA. Although only two animals of each group were tested with the mitogen phytohaemagglutinin and there were technical limitations to obtaining sufficient numbers of cells from groups D, E and F, there was a weak response in these

Table 5. Antibody titres to aminoglycan and to bovine serum albumin (BSA) and numbers of mesenteric lymph node and splenic cells with bound antibody to BSA

Group	Agglutinating antibody		Passive cutaneous anaphylaxis	No. of cells with bound Ab/10⁶ cells tested	
	Aminoglycan	BSA/IgG	(BSA/IgE)	Mesenteric lymph node	Spleen
A	4	ND	ND	24	36
B	8	256	0	812	3420
C	16	16	64	86	920
D	64	ND	ND	0	18
E	128	512	0	0	3986

ND, not done

282

groups to mitogen stimulation. Despite these changes in histology and function of the lymph nodes, there was no decrease in the amount of circulating antibody.

It follows, therefore, that tests for immune competence on lymphoid tissue must be made on the spleen and on lymph nodes from different sites or on a pool of lymphocytes from several lymph nodes.

DETECTION OF REDUCED IMMUNOCOMPETENCE IN ROUTINE TOXICOLOGICAL TESTS FOR HAZARD

It is necessary to achieve a balance between ensuring safety for persons exposed to chemicals and the amount of testing to be carried out over and above that already required by regulatory authorities, especially when more animals must be used. In tests to determine the significance of any reduced immunity, e.g., by challenge with infection, for which many animals are necessary, either as one group treated with an approximative LD_{50} or as few animals in each of three or more groups treated with a range of doses. Tests for reduced immunocompetence should rarely be required as a routine procedure. The issues to be considered are:

(1) Are test results indications of selective or significant changes in the histology of the lymphoid system, blood mononuclear cells and total or γ-globulin?
(2) Are there changes in other organs that provide evidence for acceptability for proposed use, safe handling or special restrictions?

Metals and many other chemicals induce damage in several organs that are sufficient to indicate caution on frequent exposure. It is unlikely that additional tests for reduced immunocompetence are necessary if other hazards are identified and precautions are instituted for safe handling or limited exposure.

It is possible that functional tests for immune competence are required only for therapeutic drugs intended for long-term use, and, even for these, indications of a potential adverse effect should be detected in routine tests.

When evidence of reduced immunocompetence is detected by laboratory tests, it cannot be interpreted to mean that the individual is susceptible to adverse effects, e.g., infection, autoimmunity or cancer. The system has a very large functional reserve. Of the two examples summarized above, the first showed that a harmless substance, fat, may reduce lymphocyte responsiveness to antigen and to mitogen and reduce formation of antibodies to some antigens, with no increase in susceptibility to spontaneous ill health or to experimental infections. In the second, severe histological change in a major lymph node and some changes in the spleen were not associated with decreased formation of antibody to a complex microbial antigen or to a protein. Thus, even histological change in a lymph node is not necessarily an indication for extensive immune function tests.

The above proposals are not suggestions to limit the number of tests necessary to safeguard the health of people exposed to chemicals. They are an attempt to achieve a practical balance in the amount of routine testing required for industrial chemicals, so that additional tests are needed only when there are definite indications that such tests are advisable and would be relevant to human exposure.

REFERENCES

Crevel, R.W., Friend, J.V., Goodwin, B.F.J. & Parish, W.E. (1990) High fat diets and the immune response of C57 Bl mice. (Submitted)
David, J.R., Al-Askari, S., Lawrence, H.S. & Thomas, L. (1964) Delayed hypersensitivity in vitro. I. The specificity of inhibition of cell migration by antigen. *J. Immunol.*, **93**: 264-273
De Deckere, E.M.A., Verplanke, J., Blonk, C.G. & Van Nielen, W.G.L. (1988) Effects of type and amount of dietary fat on rabbit and rat lymphocyte proliferation *in vitro*. *J. Nutr.*, **188**: 11-18
Friend, J.V., Lock, S.O., Gurr, M.I. & Parish, W.E. (1980) Effect of different dietary lipids on the immune response of Hartley strain guinea pigs. *Int. Arch. Allergy appl. Immunol.*, **62**: 292-301
Friend, J.V., Crevel, R.W.R., Parish, W.E., Humphreys, A., Carter, M. & Crowther, J.S. (1990) Reduced immunocompetence in mice fed high-level fat diets tested for resistance to infection by pathogenic bacteria and yeast. (Submitted)

Jonas, W.E., Gurner, B.W., Nelson, D.S. & Coombs, R.R.A (1965) Passive sensitization of tissue cells. 1. Passive sensitization of macrophages by guinea-pig cytophilic antibody. *Int. Arch. Allergy appl. Immunol.*, **28**: 86-104

Levis, W.R., Whalen, J.J. & Mille   A.E.(1974a) Studies on the contact sensitization of man with simple chemicals. II. Lymphokine production in allergic contact dermatitis to dinitrochlorobenzene. *J. invest. Dermatol.*, **62**: 2-6

Levis, W.R., Whallen, J.J. & Miller, A.E. (1974b) Blastogenesis of autologous, allogeneic and syngeneic (identical twins) lymphocytes in response to lymphokines generated to dinitrochlorobenzene-sensitive human leukocytes cultures. *J. Immunol.*, **112**: 1488-1493

Luster, M.I., Munson, A.E., Thomas, P.T., Hosapple, M.P., Fanters, J.D., White, K.L., Lauer, L.D., Germolc, D.R., Rosenthal, G.J. & Dean, J. (1988) Methods evaluation: development of a testing battery to assess chemical-induced immunotoxicity: National Toxicology Programs guidelines for immunotoxicity evaluation in mice. *Fundam. appl. Toxicol.*, **10**: 2-19

McConnell, I., Monro, A., Gurner, B.W. & Coombs, R.R.A. (1969) Studies on actively allergized cells. 1. Cyto-dynamics and morphology of rosette-formation with antibody to mouse immunoglobulins. *Int. Arch. Allergy appl. Immunol.*, **35**: 209-227

Mertin, J. (1976) Effect of polyunsaturated fatty acids on skin allograft survival and primary and secondary cytotoxic response in mice. *Transplantation,* **21**: 1-4

Mertin, J. & Hughes, D. (1975) Specific inhibitory action of polyunsaturated fatty acids on lymphocyte transformation induced by PHA and PPD. *Int. Arch. Allergy appl. Immunol.*, **48**: 203-210

Offner, H. & Clausen, J. (1974) Inhibition of lymphocyte response to stimulants by unsaturated fatty acids and prostaglandins. *Lancet*, **ii**: 400-401

Parish, W.E. (1971) Studies in vasculitis. I. Immunoglobulins, βIC, C-reactive protein and bacterial antigens in cutaneous vasculitis lesions. *Clin. Allergy*, **1**: 97-109

Parish, W.E. (1980) Microbial antigens in vasculitis. In: Wolff, I.L. & Winkelman, R.K., eds, *Vasculitis*, London, Lloyd-Luke, pp.129-150

Parish, W.E. & Rhodes, E.l. (1967) Bacterial antigens and aggregated gamma globulin in lesions of nodular vasculitis. *Br. J. Dermatol:*, **79**: 131-147

Tsang, W.M., Weyman, C. & Smith, A.D. (1977) The effect of fatty acids and albumin on the transformation of rodent spleen lymphocytes stimulated by phytohaemagglutinin, concanavalin A or bacterial lipopolysaccharide. *Biochem. Soc. Trans.*, **5**: 1159-1160

Vos, J.G. & Van Loveren, H. (1987) Immunotoxocity testing in the rat. In: Mehlman, M.A., ed., *Advances in Modern Environmental Toxicology*, Vol. XIII, *Environmental Chemical Exposures and Immune System Integrity*, Princeton, NJ, Princeton Scientific, pp. 147-159

THE IMMUNE SYSTEM: HUMAN STUDIES

CLINICAL ASPECTS OF POTENTIAL
IMMUNOTOXIC EFFECTS OF CHEMICALS:
DIAGNOSTIC AND EPIDEMIOLOGICAL CAUTION

A.D. Dayan

DH Department of Toxicology
St Bartholomew's Hospital Medical College
London EC1, UK

ABSTRACT

Our understanding of the mechanisms of immunity is advancing but is still limited, especially in relation to attributing particular abnormalities as causes of disease. Similarly, although many aspects of immune responses can be dissected in the laboratory, there remain areas of ignorance which hinder any attempt to correlate measured abnormality with clinical disorder, even in those few instances where reagents and assay techniques have been adequately standardized.

The concept that 'immunotoxicity' represents a general health hazard to man and animals, like any other type of target organ toxicity, is attractive, although there are few examples other than the special case of hypersensitivity. Whether working at the level of a population monitored by an epidemiologist, as a clinician concerned with individual patients, or as a scientist measuring components of the immune response, particular care is required in trying to link exposure with effect in view of the complexity and flexible responsiveness of the immune system.

GENERAL CONCERNS RAISED BY CLAIMS OF CHEMICAL IMMUNOTOXICITY

On theoretical grounds, it is reasonable to expect chemicals as a class to be able to produce any effect on the immune system, causing general or selective enhancement or depression of specific immune responses to endogenous or exogenous antigens, or of nonspecific defences, or no effect at all. The clinical culmination of such actions, producing a condition that will bring the patient to medical or veterinary attention, represents a balance between the severity of the disorder and the compensatory ability of the immune system (and possibly of other bodily functions) in response to the variable challenges of everyday life. Of no lesser importance is the ability and willingness of those affected to recognize and complain of a non-normal state, the diagnostic acumen of the clinician in recognizing the abnormal condition (disease or a lesser degree of dysfunction), the quantitative power of any diagnostic test applied to the individual, and the statistical power of any population survey of disease or laboratory finding. And, there is the skill required to demonstrate the association with exposure to the chemical at an appropriate time before or during the occurrence of the clinical abnormality.

For final proof, it would be valuable to reproduce the disease or its underlying pathogenetic mechanism in a model laboratory system.

Together, these requirements amount to the process of suspicion, detection, diagnosis and proof that applies to any disease of man and animals. They are specifically mentioned in the present context in order to stress certain points:

Immunotoxicity of Metals and Immunotoxicology, Edited by
A. D. Dayan *et al.,* Plenum Press, New York, 1990

(i) Immunotoxicity due to exposure to chemicals is unlikely to produce an entirely novel disorder. It is likely, instead, to mimic in whole or in part an existing disease complex, although the relative severity or incidence of the various abnormalities that make up recognized syndromes may well be unusual.

(ii) The broad pathophysiological possibilities represented by effects on the immune system may in principle be manifested as a specific disease, due to an excessive or a deficient response (e.g., an acquired allergy to a particular antigen or a defect in resistance to a particular infective organism), as a more general abnormality, culminating in, say, an autoimmune disorder, as neoplasia affecting the lymphoid or other body systems, or as general impairment of health revealed as a broad liability to increased conventional or atypical infections. Any tissue in the body may be the site of the noticeable effect. Any stage of development may be affected, from formation of the gonads to pre- and post-natal maturation of the succeeding generation.

(iii) An immunotoxic effect may be present as an abnormal finding in a laboratory test, with or without a clinical counterpart at that stage.

(iv) In epidemiological terms of surveillance or assessment of a population, the corresponding aspects that might come to attention would be an excess (or deficiency) or a change in the pattern of a particular disease, general ill-health (e.g., impaired growth, slowed approach to developmental milestones, an abnormal community response to infections and other challenges), or abnormality of reproductive success.

All this is so general as to be philosophical rather than practical, but the breadth of possibilities inherent in any suggestion of 'immunotoxicity' must be realized and linked with the inescapable need for caution in making such a claim, for precision in defining it, and for great care in providing sufficiently strong evidence to support it.

POSSIBLE IMMUNOTOXIC DISORDERS AND DYSFUNCTIONS

If it is accepted that induced immunotoxicity will probably mimic in whole or in part known syndromes, present medical knowledge suggests that in seeking evidence of immunotoxicity certain types of disease should be sought, and so should particular types of laboratory data. Their practical suitability as sentinel conditions or laboratory markers that alert the clinical scientist and epidemiologist raises different and very difficult questions which must probably be answered pragmatically in relation to the nature of the subjects or population involved, the background or control data already available and the feasibility of clinical or laboratory surveillance focused on appropriate changes.

The extremes of severe immunosuppression and true hypersensitivity should be relatively easy to recognize, at least in individuals; but lesser degrees of those abnormalities, for example, immunomodulation that causes a quantitatively but not qualitatively abnormal response to a normal challenge (such as an inappropriate immune reaction and slow cure of an infection, an increased incidence of autoimmune thyroiditis, a change in the response pattern to a common allergen), and a delayed consequence of exposure in development or earlier life (the 'latent' defect of teratology), would all be hard to discern and even harder to prove with present knowledge.

Similarly, at the laboratory level, ascribing 'abnormality' to a test result, or even a cluster of results, requires good foreknowledge of background variation in the population, of the accuracy and reproducibility of controlled tests, appropriate quality assurance and careful standardization of the test conditions (e.g., fasting, time, sampling collection procedure, accepted reagent). In terms of measured variables, it is important to recognize that a mixture of depression of one arm of a regulatory network and excessive activity of other pathways is likely to occur, so assessment of a range of measures is likely to be much more informative than a single estimation. Abnormal laboratory findings may not accompany a clinically apparent disorder.

TYPES OF DISORDER

In epidemiological terms, retrospective surveillance of spontaneous reports or prospective assessment of a population, the most striking aspects that seem likely to come to attention might be:

Immunosuppression

Infections. General immunosuppression will result in enhanced susceptibility to normal infectious agents, prolongation of such infections due to impairment of the normal, curative immune responses, and the related development of infections to normally non-pathogenic agents. Clinical experience has shown that the organisms involved can be viruses, bacteria, fungi, protozoa and metazoa.

Neoplasia. Although the simple hypothesis of immune surveillance is no longer accepted, there is known to be an increased incidence of several types of tumours in immunosuppressed persons and animals, whether that state is congenital or acquired. Neoplasms may occur of external epithelia (skin and gastrointestinal tract), visceral organs, the lymphoid system and haematopoietic cells.

Autoimmune disorders. Selective impairment of various components of immunity is important in the genesis of certain autoimmune reactions, which probably develop on certain genetic backgrounds, and in response to infections.

Immunopotentiation (enhancement)

This, too, may be general or specific, thereby producing a wide range of possible disorders. True allergic hypersensitivity to a single hapten or epitope is the most striking manifestation of this phenomenon, which may depend on an interplay between genetic composition and exposure to an immunogen.

It may be regarded as merging into broader syndromes of autoimmunity, which may affect just one tissue (e.g., drug-induced thrombocytopenia), or several, either by direct attack (e.g., lupus erythematosus-like syndromes) or by the 'innocent bystander' mechanism, in which immune complexes, complement units or aggressive cells damage the tissue in which they are generated or deposited (e.g., serum sickness, anaphylactic shock, polyarteritis).

Less is known about the consequences of general enhancement of all or a major part of the immune processes, so the nature and extent of the clinical conditions and the relationship between damage attributable to the classic types-I-IV reactions and, for example, the systemic effects of the cytokines is unclear. The link between neoplasia and immunopotentiation is also unclear at present, but there is an association between continued stimulation and proliferation of lymphoid cells and at least certain types of oncogenesis, as in Burkitt's lymphoma, even though other processes may also be involved, such as mutation and genomal rearrangement.

Hypersensitivity is such a striking phenomenon that it has captured much clinical attention, but it is important to be alert to less prominent syndromes attributable to more generalized enhancement or depression of immunity.

LABORATORY MEASURES OF IMMUNITY

A detailed review of individual procedures and their specific interpretation belongs elsewhere, but, at present, when knowledge is developing rapidly and understanding lags, as much caution is required in the laboratory as in the clinic. There must be tight control and careful standardization of specimen collection and assay procedures, if results are to be compared between laboratories. Reference standards are important anyway, particularly if analytes are assayed by different techniques. Populations being investigated must also be standardized, or allowance must be made for differences in, e.g., age, sex, nutrition and health status.

At the relatively simple level of measuring the total concentration or level of a specific immunoglobulin, or complement, reasonable accuracy may be anticipated, as in doing total and differential white cell counts. Once more, sophisticated measures are employed, however, there is increasing need for caution in interpretation, especially in interlaboratory comparisons, as few data have been published on such basic measures as coefficient of variation and precision. This caveat applies to specific and nonspecific mitogen-driven cell proliferation, allogenic lymphocyte responses, counting specific cell types using surface markers, resistance to infectious agents, experiments on humoral and cell-mediated immune responses, and assay of circulating cytokines and receptors.

MARKERS OF IMMUNOTOXICITY

As already stated, there seems no reason to anticipate unique clinical or laboratory markers of immunotoxicity. Instead, it will be necessary to isolate disease syndromes and disordered laboratory functions from the background noise of conventional illnesses and to associate them with exposure. Actions claimed in man or other target species should be matched against known laboratory findings and experimental results for the substance in question.

The range of possible effects and diseases that should be considered is outlined briefly in Table 1. Its breadth underlines the need for caution in attribution of a condition or

Table 1. Possible clinical aspects of immunotoxic responses

Response	Conventional clinical syndrome	Signal effect
Immunosuppression (deficiencies)		
Generalized	Combined immunodeficiency disease	Infections Maldevelopment (?)
	Neoplasia (?)	Lymphoid and systemic neoplasms
Partial	Hypogamma globulinaemia	Infections (protean) Arthritis Haemolytic anaemia
	Selective Ig class deficiency	Kidney diseases Malabsorption
	Complement system	Infections Immune complex diseases Clotting disorders (?)
	Amyloidosis	
	Chronic granulomatous disease	Infections
	Chediak-Higashi syndrome	
	Autoimmune disorders	Protean (endocrines, joints)
	Hypersensitivity disorders	Skin, gastrointestinal tract, respiratory disorders
	Neoplasia (?)	Lymphoid and systemic neoplasms
	Reproductive damage (?)	Impaired development
Immunopotentiation		
Generalized	?	Multi-system allergies (?) Multi-system damage (?)
	Neoplasia (?)	Lymphoid neoplasia (?)
Partial	Hypersensitivity syndromes	Respiratory tract, skin, gastrointestinal tract
	Autoimmune disorders	Protean (endocrines, joints) Lupus syndromes (?)
	Immune complex disorders (?)	Vasculitis (?) Lupus syndromes (?)
	Neoplasia	Lymphoid
	Amyloidosis (?)	Multi-system
	Reproductive damage	Impaired fertility Impaired development (?)

290

laboratory finding to immunotoxicity, and for equally particular vigilance in dismissing such claims.

GOVERNMENTAL REGULATION AND EVIDENCE OF IMMUNOTOXICITY

This can only be a troubled area for a while, because of the common uncertainty about whether immunological events are causal, necessary but not themselves sufficient, or reactive epiphenomena in many diseases. Until laboratory assays are better defined and generally accepted standards applied, there will be equivalent uncertainty about the meaning of changes in one or several laboratory variables, with or without a corresponding clinical disorder. More experience is required to disentangle methodological variations in test results from limited or secondary changes that remain within the range of tolerable or physiological responses, and the more sinister abnormalities that have passed beyond the limit of reaction into pathological change.

Such diagnostic and investigative uncertainty must engender caution in anyone seeking evidence of immunotoxicity and intending to use it in risk assessment. Basing regulations to prevent or limit exposure on immunotoxicity requires particular care and sensitivity because of the many possibilities for error in evaluating such risk.

CONCLUSIONS

We have only limited understanding of the role of the immune system in the pathogenesis of disease syndromes, but it is apparent that many and quite possibly all the consequences of immune disorders due to chemicals may individually match those of naturally occurring conditions. Laboratory measurements of abnormalities have yet to be standardized in most instances, which makes comparison difficult, and, for the more sophisticated assays, it is not yet possible to define the border between tolerable physiological response and definite, pathological abnormality.

Together, these concerns mean that it may be easy to hypothesize that a condition or test result is due to 'immunotoxicity' but its proof in the individual or the community is more difficult. Diagnosticians, laboratory scientists and those required to act on their findings should use caution in this field until understanding is better established.

LONG-TERM MONITORING OF HUMAN POPULATIONS FOR EFFECTS ON COMPONENTS OF THE IMMUNE SYSTEM

V. Kodat

Department of Hygiene and Epidemiology
Ministry of Health and Social Affairs, Czechoslovakia

Studies on the effects of chemical substances on the immune system point to the advantages of implementing immunological methods in resolving toxicological problems. These methods enable us to obtain important information on physiological reactions of the organism and their impairment. Also essential is a system for interpreting results, which makes it possible to evaluate differentially the significance of immunological reactions to given concentrations of chemical substances and to quantify the health hazard of long-term human exposure. On the basis of these studies, it is recommended that toxicological models be elaborated for the standard identification of the effects of toxic substances that impair immune processes, which will facilitate the use of standardized tests.

The effects of chemical substances on the defence mechanisms of the macroorganism are not yet fully known. We have information on changes in immune reactions in people who produce such chemical substances or are otherwise exposed to them in industry, agriculture or the household.

Research on the influence of chemicals on the immune system of man began in the early 1970s. Mostly occupationally exposed populations were studied, using selected indices of specific and nonspecific immunity. It is known that chemical substances modify the immune response, but it is necessary to ascertain what risk to human health these effects pose and how informative the various tests are. The effect of chemical substances depends first of all on the dose and period of exposure, the result being either a reduction in the response - immunosuppression - or an enhancement of the response - immunopotentiation or immunostimulation. The result also depends on the characteristics of the substance and its toxic properties, whether it is accumulated in the organism, and on individual differences in the person affected.

The manifestation of chemical injury of the defence system differs according to the cellular structure it affects (cell membranes, cytoplasmic structures, enzymic systems, nuclear structures). Therefore, very important in the basic assessment of immunological tests is whether their range and quality can give the information needed for the detection of immuno-toxicological effects, how reliable they are and whether it is possible on the basis of studies to deduce and set the correct strategy for the implementation of selected tests according to the immunotoxic effects of each chemical substance.

In immunological diagnostics, epidemiological data are being used in combination with specific immunological tests. Those selected for investigations of exposure to chemical substances are the following:

Blood serum: (1) IgG, IgA, IgM, IgD, IgE
(2) Alpha-I-antitrypsin
(3) Orosomucoid

Immunotoxicity of Metals and Immunotoxicology, Edited by
A. D. Dayan *et al.,* Plenum Press, New York, 1990

	(4) Caeruloplasmin
	(5) Prealbumin
	(6) Haemopexin
	(7) Lysozyme
	(8) Transferrin
	(9) C-Reactive protein
	(10) Alpha-2-macroglobulin
	(11) Alpha-2-AP-glycoprotein
	(12) Antibody response - xenoagglutinins
	(13) Antigen impulse
Saliva:	(14) IgA
	(15) IgG
	(16) IgM
	(17) Albumin
Urine:	(18) Lysozyme
	(19) 3-2-microglobulin
Capillary blood:	(20) Differential leukocyte count
	(21) Smetana N-test

These indices have been shown to be meaningful, as their values changed significantly in the presence of toxic agents, in relation to the predisposition of the human organism, and for follow-up of the effectiveness of remedial measures after long-term surveillance. The selection of indices depends on the properties of the toxin (e.g., carcinogenetic or nephrotoxic) and on the characteristics of the group studied.

Among the chemical substances of primary interest have been styrene, polycyclic aromatic hydrocarbons, epichlorohydrin, cytostatic drugs and formaldehyde (Table 1).

The aim of the studies conducted so far has been to ascertain the effect of exposure to various chemical compounds on immunological mechanisms in exposed workers. Ten years ago, we started a longitudinal epidemiological study in selected work places where the concentration of chemicals constituted a risk factor. On the basis of these results, a protocol was developed for further studies.

The results obtained by examining individuals made it is possible to assess the magnitude of the reaction of the organism to the toxic load; naturally there was a difference between exposed and nonexposed persons. The results point not only to the toxic load but also to the adaptive reactions of the organism. Often, the enhancement of immune mechanisms is not irreversible, as it is usually a consequence of a primary increase in activity as a response to a specific stimulation, or it may represent a compensatory elevation in the activity of systems supplanting the diminished function of an already altered component of immune mechanisms. Depending on the intensity of the action of the toxin and on the condition of the organism, this phase of enhanced activity is followed by a gradual decrease, either within the range of physiological values or, on the contrary, to pathological levels.

Table 1. Responses in different immunological tests of five known risk factors

Risk factor	Immunological test[a]																				
	1	2	3	4	5	6	7	8	9	10	11	12	13	14	15	16	17	18	19	20	21
Styrene	+	+		+		=			+					+							-
PAH	+	+				=		++		-	+	+		+	=	+	++	+			
Epichlorohydrin	+	+			-		+	+	++	-	+++	+	+		=			-	+		
Cytostatic drugs	++	++	++	=	=		=	+	+	-	++	++	++		=	-	-	-	+	+	-
Formaldehyde	+		++					++			++	++		-							

[a]See text for definitions.

The increased load of some carcinogenic substances due to prolonged exposure is associated with a greater risk for malignant disease. In this case, the application of immunological methods within the scope of preventive epidemiological investigations is of great significance, because the immune system is altered and it is often possible to recognize ensuing disease before the onset of clinical manifestations detectable by current routine diagnostic procedures.

The damage to immune mechanisms of long-term exposure finally leads to increased morbidity and mortality, as evidenced by epidemiological studies that show the danger of exposure to chemical substances. Immunotoxicology is one element that contributes by methods to detect incipient or already established damage with the possibility of a quantified approach. A scheme is presented for the evaluation and interpretation of such results (Table 2), which shows the horizontal course of the changes leading to a gradation from absolute health up to the critical point of origin of illness. This course is divided into four stages, although this division is theoretical.

The first stage (1a) comprises the largest group (approximately 90% of the population), with absolutely normal immunological findings (in relation to age, sex and other indices), with no inborn or acquired deficiency of any type, showing a well-preserved circadian rhythm and no necessity for activation of compensation mechanisms. In the case of such workers, no measure is necessary; they are capable of working in any environment.

Stage 1b comprises the rest (about 10%) of the population, who have either an inborn or acquired deficiency of some part of the immune reaction, necessitating a partial replacement of the immune potential through adaptative changes, leading to a swift exhaustion of the immune potential. These workers must keep in mind this dysfunction of the immune potential when choosing a job or, better still, when deciding on an apprenticeship. This group also includes people in whom the toxin (usually in combination with other, nonoccupational influences) decreases certain components of the immune potential.

The second stage expresses changes arising from stage 1a or 1b and, therefore, shows different gradations as well as different time intervals. It is difficult to define this stage precisely, as the current spectrum of immunological methods used for monitoring the

Table 2. Scheme for evaluation and interpretation of results of epidemiological studies

First stage (a) - normal physiological findings	First stage (b) - susceptible terrain, adaptation to ensure normal reaction	Second stage - signs of damage (biological beginning of illness)	Third stage - preclinical stage	Fourth stage - clinical stage
Characteristics: Findings in cell and humoral immune response in specific and non-specific elements within the norm, corresponding to age and sex	Genetically predisposed population with manifestations of humoral cell immunity deficiency, suspect disorders in immune reactions or predisposition to lower resistance (enzyme deficiency, regulatory proteins)	Population with temporarily positive indices in the investigated spectrum without clinical expression	Population with irreversible positive markers in immunological investigations without clinical expression	Beginning of clinical changes
Investigation: First check-up	First check-up	Regular check-ups	Regular check-ups	Regular check-ups
Steps taken:	Immunology dispensary	Immunology dispensary	Clinical dispensary	Preventive examinations
	Choice of job			
		Biological beginning of illness	Manifestation of immunological changes	Usual diagnosis

population is not as yet capable of defining with precision the point of the biological beginning of illness. The aim is to approach this point as closely as possible, and this will differ for different groups of diseases, primarily because various degrees of attention are paid to different ailments and diseases. A chance to verify or record a gradation in the changes is offered through regular check-ups with immunological tests undertaken at set intervals (once a year). In many cases, the findings disappear after repeated tests, and can be attributed mostly to nutritional compensation or decreased exposure to the toxin. Erroneous judgements can sometimes be made if an acute viral or other ailment (subclinical or preclinical) is present when the test samples are taken.

When the finding is repeated or when gradation occurs, these cases are moved into the third stage, which includes irreversibly changed findings with time gradation, without clinical change or subjective complaints. For these persons, we recommend special care, with testing twice a year and clinical monitoring aimed at following up the basic illness. A positive effect should be seen in these persons when compensatory measures are taken against the toxin that caused the changes. A transfer into the next stage can take years, and it may be years from the critical point to clinical diagnosis of the fourth stage - the clinical stage of the illness. Even in this phase, the period between the critical point (the origin of the illness) and the moment of diagnosis differs. This depends primarily on: the quality of diagnostics as a whole and the clinical manifestation of the symptoms in the patient. Approaching the critical point will, of course, be easier with knowledge about the frequency of the illness in relationship to exposure to various types of agents gained through model experiments as well as by an epidemiological approach.

Although this method of evaluating a patient's state of health is in its beginnings, many results already demonstrate the significant contribution of immunological methods to early recognition of inflicted damage. Information about the changes that indicate injury (damage) will increase through a suitable broad spectrum of immunological tests reflecting all the elements of the immune response. This spectrum of tests, although relatively accessible in clinical-immunological diagnostics for individual cases, is very difficult to apply *en masse*.

For large-scale testing, it is indispensable that automated cell and humoral investigations be used, at least in the key laboratories working on these problems. The subject of such tests is primarily the values for the individual immunological indices in relation to age, sex, season of the year, circadian rhythm, etc. Only with perfect knowledge of the physiology of these immunological indices will it be possible to interpret correctly the findings in the horizontal change from health to illness. Moreover, these changes are much smaller over a much longer period than the actual period of clinical manifestation, which has a strong gradation of indices in a relatively short time. It is essential that computer systems be applied to these group and individual evaluations.

For individual groups, a special classification of immunological indicators was prepared, divided according to age group and sex. For example, the third group includes strongly irritated populations with subclinical findings; in this group, we place the individuals in whom the normal limit values are increased or decreased by a specific quantity. Into group 4 we place those individuals in whom the limits are increased by higher values of one or more indices and in whom the results of laboratory tests can be verified by clinical manifestation.

On the basis of these studies, toxicological models can be developed for standard identification of the effects of toxic substances that impair immune processes and for elaborating standardized tests.

RELEVANCE OF ATOPY TO THE
IMMUNOTOXIC EFFECTS OF METALS

R. Cattaneo

Associate Professor of Clinical Immunology
Head of Clinical Immunology Unit
University of Brescia, Italy

ABSTRACT

Relationships between atopy and hypersensitivity reactions to heavy metals are discussed. Atopic subjects have an inherited predisposition to develop IgE-mediated hypersensitivity to environmental agents. Occupational exposure to heavy metals has been shown to induce respiratory symptoms, namely asthma, compatible with type-I, IgE-mediated reactions. To date, however, specific IgE have been consistently demonstrated only in workers exposed to platinum salts. Asthma induced by cobalt, chromium and nickel is apparently IgE-mediated, but specific IgE have been reported only in single cases. Evaluation of a potential predisposing role of atopy is therefore impossible. Studies on the relationship between atopy and immunotoxic effects of metals must also take into account potential effects of metals on the mechanisms that mediate the allergic reaction. This suggestive hypothesis, however, requires experimental support.

INTRODUCTION

Atopy may be defined as the inherited tendency to enhanced production of specific IgE antibodies in response to ordinary exposure to common antigens of the subject's environment. It is now generally accepted that susceptibility to atopy is inherited along multiple genetic loci: there is evidence for at least two types of genetic control of IgE responsiveness in humans, namely, HLA-linked control of specific antibody responses and non-HLA-linked control of the overall production of IgE, in which high IgE is inherited as a recessive trait (Marsh, 1988). Expression of the atopic phenotype, characterized by the production of specific IgE, requires exposure of the genetically predisposed individual to the relevant environmental allergen.

Atopic status, defined in immunological terms (presence of specific IgE to common allergens) and without clinical implications, is relatively common, affecting 25-30% of the general population (Mygind, 1986). Only a proportion of atopic subjects (50-60% of the total) develop clinical disease after exposure to a sensitizing allergen. The significance of asymptomatic atopy is debatable. It has been shown (Hagy & Settipane, 1971) that a proportion of these subjects will develop clinical allergy in subsequent years; others may have recovered from mild disease in the past or suffer from a current subclinical disease. Atopic status, independently of presence or absence of actual clinical disease, may predispose to further sensitization to other allergens and possibly to disease.

DIAGNOSIS OF ATOPY

Diagnostic tests

Methods for detecting specific IgE sensitization can be divided into those that challenge the patient's tissues with allergens (in-vivo tests) and those that detect IgE antibodies in serum or body secretions (in-vitro tests).

The diagnostic significance of in-vivo tests relies on the elicitation of a type-I (immediate) reaction, which is indirect evidence of a specific IgE antibody. The immediate response may be followed, 6-12 h later, by a delayed reaction (late reaction), which too is considered an expression of IgE antibodies, being mediated by the release of chemotactic factors by degranulating basophils and subsequent cell migration into the target organ.

In-vivo tests include skin tests (scratch, prick and intradermal tests) and tests for the provocation of target organs (bronchi, nose). Skin testing, preferably with the prick technique, is still the primary tool for diagnosing allergy. Because IgE sensitization is generalized, a positive result in a skin test reflects the presence of specific IgE in the blood and in the respiratory and gastrointestinal tracts.

In-vitro tests (radioallergosorbent test (RAST) or enzyme-linked radioimmunoassay (ELISA)) have a theoretical advantage over skin tests, inasmuch as they provide direct evidence of IgE antibody. They also have some drawbacks, which limit their specificity and sensitivity. First, non-specific IgE binding to the allergosorbent, dependent on the quantity of total IgE, may decrease the specificity of a test. A second problem is interference of IgG antibodies with the same allergen specificity as the IgE antibodies, which can occupy the allergen on the paper disc. Finally, many commercial allergen extracts are not yet sufficiently purified and standardized. Although these technical inconveniences may be obviated by accurate performance of tests on a suitable allergosorbent, this is often not possible in practice, especially when one must examine a great number of specimens. Under these conditions, RAST (or ELISA) offers no clear advantage in terms of specificity and sensitivity over skin tests, which are preferable, at least in terms of cost effectiveness. RAST is clearly indicated only in certain conditions, where skin testing is unsatisfactory, particularly where there is dermographism or widespread skin disease. RAST is, however, an important research tool, especially when one needs confirmation that an immediate reaction to a still unknown antigen is IgE-mediated.

In selected cases, the results of skin testing or RAST may need confirmation by provocation tests. These tests have the theoretical advantage of being the only way to prove a direct cause-effect relationship between exposure to an allergen and development of symptoms in the target organ; however, for practical purposes and for safety, this is usually not necessary. With regard to common environmental allergens, especially the inhalants, provocation tests (nasal, bronchial) have limited value, because a significant correlation is found between positive skin testing (or RAST) and provocation tests. This makes it unnecessary to perform a test which is time-consuming, difficult to standardize and interpret, and, more importantly, potentially hazardous for the patient. Provocation tests do have an important place in identifying new allergens and haptens, which cannot yet be detected by skin testing or RAST, as in most cases of food allergies and occupational allergies. It is, however, worth noting that provocation tests also give no information on the pathogenetic mechanism involved, whether immunological or nonimmunological, and this requires further investigation by in-vitro tests.

Diagnosis of atopic disease

This requires a combined clinical and immunological approach. Clinical history is by far the most important single diagnostic tool. IgE-mediated reactions, through the effects of mediators liberated by basophils and mast cells, are responsible for a limited set of clinical manifestations, which vary according to the route of exposure to the allergen, whether respiratory (rhinoconjunctivitis and/or asthma) or alimentary (urticaria and gastro-intestinal symptoms). Atopic eczema is another well-known clinical manifestation, the pathogenesis of which is, however, still not completely understood. Nasal polyps, sinusitis and otitis media, although not directly IgE-mediated, may be the consequence of allergic rhinitis. It should be kept in mind that the same clinical diseases can be caused by non-IgE-mediated mechanisms. The primary purpose of an allergy evaluation should be to determine if the symptoms are compatible with an allergic pathogenesis and to find clues to the allergen that is potentially involved. The last, most important step in the diagnostic procedure is to establish strict temporal and spatial links between onset of symptoms and exposure to the allergen to which specific IgE have been identified.

Diagnosis of atopic status

This is independent of current clinical problems and relies on identification of specific IgE by in-vivo or in-vitro tests. As yet, there are no established criteria. For practical purposes, in the absence of clinical indications, skin testing (or RAST) with a small number of allergens appropriate for the particular environment may suffice. According to a pragmatic definition, atopic individuals show at least one positive skin test when tested with five common allergens (Pepys, 1975). The allergens initially proposed were: grass pollen, *Dermatophagoides pteronyssinus*, cat (or dog) dander, tree pollen and one of the fungi. It is worth noting that the commonest allergens may not be the same all over the world. For instance, in Mediterranean countries, parietaria should be substituted for tree pollen. It is also questionable whether to include the commonest food allergens, e.g., milk and egg proteins. The choice between skin testing and in-vitro tests depends on practical considerations, such as number and geographical distribution of subjects to be tested, local availability of allergy services and, last but not least, cost effectiveness. This last parameter must be calculated not only on the basis of the cost of reagents and equipment but also taking into account cost of personnel. Recently available multi-RAST procedures, which allow simultaneous determination, on a single allergosorbent, of specific IgE to numerous allergens, may significantly reduce cost differences between in-vivo and in-vitro tests, at least for screening purposes. The degree of sensitization (number of positive tests) seems to be an important indicator of predisposition to further sensitization. A single positive result (low atopic status) implies a low risk, and multiple allergic reactions (high atopic status) a high risk (Mygind, 1986).

Diagnosis of atopic predisposition

This would be important for early preventive measures; however, it can be only presumptive. A family history of atopic disease, a high neonatal serum IgE concentration and a low T-cell function at one month of age all indicate a significantly increased risk for atopy (Kjellman, 1988). The importance of these risk factors decreases with advancing age. In particular, raised IgE levels in adults may be due to a number of causes, independent of atopic predisposition.

RELEVANCE OF ATOPY TO THE IMMUNOTOXICITY OF METALS

This topic may be considered from two points of view; in theory, atopy might predispose to sensitization to metals; alternatively, metals might modify a preexisting atopic status by acting on the immunocompetent system or on its mediators. To date, only the first possibility is explorable inasmuch as it is supported by sufficient clinical and experimental data. Studies on the potential effects of metals on the immune response are still in a preliminary (although extremely promising) phase, and only studies on the effects of zinc deficiency may be of relevance to our topic. It has been shown that zinc inhibits histamine release from rat peritoneal mast cells (Kazimierczak & Maslinski, 1974) and on degranulation of human basophils (Marone *et al.*, 1981). Preliminary clinical studies have demonstrated that atopic subjects have significantly lower plasmatic zinc levels than non-atopic subjects (Guerrier *et al.*, 1987). To our knowledge, no report has been made about similar effects of other metals. We therefore limit our discussion to the first possibility.

Does atopy predispose to sensitization to metals?

Exposure to heavy metals can induce clinical manifestations compatible with an allergic pathogenesis. Identification of a population at risk would be advisable, as this would allow early adoption of preventive measures. In order to respond to the question raised, certain conditions must be verified.

It is well known that atopy predisposes to further sensitization, but only in the context of IgE-mediated reactions. As a consequence, atopy does not predispose to type-IV allergy, such as allergic contact dermatitis (Blondeel *et al.*, 1987), which is one of the commonest forms of metal-induced allergy. A preliminary condition, therefore, is to consider IgE-mediated allergy to metals. Some metals (platinum, nickel, chromium, cobalt) have been implicated as responsible for respiratory symptoms, namely asthma, compatible with a type-I reaction.

As in the case of other low-molecular-weight components, the demonstration of IgE-mediated allergy presents certain technical problems. Metals salts are highly reactive and can induce both irritant and hypersensitivity reactions. For skin testing, an appropriate, nonirritative dose must be assessed by testing serial dilutions in volunteers, starting with very dilute concentrations and gradually increasing them. The problem is best exemplified by studies performed with platinum salts. It has been shown (Pepys et al., 1972) that virtually all nonexposed subjects skin-tested with halide salts of platinum give positive reactions at low dilutions of salt (10^{-2} to 10^{-1} g/ml), whereas only affected subjects reacted to concentrations of less than 10^{-3} g/ml.

Skin testing with protein conjugates is theoretically preferable, because there is more effective IgE bridging by larger molecules, such as hapten (metal)-carrier (protein) conjugates; however, the suitability of different metal-protein conjugates has not yet been established. Pepys (1984) found that use of platinum-protein conjugates gives, paradoxically, negative results. He suggested that, while carrier molecules are needed for sensitization, this may not necessarily be the case for elicitation of type-I reactions. Similar finding were reported for other low-molecular-weight substances, such as azo and anthraquinone dyes (Alanko et al., 1978), ammonium salts (Pepys et al., 1976) and chloramine T (Bourne et al., 1979). Provocation tests, which remain the tests of choice for identification of specific etiological agents, present the same problems, with the additional disadvantage of severe untoward reactions. Problems also exist with in-vitro tests (RAST or ELISA), which are the necessary complement of in-vivo tests if one is to obtain direct evidence of the presence of IgE antibodies. A major drawback of in-vitro tests is the high protein affinity of many low-molecular-weight components, which results in nonspecific positivity. This inconvenience may be reduced by using protein conjugates. Studies with platinum salts (Pepys, 1984) demonstrated that not all protein conjugates are suitable; moreover, even with the best conjugate, there are problems in the presence of high levels of total IgE, so that it is advisable to test serial dilutions of sera. These problems must be solved individually for each metal studied.

Despite these technical difficulties, IgE-mediated allergy has been demonstrated conclusively for some metals, in particular for platinum salts. Exposure to the complex salts of platinum frequently induces allergic reactions involving the skin, mucosae and respiratory tract. While skin manifestations are the result of cell-mediated hypersensitivity, respiratory symptoms are caused by typical immediate (type-I) reactions (Pepys et al., 1972). Studies from the group of Pepys (Pepys et al., 1972; Cromwell et al., 1979) have provided both indirect (in-vivo tests) and direct (RAST) evidence of IgE-mediated reactions. These reports have outlined many of the difficulties encountered in studying allergy to low-molecular-weight substances and have provided clues to the solution of many technical problems.

Epidemiological studies have demonstrated that IgE-mediated allergy is a major problem in workers exposed to platinum salts, involving up to 70% of subjects (Parrot et al., 1969). Occupational exposure to other metals (chromium, nickel, cobalt, mercury, vanadium, tungsten carbide) has also been shown capable of inducing asthma, although at a significantly lower incidence than in platinum workers. To date, IgE-mediated reactions have been clearly demonstrated only in single cases of asthma induced by chromium (Novey et al., 1983) and nickel salts (Malo et al., 1982; Novey et al., 1983; Cirla, 1985). With regard to cobalt-induced asthma, only IgE antibodies had been detected until recently and in a limited number of cases (reviewed by Cirla, 1985). Shirakawa et al. (1988), however, detected specific IgE antibodies to cobalt-conjugated human serum albumin in six out of 12 asthmatic workers. Asthma that occurs in workers exposed to aluminium solder flux is not caused by aluminium fumes but by amino-ethylenethanolamine coming from the solder flux (Pepys & Pickering, 1972); consequently, it is not directly related to the metal. Finally, no immunological study has yet been performed on asthma caused by other metals, such as vanadium (Browne, 1955) and tungston carbide (Bruckner, 1967).

The demonstration that some metals can induce IgE-mediated allergy does not, in itself, necessarily imply that atopic subjects are at a greater risk of developing IgE sensitization to these metals. It is generally accepted that the main difference between atopic and normal subjects is that atopic subjects are predisposed to produce specific IgE antibodies in response to ordinary exposure to common antigens in their environment. In other words, part of the atopic predisposition appears to be weaker suppression (allowing greater than normal production of IgE) of the local (mucosal) immune response to repetitive small quantities of inhaled or ingested antigen (Platts-Mills, 1982). The importance of the route of exposure is best exemplified by allergies to injected penicillin and to bee sting, which are not more frequent in atopic than in non-atopic subjects (Kraft *et al.*, 1977). Similarly, there is no difference in the production of specific IgE in response to ascaris infestation, which is an abnormal and peculiarly potent allergenic exposure (Strejan, 1975). Finally, almost all subjects produce specific IgE antibodies when exposed to highly allergizing substances, such as the dust of castor beans (Pepys, 1975). Platts-Mills (1982) has proposed that these allergies be referred to simply as being IgE mediated. In fact, they should not be regarded as atopic, because a large proportion of the exposed population develops hypersensitivity. Occupational studies offer other examples (reviewed by O'Neil & Salvaggio, 1988) of IgE-mediated allergies that are not influenced by the atopic state, such as asthma resulting from exposure to western red cedar, toluene diisocyanate and trimellitic anhydride. With respect to allergy to metals, only allergy to platinum salts has been evaluated from this point of view. There is evidence (Pepys, 1984) that atopy is a predisposing factor to a more rapid rate of sensitization. No definite conclusion could be drawn from earlier studies about the difference in incidence of sensitization between atopic and non-atopic subjects, owing to the high intrinsic allergenicity of platinum salts, which, at high concentrations, sensitized up to 70% of workers (Parrot *et al.*, 1969). A lower incidence of sensitization (30% of exposed subjects) was found in a recent survey (Merget *et al.*, 1988), probably due to the adoption of a threshold limit value for soluble platinum salts. This situation will allow a clearer approach to the problem. Thus, Venables *et al.* (1988) have demonstrated that, although atopy is a risk factor for platinum sensitization, it is less important than smoking. No reliable data are yet available on allergy to other metals, owing to scarcity of reports, most of which are on single cases.

CONCLUSIONS

On the basis of available data, it is not yet possible to give a clear-cut response to the question of whether atopy predisposes to sensitization to metals. At present, however, the problem is of only theoretical interest because of the modest relevance of IgE-mediated allergy to metals. A notable exception is represented by allergy to platinum salts, but its importance has lessened markedly recently, owing to reduced possibilities of exposure and the adoption of precautionary measures. Further studies are therefore needed to verify the real incidence of IgE-mediated allergy to other metals, in particular to chromium, nickel and cobalt, which appear the most likely candidates as sensitizing agents. Better knowledge about the hypothesis is a necessary prerequisite to justify costly and time-consuming epidemiological studies aimed at investigating the potential predisposing role of atopy.

REFERENCES

Alanko, K., Keskinen, H., Bjorksten, F. & Ojanen, S. (1978) Immediate-type hypersensitivity to reactive dyes. *Clin. Allergy*, **8**: 25

Blondeel, A., Achten, G., Dooms-Goossens, A., Bucknes, P., Broeckx, W. & Oleffe, J. (1987) [Atopy and contact allergy.] (in French) *Ann. Dermatol. Venereol.*, **114**: 203-209

Bourne, M.D., Flindt, M.H.L. & Miles-Walker, J. (1979) Asthma due to industrial use of chloramine. *Br. med. J.*, **iii**: 10

Brown, R.C. (1955) Vanadion poisoning from gas turbine. *Br. J. ind. Med.*, **12**: 57-59

Bruckner, H.C. (1969) Extrinsic asthma in a tungsten carbide worker. *J. occup. Med.*, **9**: 518-519

Cirla, A.M. (1985) Asthma induced by occupational exposure to metal salts. *Folia Allergol. Immunol. Clin.*, **32**: 21-28

Cromwell, O., Pepys, J., Parish, W.E. & Hughes, E. G. (1979) Specific IgE antibodies to platinum salts in sensitized workers. *Clin. Allergy*, **9**: 107-117

Guerrier, G., Veysseyre, C., Nourian, A., Graveriau, D. & Carron, R. (1987) [Inhibition *in vitro* by zinc gluconate of the degranulation of human basophils sensitized to grass pollen.] (in French) *Rev. fr. Allergol.*, **27**: 1-5

Hagy, G.W. & Settipane, G.A. (1971) Prognosis of positive allergy skin tests in an asymptomatic population. *J. Allergy*, **48**: 200

Kazimierczak, W. & Maslinski, C. (1974) Histamine release from mastcells by compound 48/80. The membrane action of zinc. *Agent Action*, **4**: 320-323

Kjellman, N.I.M. (1988) Epidemiology and prevention of allergy. *Allergy*, **43** (Suppl. 8): 39-40

Kraft, D., Roth, A., Mischer, P., Pichler, H. & Ebner, H. (1977) Specific and total serum IgE measurements in diagnosis of penicillin allergy. A long term follow-up study. *J. Allergy clin. Immunol.*, **55**: 241

Malo, J.L., Cartier, A., Doepner, M., Nieboer, E. & Dolovich, J. (1982) Occupational asthma caused by nickel sulfate. *J. Allergy clin. Immunol.*, **69**: 55

Marone, G., Findlay, S.R. & Lichtenstein, M. (1981) Modulation of histamine release from human basophils *in vitro* by physiological concentration of zinc. *J. Pharmacol. exp. Ther.*, **217**: 292-298

Marsh, D.G. (1988) Molecular studies of human immune recognition of allergens. *Allergy*, **43** (Suppl. 8): 7-8

Merget, R., Schultze-Werninghaus, G., Muthorst, T., Friedrich, W. & Meier-Sydow, J. (1988) Asthma due to the complex salts of platinum - a cross-sectional survey of workers in a platinum refinery. *Clin. Allergy*, **18**: 569-580

Mygind, M. (1986) *Essential Allergy*, Oxford, Blackwell Scientific Publications

Novey, H.S., Habib, M. & Wells, I.D. (1983) Asthma and IgE antibodies induced by chromium and nickel salts. *J. Allergy clin. Immunol.*, **72**: 407

O'Neil, C.E. & Salvaggio, J.E. (1988) The pathogenesis of occupational asthma. *Baillière's clin. Immunol. Allergy*, **2**: 143-175

Parrot, J.L., Herbert, R., Saindelle, A. & Ruff, R. (1969) Platinum and platinosis. Allergy and histamine release due to some platinum salts. *Arch. environ. Health*, **19**: 685-691

Pepys, J. (1975) Atopy. In: Gell, P.G.H. & Coombes, R.R.A., eds, *Clinical Aspects of Immunology*, 3rd ed., Oxford, Blackwell Scientific Publications, p. 877

Pepys, J. (1984) Occupational allergy due to platinum complex salts. *Clinics Immunol. Allergy*, **4**: 131-157

Pepys, J. & Pickering, C.A. (1972) Asthma due to inhaled chemical fumes: aminoethylenethanolamine in aluminium soldering flux. *Clin. Allergy*, **2**: 197

Pepys, J., Pickering, C.A. & Hughes, E.G. (1972) Asthma due to inhaled chemical agents - complex salts of platinum. *Clin. Allergy*, **2**: 391-396

Pepys, J., Hutchcroft, B.J. & Breslin, A.B. (1976) Asthma due to inhaled chemical agents - persulphate salts and henna in hairdressers. *Clin. Allergy*, **6**: 399

Platts-Mills, T.A.E. (1982) Type I or immediate hypersensitivity: hay fever and asthma. In: Lackman, P.J. & Peters, D.H., eds, *Clinical Aspects of Immunology*, 4th ed., Oxford, Blackwell Scientific Publications, p. 579

Shirakawa, T., Kusaka, Y., Fujimura, N., Goto, S. & Morimoto, K. (1988) The existence of specific antibodies to cobalt in hard metal asthma. *Clin. Allergy*, **18**: 451-460

Strejan, G.H. (1975) Reagin mediated hypersensitivity: the ascaris model. *Immunochemistry*, **12**: 569

Venables, K.M., Stevens, J., Nunn, A.J., Stevens, R.J., Farrer, N.M., Stewart, M., Hughes, E.G. & Newman Taylor, A.J. (1988) Increased risk of occupational allergy in smokers working in a platinum refinery. *Thorax*, **43**: 264

PARTICIPANTS

J. Althoff
Winthrop Sterling, 5, boulevard Eiffel, 21602 Longvic/Dijon, France

R.A. Andersen
Department of Immunology, National Institute of Public Health, Geitmyrsvn. 75,
0462 Oslo 4, Norway

J. Arts
CIVO-TNO Institutes, PO Box 360, 3700 AJ Zeist, Utrechtseweg 48, 3704 HE Zeist,
Netherlands

T. Auf der Heide
Medical High School, Hanover, FRG

A. Berlin
Head, Specialized Service, Health and Safety Directorate, Commission of the European
Communities, Bâtiment Jean Monnet, Plateau de Kirchberg, BP 1907, 2920 Luxembourg

M. Berlin
Institute of Environmental Medicine, University of Lund, Sölvegatan 21, 223 62 Lund,
Sweden

D.M. Blackburn
Imperial Chemical Industries PLC, Central Toxicology Laboratory, Alderley Park,
Macclesfield, Cheshire SK10 4TJ, UK

P.A. Botham
Imperial Chemical Industries PLC, Central Toxicology Laboratory, Alderley Park,
Macclesfield, Cheshire SK10 4TJ, UK

R. Cattaneo
Head, Clinical Immunology Unit, University of Brescia, 25125 Brescia, Italy

T.W. Clarkson
University of Rochester, School of Medicine and Dentistry, Rochester, NY 14642, USA

M. Crippa
Institute of Occupational Health, University of Brescia, P. le Spedali Civili 1, 25100 Brescia,
Italy

A.D. Dayan
Director, DHSS Department of Toxicology, St Bartholomew's Hospital Medical College,
University of London, 59 Bartholomew Close, London EC1 7ED, UK

J. Descotes
Laboratory of Fundamental and Clinical Immunotoxicology, INSERM U80/CNRS URA1177/
UCBL, Faculty of Medicine Alexis Carrel, 69008 Lyon, France

I. Desi
Department of Hygiene and Epidemiology, University Medical School Szeged, Dom ter 10, 6720 Szeged, Hungary

P. Druet
INSERM U28, Hôpital Broussais, 96 rue Didot, 75674 Paris Cédex 14, France

D. Ende
Society for Radiation and Environmental Studies Ltd, Kühbachstrasse 11, Munich 90, FRG

S. Eneström
Department of Pathology, University of Linköping, 581 82 Linköping, Sweden

J.H. Exon
Department of Veterinary Medicine & WOI Regional Program, University of Idaho, Veterinary Science Building, Moscow, ID 83843, USA

V. Fao
Institute of Occupational Medicine, University of Milan, via San Barnaba 8, 20122 Milan, Italy

J. Franek
Head, Department of Immunology, Czechoslovak Academy of Sciences, Institute of Experimental Medicine, Lidovych Milici 61, 120 00 Praha 2, Czechoslovakia

L. Friberg
The Karolinska Institute, Department of Environmental Hygiene, 104 01 Stockholm, Sweden

E. Gleichmann
Division of Immunology, Medical Institute for Environmental Health, University of Düsseldorf, Postfach 5634, 4000 Düsseldorf 1, FRG

M. Goldman
Medico-Surgical Department of Nephrology, Dialysis and Transplantation, Hôpital Erasme, Free University of Brussels, route de Lennik 808, 1070 Brussels, Belgium

P. Grandjean
Odense University, Institute of Community Health, Department of Environmental Medicine, J.B. Winslows vej 19, 5000 Odense C, Denmark

P. de Haan
Department of Dermatology, University Hospital, Free University, de Boelelaan 1117, 1081 HU Amsterdam, Netherlands

S. Hernberg
Institute of Occupational Health, Topeliuksenkatu 41aA, 00250 Helsinki, Finland

R.F. Hertel
Fraunhofer Institute of Toxicology and Aerosol Research, Nikolai-Fuchs-Str. 1, 3000 Hanover 61, FRG

E. Heseltine
Lajarthe, St Léon-sur-Vézère, 24290 Montignac, France

R. Hess
Ciba Geigy AG, 4002 Basel, Switzerland

B. Hildebrand
BASF Aktiengesellschaft, Department of Toxicology, ZST - Z 470, 6700 Ludwigshafen, FRG

Federal Ministry for Environment, Nature and Conservation and Nuclear Safety, Haus 8 im BMI, Graurheindorfer Str. 198, 5300 Bonn, FRG

P. Ibsen
National Food Agency, Ministry of the Environment, 19 Morkhoj Bygade, 2860 Soborg, Denmark

M.E. Kammuller, Sandoz AG, 4002 Basel, Switzerland

F. Kayama
School of Medicine, University of Occupational and Environmental Health, Yahata nishi ku, Kitakyushu 807, Japan

D. Kayser
Bundesgesundheitsamt, Max von Pettenkofer Institute, Thielallee 88-92, Postfach 330013, 1000 Berlin (West) 33

G. Kazantzis
Professor, Occupational Medicine, Department of Public Health and Policy, London School of Hygiene and Tropical Medicine, Keppel Street, London WC1E 7HT, UK

I. Kimber
Imperial Chemical Industries PLC, Central Toxicology Laboratory, Alderley Park, Macclesfield, Cheshire SK10 4TJ, UK

V. Kodat
Director, Department of Hygiene and Epidemiology, Ministry of Health and Social Affairs of the Czech Socialist Republic, 2 Palackeho nam. 4, 120 37 Praha 10, Czechoslovakia

L.D. Koller
Dean, College of Veterinary Medicine, Oregon State University, Corvallis, OR 97331-4802, USA

M.A.M. Krajnc-Franken
National Institute of Public Health and Environmental Protection, Antonie van Leeuwenhoeklaan 9, PO Box 1, 3720 BA Bilthoven, Netherlands

F. Kuper
CIVO-TNO Institutes, PO Box 360, 3700 AJ Zeist, Utrechtseweg 48, 3704 HE Zeist, Netherlands

K. Kuttler
BASF, Department of Toxicology, ZST - Z 470, 6700 Ludwigshafen, FRG

R. Lauwerys
Faculty of Medicine, Unit of Industrial and Occupational Medical Toxicology, Catholic University of Louvain, Clos Chapelle-aux-Champs 30-54, 1200 Brussels, Belgium

J. Lewalter
Medical Department, Geb. L. 9, Bayerwerk, 5090 Leverkusen, FRG

M.-L. Lohmann-Matthes
Department of Immunology, Fraunhofer Institute of Toxicology and Aerosol Research, Nikolai-Fuchs-Str. 1, 3000 Hanover 61, FRG

M. Lovik
Department of Immunology, National Institute of Public Health, Geitmyrsvn. 75, 0462 Oslo 4, Norway

R. Luebke
Pulmonary Toxicology Branch (MD-82), US Environmental Protection Agency, Health Effects Research Laboratory, Research Triangle Park, NC 27711, USA

K. Lundberg
Department of Toxicology, Uppsala University, PO Box 594, 75124 Uppsala, Sweden

C. Madsen
National Food Agency, Ministry of the Environment, 19 Morkhoj Bygade, 2860 Soborg, Denmark

T. Maurer
Ciba Geigy AG, Toxicology PS, 4002 Basel, Switzerland

T. Menné
Department of Dermatology, Gentofte Hospital, 2900 Hellerup, Denmark

M. Mercier
International Programme on Chemical Safety, World Health Organization, 1211 Geneva 27, Switzerland

R. Merget
Hospital of the Johann Wolfgang Goethe University, Department of Internal Medicine, Division of Pneumonology, 6000 Frankfurt/Main, FRG

K. Miller
British Industrial Biological Research Association, Woodmansterne Road, Carshalton, Surrey SM5 4DS, UK

U. Mohr
Fraunhofer Institute of Toxicology and Aerosol Research, Nikolai-Fuchs-Str. 1, 3000 Hanover 61, FRG

T. Morrow
Unilever Research and Engineering, Colworth House, Sharnbrook, Bedford MK44 1LQ, UK

M. Murray
Procter and Gamble Co., Miami Valley Laboratories, PO Box 398707, Cincinnati, OH 45239-8707, USA

A. Mutti
Institute of Clinical Medicine and Nephrology, Laboratory of Industrial Toxicology, University of Parma, Parma, Italy

S. Nicklin
Department of Immunotoxicology, British Industrial Biological Research Association, Woodmansterne Road, Carshalton, Surrey SM5 4DS, UK

G. Nordberg
Department of Environmental Medicine, University of Umeå, 901 87 Umeå, Sweden

T. Ockhuizen
CIVO-TNO Institutes, PO Box 360, 3700 AJ Zeist, Utrechtseweg 48, 3704 HE Zeist, Netherlands

S. Ollive
Elida Gibbs Ltd, Coal Road, Seacroft, Leeds, Yorkshire L514 2AR, UK

D.P. Olson
Department of Veterinary Medicine & WOI Regional Program, University of Idaho, Veterinary Science Building, Moscow, ID 83843, USA

B. Oredsson
National Chemicals Inspectorate, Box 1384, 171 27 Solna, Sweden

G.S. Panayi
Rheumatology Unit, Division of Medicine, Shepherds House, Guy's Hospital, London SE1 9RT, UK

W.E. Parish
Unilever, Colworth House, Sharnbrook, Bedford MK44 1LQ, UK

A.H. Penninks
Research Institute of Toxicology, Section Immunotoxicology, University of Utrecht,
PO Box 80 176, 3508 TD Utrecht, Netherlands

O.P. Preuss
1393 Coyote Road, Prescott, AZ 86303, USA

J. Prochazkova
Head, Department of Medical Immunology and Reference Laboratory for Immunotoxicology,
Regional Institute of Hygiene, 500 36 Hradec Kralové, Czechoslovakia

A.L. Reeves
Department of Occupational and Environmental Health, College of Pharmacy and Allied
Health Professions, Wayne State University, 625 Mullet, Detroit, MI 48226, USA

B. Remandet
Sanofi Research, rue T.J. Blayac, 34082 Montpellier Cedex, France

J.P. Revillard
Director, Unit of Research on Nephro-urology, Transplantation and Clinical Immunology,
Pavillon P, Hôpital Edouard Herriot, 69374 Lyon Cédex 08, France

J. Richter
Department of Immunology, Regional Institute of Hygiene, Moskavska 15,
400 48 Usti nad Labem, Czechoslovakia

H.B. Richter-Reichhelm
Bundesgesundheitsamt CV3, Postfach 330013, 1000 Berlin (West) 33

L. Rosival
Director, Centre of Hygiene of the Research Institute of Preventive Medicine, Limbova 14,
83301 Bratislava, Czechoslovakia

G. Rosner
Fraunhofer Institute of Toxicology and Aerosol Research,
Nikolai-Fuchs-Str. 1, 3000 Hanover 61, FRG

B. Rushton
Roche Products Ltd, PO Box 8, Broadwater Road, Welwyn Garden City, Hertfordshire, UK

K. Schilling
BASF, Department of Toxicology, ZST - Z 470, 6700 Ludwigshafen, FRG

A. Schleusener
Bundesgesundheitsamt C IV 3, Thielallee 88-92, 1000 Berlin (West) 33

E. Schmidt
Bundesgesundheitsamt C IV 6, Max von Pettenkofer Institute, Postfach 330013,
1000 Berlin (West) 33

A. Simoes de Carvalho
Abel Salazar Institute of the Biomedical Sciences, University of Oporto, 4000 Porto, Portugal

S. Skerfving
Department of Occupational and Environmental Medicine, University Hospital,
221 85 Lund, Sweden

R. Smialowicz
MD - 82, Health Effects Research Laboratory, US Environmental Protection Agency,
Research Triangle Park, NC 27711, USA

E.M. Smith
International Programme on Chemical Safety, Division of Environmental Health, World
Health Organization, 1211 Geneva 27, Switzerland

N.J. Snoeij
Department of Toxicology, Duphar BV, PO Box 2, 1380 AA Weesp, Netherlands

A. Somogyi
Bundesgesundheitsamt, Max von Pettenkofer Institute, Thielallee 88-92, Postfach 330013,
1000 Berlin (West) 33

B. Steiniger
Centre of Anatomy, Anatomy Department, Medical High School, Hanover, FRG

V. Stejskal
Head, Immunotoxicology, Safety Assessment, AB Astra, 151 85 Södertälje, Sweden

M. Stewart
Group Occupational Physician, Materials Technology Division, Johnson Matthey, Orchard
Road, Royston, Hertfordshire SG8 5HE, UK

H. Tryphonas
General Toxicology Section, Toxicology Research Division, Bureau of Chemical Safety, Food
Directorate (2nd floor East), Sir Frederick G. Banting Building, Tunney's Pasture, Ottawa,
Ontario, Canada K1A OL2

M.-T. Van der Venne
Health and Safety Directorate, Commission of the European Communities, Bâtiment Jean
Monnet, Plateau de Kirchberg, BP 1907, 2920 Luxembourg

H. Van Loveren
Laboratory for Pathology, National Institute of Public Health and Environmental Protection,
Antonie van Leeuwenhoeklaan 9, PO Box 1, 3720 BA Bilthoven, Netherlands

H.W. Vohr
Bayer AG, Pharmaforschungszentrum, Aprather weg, Tox. LW, 5600 Wuppertal, FRG

J.G. Vos
Director of Immunology, National Institute of Public Health and Environmental Protection,
Antonie van Leeuwenhoeklaan 9, PO Box 1, 3720 BA Bilthoven, Netherlands

J.J. Weening
Department of Pathology, State University of Groningen, Oostersingel 63, 9713 EZ
Groningen, Netherlands

K.I. Welsh
Senior Lecturer in Immunogenetics, NGH 3, Guy's Hospital, London
SE1 9RT, UK

K. White
Department of Pharmacology and Toxicology, Medical College of Virginia, Box 613, Richmond, VA 23298, USA

R.J.P. Williams
Inorganic Chemistry Laboratory, University of Oxford, South Parks Road, Oxford OX1 3QR, UK

W. Zachgo
ZIM, Division of Pneumology, Clinic of the J.-W. Goethe University, Theodor Stern Kai 7, 6000 Frankfurt/Main 70, FRG

SUBJECT INDEX

Macrophage (continued)
    migration inhibition test, 8, 48, 51, 70,
           73, 183, 185, 187, 275-276
    production, 32
Magnesium, uptake of, 63
Major histocompatibility complex (MHC), 19
    antigens
        class-I, 22, 26, 33, 106, 110
        class-II, 6, 7, 9, 21, 22, 26, 33, 105-
           107, 110, 129
        genes linked to, 6, 10, 38-40
        interaction with, 22
        recognition of, 246
Manganese
    and enhancement of nonspecific
           immunity, 7
    uptake of, 63
Marker of immunotoxicity, 34, 290-291
Maximization test (see Guinea-pig
           maximization test)
Mercury
    and asthma, 300
    and autoimmune reactions, 7, 9, 10, 39,
           122-127, 158
    binding of, 121-122
    in dental amalgam, 8, 9, 163, 168-170
    dose-response relationships, 164-168
    genetic control of effects of, 22, 38
    and hypersensitivity reactions, 7, 8, 38,
           69, 71, 124
    and immune complex formation, 9
    immunosuppressive effects of, 7,135
    induction of anti-Ia T cells by, 129
    induction of interferon gamma by, 132
    occupational exposure to, 8, 71, 163
    toxicology of, 163-170
Metals (see also individual metals)
    heavy
        and activation of B cells, 7
        sensitization to, 139-150
        toxic effects of, 209
    immunotoxicity of, 3, 6-10, 121-135, 297-
           301
    recognition of by proteins, 57-64
Mitogen
    -induced lymphocyte transformation, 51
    response to, 12, 51, 196-197, 201, 235,
           238, 242, 282
Mixed leukocyte response, 12, 197
Mixed lymphocyte reaction, 20, 32-33, 234,
           235, 237, 267
Molybdenum
    and hypersensitivity, 72
    uptake of, 63
Monitoring of human populations, 293-296
Mouse, as experimental model, 5, 11, 32, 34,
           75, 76, 78-81, 108-111, 134,
           146-149, 236, 277-278
Mouse ear swelling test (MEST), 5, 80-81,
           148-149, 277-278

Mouse ear swelling test (continued)
    with vitamin A acetate, 80-81, 149
Multiple sclerosis, and exposure to zinc, 227

Natural killer cell, 12, 30, 197, 201, 219,
           234
    activity, 32, 106, 175, 242, 245, 268
    effect of lead on, 219
    effect of zinc on, 223, 226
    susceptibility to cyclophosphamide, 49
Nephropathy
    induced by gold, 71, 124
    induced by lithium, 124
    induced by mercury, 71, 124, 164-167
    induced by nickel, 124
Nickel
    allergy, prevalence of, 8
    and contact dermatitis, 69-70, 83-90,
           124, 132-133
    dose-response relationships of, 10
    and hypersensitivity reactions, 7-10, 38-
           39, 69-70, 124, 297-301
    immunosuppressive effects of, 133
    induction of anti-Ia T cells by, 129-134
    and lymphocyte proliferation, 177
    and respiratory tract hypersensitivity, 9,
           297, 299-301
    uptake of, 63

Occupation
    and asthma, 75
    and contact dermatitis, 75, 84
    epidemiological studies of, 14, 293-296
    and exposure to beryllium, 9
    and exposure to cobalt, 70
    and exposure to chromium, 70, 84, 87-89
    and exposure to lead, 219
    and exposure to mercury, 8, 71, 163
    and exposure to nickel, 84
    and exposure to platinum, 72, 93-99, 145
    and hypersensitivity reactions, 30
Open epidermal test, 79
Optimization test, 79, 176
Organotin compound
    and suppression of specific immunity, 7
    disubstituted, 7, 191-198, 200, 202-204
    effect on lymphoid organs and lymphoid
           functions, 191-204, 249-253
    exposure to, 191-192
    immunosuppressive effects of, 7, 52-53
    trisubstituted, 7, 191-192, 197-204

Paratope, 19-22
Passive cutaneous anaphylaxis, 96
Patch test, 6, 70, 73, 149, 168, 183-184,
           187
Peptide, binding to, 19, 22
Phagocytosis, 12
    assessment of, 237-238, 242
    effect of cadmium on, 211

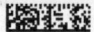